# Assessment and Diagnosis Review for APRN Certification Exams

**Alice M. Teall, DNP, APRN-CNP, FAANP,** is Director of Graduate Wellness Academic Programming, Director of Innovative Telehealth Services, and an Assistant Professor of Clinical Nursing at The Ohio State University. She was a founding member of the College of Nursing's team delivering distance education and served as Director of the online Family Nurse Practitioner program. Dr. Teall has published and presented nationally about innovation in online education, the incorporation of wellness coaching techniques in clinical practice, and the use of telehealth as an evaluation strategy for distance students. She has received leadership, alumni, teaching, and practice awards, including the Provost's Award for Distinguished Teaching at The Ohio State University. Dr. Teall is a Fellow of the American Academy of Nurse Practitioners. As a certified nurse practitioner and an integrative nurse coach, her areas of clinical practice expertise include adolescent health, primary care of at-risk children and families, college health, and recovery from substance use disorder. Her favorite quote is from Brené Brown, "I don't have to chase extraordinary moments to find happiness—it's right in front of me if I'm paying attention and practicing gratitude." Dr. Teall is co-editor and author of *Evidence-Based Physical Examination: Best Practices for Health and Well-Being Assessment* and *Evidence-Based Physical Examination Handbook* and is a former item-writer for the American Nurses Credentialing Center.

**Kate Sustersic Gawlik, DNP, APRN-CNP, FAANP,** graduated with her Doctorate of Nursing Practice from The Ohio State University and is certified by the American Nurses Credentialing Center as a family nurse practitioner. She also serves as the Director of Undergraduate Health and Wellness Academic Programming, the Co-Director of Health and Wellness Innovation in Healthcare program, and the project manager for the Million Hearts initiatives at The Ohio State University College of Nursing. She has experience in family practice, college health, urgent care, and reproductive care with clinical interests in population health, preventive medicine, clinician well-being, education of health professionals, wellness, parental burnout, and cardiovascular disease prevention. Dr. Gawlik is an associate professor of clinical nursing at The Ohio State University. She has taught a variety of undergraduate and graduate nursing courses and serves as a clinical preceptor for advanced practice nursing students. Dr. Gawlik was awarded the Outstanding Faculty Award in 2013 and the Outstanding Leadership Award in 2017. In 2018 she received the American Association of Nurse Practitioners State Award for Excellence for Ohio and was inducted as a Fellow of the American Association of Nurse Practitioners. She is co-editor and author of *Evidence-Based Physical Examination: Best Practices for Health and Well-Being Assessment* and *Evidence-Based Physical Examination Handbook*. She enjoys chasing after her four children, summer, being outdoors, yoga, making s'mores, and helping nursing students to realize their amazing abilities and true potential.

**Bernadette Mazurek Melnyk, PhD, APRN-CNP, FAANP, FNAP, FAAN,** is the Vice President for Health Promotion, University Chief Wellness Officer, and Helene Fuld Health Trust Professor of Evidence-Based Practice and Dean of the College of Nursing at The Ohio State University. She also is a Professor of Pediatrics and Psychiatry at the College of Medicine and Executive Director of the Helene Fuld Health Trust National Institute for Evidence-based Practice in Nursing and Healthcare. Dr. Melnyk is a nationally and internationally recognized expert in evidence-based practice, intervention research, child and adolescent mental health, and health and wellness. She is both a pediatric nurse practitioner and psychiatric mental health nurse practitioner, and co-editor of eight books, including *Evidence-Based Physical Examination: Best Practices for Health and Well-Being Assessment; Evidence-Based Physical Examination Handbook; Implementing the Evidence-Based Practice (EBP) Competencies in Healthcare: A Practical Guide for Improving Quality, Safety, and Outcomes; Evidence-Based Practice in Nursing and Healthcare: A Guide to Best Practice* (Fourth Edition); *Implementing EBP: Real World Success Stories; A Practical Guide to Child and Adolescent Mental Health Screening, Early Intervention and Health Promotion* (Third Edition); *Intervention Research and Evidence-Based Quality Improvement: Designing, Conducting, Analyzing and Funding* (Second Edition); and *Evidence-Based Leadership, Innovation and Entrepreneurship in Nursing and Healthcare*. Dr. Melnyk has over $33 million of sponsored funding from federal agencies and foundations and has authored over 450 publications. She is an elected fellow of the National Academy of Medicine, the American Academy of Nursing, the National Academies of Practice, and the American Association of Nurse Practitioners, and serves as Editor of the journal *Worldviews on Evidence-based Nursing.* Dr. Melnyk served a 4-year term on the U.S. Preventive Services Task Force and recently served on the mental health standing committee of the National Quality Forum. She is currently a member of the board of directors for the National Forum for Heart Disease and Stroke Prevention and a member of the National Academy of Medicine's Action Collaborative on Clinician Well-being and Resilience. She has received numerous national and international awards, including being named an edge-runner three times by the American Academy of Nursing.

# Assessment and Diagnosis Review for APRN Certification Exams

Alice M. Teall, DNP, APRN-CNP, FAANP
Kate Sustersic Gawlik, DNP, APRN-CNP, FAANP
Bernadette Mazurek Melnyk, PHD, APRN-CNP, FAANP, FNAP, FAAN

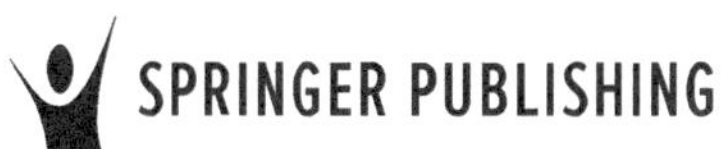

First Springer Publishing edition 2022



Springer Publishing Company, LLC
11 West 42nd Street, New York, NY 10036
www.springerpub.com
connect.springerpub.com
ExamPrepConnect.com

*Acquisitions Editor*: Adrianne Brigido
*Developmental Editor*: Lucia Gunzel
*Compositor*: Integra

*ISBN*: 9780826164674
*ebook ISBN*: 9780826164681
*DOI:* 10.1891/9780826164681

21 22 23 24 / 5 4 3 2 1

The author and the publisher of this Work have made every effort to use sources believed to be reliable to provide information that is accurate and compatible with the standards generally accepted at the time of publication. Because medical science is continually advancing, our knowledge base continues to expand. Therefore, as new information becomes available, changes in procedures become necessary. We recommend that the reader always consult current research and specific institutional policies before performing any clinical procedure or delivering any medication. The author and publisher shall not be liable for any special, consequential, or exemplary damages resulting, in whole or in part, from the readers' use of, or reliance on, the information contained in this book. The publisher has no responsibility for the persistence or accuracy of URLs for external or third-party Internet websites referred to in this publication and does not guarantee that any content on such websites is, or will remain, accurate or appropriate.

**LCCN:** 2021912936

***Publisher's Note:*** **New and used products purchased from third-party sellers are not guaranteed for quality, authenticity, or access to any included digital components.**

Printed in the United States of America.

*In loving memory of my parents, Joseph and Lucille Dubina, who used to call me just to have a good argument, taught me about resilience and grit, and would introduce me as "my daughter, who is almost a doctor" long before I entered a doctoral program. I will always love and miss you. To my husband, Tom, thank you for your unwavering support, true partnership, and amazing sense of humor. To Amy, Mallory, Kevin, and Dominique, you are exceptional, and I am so proud of you. To my grandchildren, Noah, Aiden, Evan, Sebastian, Emma, and August, you are unconditionally loved.*

—ALICE M. TEALL

*This book is dedicated to my sisters, Jennifer and Rebecca. Through all the years of playing Little House on the Prairie, watching Anne of Green Gables, eating Cameo pizzas, and catching lightning bugs on cottage summer nights, there was you. May we always be the constant, the compass, and the mirror each other's needs. The greatest gift Mom and Dad ever gave us was each other. In childhood, now, and always. We are the lucky ones.*

—KATE SUSTERSIC GAWLIK

*I dedicate this book to my loving husband, John, who has supported me throughout the past 3 decades to pursue my dreams; my three wonderful daughters Kaylin, Angela, and Megan who have provided understanding and support to me to fuel my passions, and my two awesome grandsons, Alexander and Bradley, who I will continue to encourage to dream, discover, and deliver throughout their life's journeys. In addition, I would like to devote this book to all my past and current students who have kept my "spirit of inquiry" thriving through their quest to become the best evidence-based providers to ultimately transform health and improve lives throughout the nation and world.*

—BERNADETTE (BERN) MAZUREK MELNYK

# Contents

# Preface

*"Tell me and I will forget, teach me and I may remember, involve me and I learn."*
*—Benjamin Franklin*

Active learning is an approach to instruction that involves engagement with content through case studies, discussion, problem-solving, and reflection. As experienced faculty who have taught advanced assessment, diagnostic reasoning, leadership, evidence-based practice, and clinical management courses across educational programs, we recognize that students who are actively engaged in learning evidence-based techniques and approaches are better prepared to deliver safe, effective, patient-centered, quality clinical care. Engagement in learning requires review and feedback to integrate the skills of history taking, physical examination, and diagnostic decision-making within the context of evidence-based clinical practice.

The process of learning is complex. Throughout our teaching careers, advanced practice nursing graduate students have consistently asked for additional opportunities to engage in content review, and to practice answering the type of questions that they might find on certification exams. While certification exam review books were available for their review, students who were enrolled in advanced assessment and early clinical management courses consistently sought review questions focused on assessment and diagnostic decision-making, the foundation of advanced nursing practice. Our text was developed in response to this gap in availability of review books focused on assessment and diagnosis, and in response to their requests for additional opportunities for active learning and engagement.

*Assessment and Diagnosis Review for APRN Certification Exams* is intended for students and program graduates who are interested in reviewing the foundational knowledge needed for advanced clinical practice. Each chapter has a concise review of advanced assessment and diagnostic content and includes practice questions with rationale to aid in learning. This book offers an opportunity to gain and synthesize critical knowledge needed for advanced nursing practice, including challenges that require engagement in problem-solving and diagnostic reasoning. This book includes a review of how to approach individuals across the life span, prioritizes a broad understanding of wellness, presents evidence-based recommendations for assessments, and systematically reviews the physical examination components required to inform clinical decision-making.

## GOALS OF THIS REVIEW BOOK

The overall goal of this book is to provide a review of evidence-based advanced assessment and diagnostic decision-making, integrating wellness, health promotion, and disease prevention to successfully prepare for advanced practice certification exams developed and administered by the American Academy of Nurse Practitioners Certification Board (AANPCB), American Nurses Credentialing Center (ANCC), and the Pediatric Nursing Certification Board (PNCB). Additional goals of this text include:

1. Review of evidence-based practice at the assessment and diagnostic levels
2. Incorporation of a practice approach that encompasses cultural humility and determinants of health, and keeps a wellness perspective at the center of all patient interactions
3. Information provided on specific assessment skills that are often overlooked or misunderstood
4. Summaries of abnormal findings for common disease states across the life span
5. Feedback that enhances learning through detailed rationale accompanying each practice question

## DISTINGUISHING FEATURES TO SUPPORT STUDENT LEARNING

*Assessment and Diagnosis Review for APRN Certification Exams* strives to incorporate the latest and best clinical evidence for physical examination assessment skills and findings that are valuable in everyday clinical practice. It includes assessment of the dimensions of wellness and health behaviors as a routine component of history taking and involves when and how to incorporate specific physical examination techniques. Evidence-based national guidelines are integrated into the recommendations for the history and physical examination for individuals across the life span.

The review book incorporates format and content of practice questions based on AANPCB, ANCC, and PNCB certification exams. It features alternate-format questions such as photos of skin, eye, and ear conditions; body system diagrams; EKGs, and more challenging drag-and-drop and multiple-response questions. This review text covers the entire life span and is organized by both body systems and population health. It includes end-of-chapter questions to assess knowledge retention, a 150-question practice exam that covers all populations across the life span, and a bonus 50-question mini practice exam focused on the pediatric population. Each of the 350 questions includes a comprehensive remediating rationale that addresses both correct and incorrect answer options. These questions offer an opportunity to critically consider normal and abnormal assessment findings, growth and development, lab findings, signs and symptoms of emergent problems, risk factors for developing acute and chronic health problems, evidence-based guidelines, and indicators of threats to health and wellness.

Purchase includes 6 months' free digital access to the interactive digital version on ExamPrepConnect (see access details on inside front cover). Features include:

- Personalized study plan based on exam date
- Lessons based on the review content in each chapter
- Practice questions categorized by body system
- Timed practice tests and untimed mini-tests
- Analytics to strengthen test performance, including identification of strengths and weaknesses, test performance over time, and rank against other users
- Game center and discussion board

## INTENDED AUDIENCE

This textbook is intended for advanced practice nursing students across specialties who strive to expand their knowledge of evidence-based assessment and practice. This is the first review book to solely focus on the foundation of advanced assessment and diagnostic decision-making.

Graduates of advanced practice nursing programs who are preparing for certification exams will benefit from this detailed review of assessment and diagnosis, as understanding the importance of history, risk factors, and signs and symptoms of disease processes provide the basis for evidence-based clinical management. The review book incorporates format and content based on AANPCB, ANCC, and PNCB certification exams, of which more than 50% of these exams test knowledge and competency in the areas of assessment and diagnostic decision-making.

Educators who provide instruction to students enrolled in graduate, baccalaureate, and associate degree health science programs who aspire to provide an evidence-based advanced assessment approach to individuals across the life span will also appreciate the review content and the question test bank, which can be integrated into course syllabi.

## CONTENT ORGANIZATION

### PART I: EVIDENCE-BASED STRATEGIES FOR SUCCESS

The first two chapters of this text identify approaches to test-taking and evidence-based assessment.

Chapter 1 includes strategies for optimal test performance, including tips on maintaining wellness, practicing stress reduction, and test day success. Chapter 2 reviews the fundamentals of evidence-based assessment and clinical practice. Both chapters reinforce the importance of preparation and practice and review foundational concepts of advanced practice.

### PART II: EVIDENCE-BASED ASSESSMENT AND DIAGNOSIS

Chapters 3 through 14 focus on body systems. Each of these chapters includes a review of advanced assessment as a foundation for interpreting examination findings. Each chapter includes a listing of pertinent components of key history considerations, examination techniques organized by normal and abnormal findings, life-span considerations, and potential differential diagnoses. Body systems reviewed include mental health assessment, as mental and physical health are inextricably combined.

### PART III: EVIDENCE-BASED CONSIDERATIONS FOR POPULATION HEALTH

Chapters 15 through 18 review the determinants of health that impact the provision of care for specific populations. Chapters address assessment and diagnostic considerations for individuals experiencing disparities, pediatric and adolescent populations, pregnant individuals, and older adult populations. While each chapter includes life-span considerations, these final chapters are intended to highlight evidence-based practice considerations.

### PART IV: PRACTICE TESTS

Part IV includes a 150-question practice test with questions that address the assessment and diagnosis of patients across the life span and a 50-question test specific to the pediatric population. Each test includes answers with comprehensive rationales.

We have enjoyed creating this review and hope that you will find it useful, practical, and engaging. We wish you the best of success on your certification exams.

*Alice M. Teall, Kate Sustersic Gawlik, and Bernadette Mazurek Melnyk*

## ACKNOWLEDGMENTS

To all of the advanced practice nurses who we have had the opportunity to teach as students, thank you. Across decades, our students have demonstrated a willingness to learn, have provided feedback to us about our teaching and evaluation methods, and have shaped our ability as educators to implement effective strategies to teach the tenets of evidence-based practice. We are so proud of our graduates who are practicing in advanced practice across this country. Even as students, we respected your dedication to providing the highest quality, patient-centered care for individuals, families, and communities. Your exceptional contributions to care as advanced practice nurses are transforming healthcare delivery.

Special thanks to our family, friends, and colleagues. The value of having someone who believes in you is impossible to measure. You have supported us through character-building challenges and encouraged us to find joy in our work. Thank you to Rosie Zeno for contributing to our pediatric content; the impact of your expertise is evident in this text and within the minds and hearts of countless pediatric nurse practitioner program graduates.

We are grateful for our team at Springer Publishing. Thank you, Adrianne Brigido, your confidence in this project has been invaluable. Lucia Gunzel, welcome to the team! We are grateful to each of you for your work to bring this text to publication.

# Part I
# Evidence-Based Strategies for Success

# Evidence-Based Strategies for Successful Test Performance

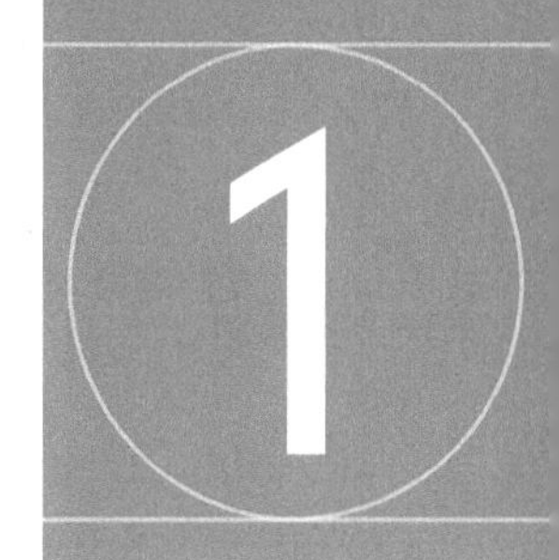


## THE IMPORTANCE OF PRACTICE

Practice is critical to learning and to successful test performance. Retrieving information through repeated testing of knowledge and understanding, with feedback and review, has been found to be the most effective strategy for long-term memory retention (Abel & Roediger, 2017; Roediger & Butler, 2011). To gain and reinforce the knowledge and skills needed to pass exams, whether course exams or a certification exam, it is critical to set aside and block times in your schedule for review and retrieval practice, including practice questions. Break up information into manageable sections to review. Take note of the rationale for practice questions missed, as well as those that you answered correctly. The benefits of retrieval practice are not only limited to the learning of specific content; review and retrieval practice produces knowledge that can be transferred and applied to different contexts (Abel & Roediger, 2017; Roediger & Butler, 2011). Practice frequently. Challenge yourself. Practice retrieving information for new and previously covered concepts, allowing time for reflection.

Preparing to take any major exam tends to be stressful. High stress disrupts learning and diminishes memory construction, storage, and retrieval. However, there are evidence-based strategies that you can implement along with review and retrieval practice to increase your probability of performing well and achieving a successful outcome. The strategies reviewed in this chapter are intended to support you in achieving success and building confidence, a positive perspective, and physical and mental well-being.

## VISUALIZE AND BELIEVE IN YOUR SUCCESS

*"Whatever your mind can conceive and believe, it can achieve!"*—Napoleon Hill

As you prepare for exams, it is critical to envision a successful outcome. Weeks before your certification examination, or any high-stakes test, visualize yourself taking the exam with confidence and passing it. If you are not feeling confident about the test, it is critical to get up every morning and say one or two self-affirmation statements; consider saying these affirming statements aloud, minimally ten times. Example affirmations include: "I have the knowledge needed to pass this exam"; "I am going to pass my test with flying colors"; "I believe I have the skills to ace my test"; and "I have learned what I need to know to be successful." The practice of daily self-affirmations has been shown through research to increase academic performance and decrease stress (Critcher & Dunning, 2015; Layous et al., 2017).

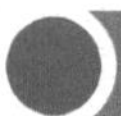

## TAKE CARE OF YOUR MIND AND BODY

Healthy lifestyle behaviors are important to keep your mind and body in optimal well-being for best performance. Prevention of chronic disease, robust learning, and academic performance, and all nine dimensions of wellness (intellectual, physical, emotional, spiritual, career, creative, financial, environmental, and social wellness) are tied to five key healthy lifestyle behaviors (Melnyk, Gawlik, & Teall, 2020). Make a commitment to achieve these key behaviors:

- Get 30 minutes of moderate-intensity physical activity 5 days per week
- Eat five fruits and vegetables per day
- Avoid smoking
- Sleep 7 to 9 hours a night
- Drink alcohol in moderation, if at all

Regarding healthy eating, keep in mind the "80/20 rule" (i.e., consume 80% healthy foods and 20% "want" foods). Eating foods high in sugar, especially prior to tests or exams, causes insulin to rise, which then causes your blood sugar to decline. When your blood sugar level crashes, the result is often a headache and feeling anxious, irritable, and fatigued. To maintain steady insulin levels, eat fewer carbohydrates and when you do, consume whole foods and complex carbohydrates, such as brown rice and whole-grain bread.

Hydrate for maximal wellness. Even mild dehydration causes headaches and fatigue, so make sure you are drinking approximately 15.5 cups of fluid a day if you are a man and 11.5 cups of fluid a day if you are a woman (National Academies of Sciences, Engineering, and Medicine, 2020). If you feel thirsty, your body is telling you it needs fluids; water instead of a sugary beverage is a much better choice. Too much caffeine also can make you feel irritable and anxious, so drink caffeinated beverages in moderation before exams. Up to 400 milligrams (mg) of caffeine (approximately four cups of brewed coffee) a day seems to be safe for most healthy adults. Some people are more sensitive to caffeine than others, so if you start to experience headaches, nervousness, insomnia, irritability, or a fast heartbeat, it is time to reduce your caffeinated beverages.

Physical activity is vital for sustained energy and optimal well-being. The recommended amount of physical activity is 30 minutes of moderate activity 5 days a week. For a person who is inactive, even small increases in moderate-intensity physical activity (e.g., 11 minutes a day) have health benefits (Powell et al., 2019). There is no threshold that has to be exceeded before benefits occur. For more energy, it also is important to sit less and move more (Melnyk, Gawlik & Teall, 2020). Several chronic diseases and conditions result from prolonged sitting. One recent study found that prolonged sitting (i.e., 6 or more hours a day versus less than 3 hours per day) was related to a higher risk of mortality from all causes, including cardiovascular disease, cancer, diabetes, kidney disease, suicide, chronic obstructive pulmonary disease, pneumonitis due to solids and liquids, liver, peptic ulcer and other digestive diseases, Parkinson disease, Alzheimer disease, nervous disorders, and musculoskeletal disorders (Patel, Maliniak, Rees-Punia, Matthews, & Gapstur, 2018). Try standing and studying for your exam instead of sitting and studying and see how much more alert you are when standing than sitting. Instead of waiting until January 1 to set a new healthy lifestyle behavior goal, consider today your January 1. Remember, it takes 30 to 60 days to make or break a new health habit (Melnyk, Gawlik & Teall, 2020). It is important to write down your new healthy lifestyle behavior goal and place that goal where you can see it every day (e.g., by where you brush your teeth or at your computer). If you do fall off track, just start again the following day. Habits take consistent practice to make or break.

Engaging in strength training at least twice a week provides benefits that include increased muscle mass, increased bone strength, better stability, and lower blood pressure. Resistance bands are an ideal convenient way to build strength as you can keep them at your desk and take them with you at work or school.

Sleep is essential for optimal health and well-being all year long, but especially the week prior to your exam. It is critical to get at least 7 hours of sleep a night to avoid excess cortisol from being released. Do not pull "all-nighters" to study before exams, as it will lead to decreased alertness and fatigue during the exam. If you have insomnia or problems with sleep, assess the amount of caffeinated beverages that you are drinking during the day. Avoid consuming caffeinated beverages or foods (e.g., chocolate candy or ice cream) 6 hours before you plan to go to sleep. Eating too heavy a meal or exercising vigorously at night also can exacerbate sleep problems. One of the best strategies for a restful night's sleep is to create a habit of going to sleep and waking up at the same time every day. In addition, limiting screen time to at least an hour or two before bedtime is helpful. If you have difficulty falling asleep, try a white noise machine that plays soothing sounds, such as an ocean or rainfall.

## PRACTICE DAILY STRESS-REDUCTION TACTICS

There is a wise saying: change your thinking; change your life! Cognitive-behavioral therapy (CBT) or cognitive-behavioral skills building is the recommended, gold standard, first-line treatment for mild to moderate depression, anxiety, and chronic stress, yet so few people suffering from these symptoms receive or have access to treatment. In CBT, individuals are taught that how they think is related to how they feel and how they behave. The ABCs are taught in CBT: An activating event (A) triggers a negative belief (B), and the consequence (C) of the negative thought includes emotional and behavioral responses (i.e., feeling stressed, anxious, or depressed; or acting in unhealthy ways).

Monitoring for activating events and recognizing negative beliefs can allow an individual to change thought patterns, which results in a change in consequences to more positive emotions and healthier behaviors. The next time that you feel stressed, anxious, angry, or depressed, ask yourself, "What was I just thinking?" Chances are it was a negative thought. Monitoring for these activating events and replacing negative beliefs are key to experiencing more positivity and gaining perspective (Melnyk, Gawlik & Teall, 2020). For example, as the day for an exam is approaching, you might be feeling more stressed because you are thinking, "I don't have many days left to study, and I might fail." It is important to notice that thought and challenge it, saying to yourself, "Is this thought really true?" or "Is this thinking helpful?" The answer is typically no, so change the thinking by saying, "I know what I need to pass the exam, and I am confident I will pass." As a result of catching the thought, checking it, and changing it, your stress level will decline. Also, recognize and remember that worry is part of negative thinking and wastes energy. When you start to worry, bring yourself back to the present moment. Turn your head slowly from left to right, taking note of what you are seeing, feeling, and sensing. Mindfulness allows you to develop a positive perspective and helps to reduce stress and anxiety.

A recent randomized controlled trial with new nurse residents in a large academic medical center in the Midwest tested a CBT-based program, MINDSTRONG, and revealed that those who received the MINDSTRONG program had less stress, anxiety, and depression as well as healthier behaviors and job satisfaction compared to those who received an attention-control program (Sampson, Melnyk, & Hoying, 2020). Consistent with this finding, try monitoring your thoughts for the next 30 days by keeping a journal of negative thought patterns and the emotions that come with them and write down how you would choose more positively to respond the next time in a similar situation. With time and practice, you can actually change your response to the stressors in your life (Melnyk & Neale, 2018).

Box 1.1 provides strategies to enhance your emotional well-being as you prepare for exams. If symptoms of anxiety, stress, or depression persist for more than 2 weeks and interfere with your daily functioning, do not wait; seek help from a qualified therapist or your healthcare provider. Emotional wellness includes seeking help when needed (Melnyk & Neale, 2018).

### Box 1.1 Strategies to Enhance Emotional Well-Being

- Engage in some physical activity each day; even small amounts can increase your energy and decrease fatigue.
- Keep a journal of what causes you stress and strategies that help to reduce it.
- Practice mindfulness—the ability to stay in the present moment. Mindfulness decreases worry about the future and guilt about the past, which are two energy-draining emotions.
- Manage your energy by taking short recovery breaks throughout the day (even 5 minutes of activity every hour can increase your level of energy).
- Read 5 minutes in a positive thinking book of your choice every morning to elevate your mood and protect yourself against negativity that can arise each day.
- When stressed, take just five slow deep breaths in and out to decrease stress and lower blood pressure. As you breathe in, say "I am calm." As you breathe out, say "I am blowing all stress out."
- Help others and be kind; compassion for others helps you to feel good.
- Talk to someone you trust about how you feel.
- Practice daily gratitude. Naming or writing down three people or things you are grateful for every morning and evening can help you to maintain a positive perspective, boost your mood, and relieve stress (Melnyk, Gawlik & Teall, 2020).

## TEST-DAY STRATEGIES

On the day of your exam, practice the mindfulness strategies, calm breathing exercises, and stress-busting affirmations that you have practiced during the preparation for the exam. You will want to activate these before and during exams when you are feeling stressed.

Make sure that you arrive early at the exam site, as being rushed will contribute to a stressful start to the exam. Wear comfortable clothes and dress in layers in case the temperature of the room is too hot or cold. Say a positive self-affirmation statement as you are getting ready to start the exam, such as "I'm going to do well!" and take a few, slow abdominal deep breaths saying "I am calm" as you breathe in and "I am blowing stress out" as you breathe out.

Review all instructions and directions. If you have access to scrap paper or an electronic note-taking application, begin the exam by writing the most important points, formulas, mnemonics, or other information that you would like to access during the test, as this allows your working memory to focus on the test questions.

Read each question carefully and focus on answering the individual question. Do not panic if you do not know an answer with certainty. Choose the best answer and mark the question for later review. Maintain positive self-talk, even if you notice that a series of questions has been difficult or challenging, as this will allow you to move through the questions with less stress and more mental clarity.

## CELEBRATE YOUR SUCCESS

Recognize your progress as you study, practice retrieving information, and meet your goals for exam review. Allow yourself to notice that you are building confidence and celebrate!

Celebration is a motivator for continuing work to meet goals. Understand that challenging questions, even those that you answer incorrectly, are opportunities to learn, recall, apply, and analyze content. Consider studying both individually and in small groups and celebrate with your team when study goals are successfully met. Once you pass your exam, celebrate your success. Recognize your accomplishment by treating yourself to something special or engaging in an activity that you enjoy. Congratulations! You have studied, prepared, and practiced to achieve success. You deserve to celebrate!

## REFERENCES

Abel, M., & Roediger, H. L. (2017). Comparing the testing effect under blocked and mixed practice: The mnemonic benefits of retrieval practice are not affected by practice format. *Memory and Cognition*. https://doi.org/10.3758/s13421-016-0641-8

Critcher, C. R., & Dunning, D. (2015). Self-affirmations provide a broader perspective on self-threat. *Personality and Social Psychology Bulletin*. https://doi.org/10.1177/0146167214554956

Ford, E. S., Zhao, G., Tsai, J., & Li, C. (2011). Low-Risk lifestyle behaviors and all-cause mortality: Findings from the national health and nutrition examination survey III mortality study. *American Journal of Public Health*. https://doi.org/10.2105/AJPH.2011.300167

Layous, K., Davis, E. M., Garcia, J., Purdie-Vaughns, V., Cook, J. E., & Cohen, G. L. (2017). Feeling left out, but affirmed: Protecting against the negative effects of low belonging in college. *Journal of Experimental Social Psychology*. https://doi.org/10.1016/j.jesp.2016.09.008

Melnyk, B. M., Gawlik, K., & Teall, A. M. (2020). Evidence-based assessment of personal health and well-being for clinicians: key strategies to achieve optimal wellness. *Evidence-Based Physical Examination*. https://doi.org/10.1891/9780826164544.0028

Melnyk, B. M., & Neale, S. (2018). 9 dimensions of wellness. *American Nurse Today, 13*(1), 10–11. Retrieved from https://www.myamericannurse.com/9-dimensions-wellness/

National Academies of Sciences, Engineering, and Medicine. (2020). Leading Health Indicators 2030: Advancing Health, Equity, and Well-Being. Washington, DC: The National Academies Press. https://doi.org/10.17226/25682

Patel, A. V., Maliniak, M. L., Rees-Punia, E., Matthews, C. E., & Gapstur, S. M. (2018). Prolonged leisure time spent sitting in relation to cause-specific mortality in a large us cohort. *American Journal of Epidemiology*. https://doi.org/10.1093/aje/kwy125

Powell, K. E., King, A. C., Buchner, D. M., Campbell, W. W., DiPietro, L., Erickson, K. I., . . . Whitt-Glover, M. C. (2019). The scientific foundation for the physical activity guidelines for Americans, 2nd edition. *Journal of Physical Activity and Health*. https://doi.org/10.1123/jpah.2018-0618

Roediger, H. L., & Butler, A. C. (2011). The critical role of retrieval practice in long-term retention. *Trends in Cognitive Sciences*. https://doi.org/10.1016/j.tics.2010.09.003

Sampson, M., Melnyk, B. M., & Hoying, J. (2020). The MINDBODYSTRONG intervention for new nurse residents: 6-month effects on mental health outcomes, healthy lifestyle behaviors, and job satisfaction. *Worldviews on Evidence-Based Nursing*. https://doi.org/10.1111/wvn.12411

# Evidence-Based Approach to History and Physical Exam

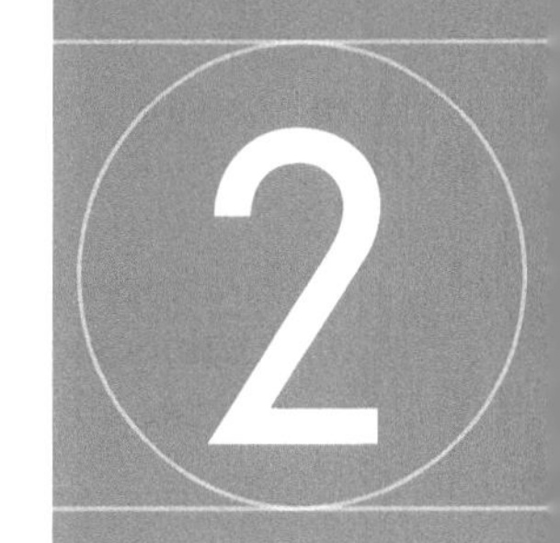


## EVIDENCE-BASED ASSESSMENT

History and physical examination are the cornerstones of advanced assessment, and advanced assessment is the cornerstone of clinical practice. To effectively implement advanced assessment skills in clinical practice involves a complex series of steps, a foundation of knowledge, an ability to appreciate the information shared by an individual/patient/family, and clinical interpretation of the assessments of health and well-being. Clinicians use advanced assessment skills as the foundation for delivering quality care. To deliver the highest quality of healthcare and ensure the best patient outcomes, there has been a dramatic shift in clinical practice to incorporating the latest research or best evidence, and to questioning the processes and systems that have been in place for years to determine whether they are the most effective and efficient methods.

Evidence-based practice (EBP) is a life-long problem-solving approach to the delivery of care that incorporates the current best evidence with a clinician's expertise and patient/family preferences and values. When implemented consistently, EBP results in the highest quality of care, improved population health outcomes, decreased costs, and clinician empowerment, otherwise known as the "quadruple aim in healthcare." However, even with all its positive benefits, EBP is not standard of care in many healthcare systems due to multiple barriers, including inadequate EBP skills in clinicians and cultures that promote a philosophy of "that is the way we do it here."

Implementing the best practices of evidence-based assessment begins with being patient-centered. To be patient-centered regarding health and well-being involves having a broad understanding of the dimensions of wellness. An individual's understanding of health, experience of well-being, ability to implement a healthy lifestyle, and achieve health in all dimensions can change over time, and is affected by their family, community, and culture. Clinicians practicing today need to holistically approach patients and help them meet their optimal wellness goals by addressing the multiple aspects affecting their health and well-being.

Fully integrating an assessment of wellness into practice involves understanding that being healthy involves more than physical health. Well-being assessment should include the nine dimensions of wellness: physical, emotional, financial, intellectual, career, social, creative, environmental, and spiritual (Figure 2.1). Clinicians need to take each of these dimensions into consideration when assessing individuals and families.

Each dimension can impact the other dimensions. Failing to take into account all nine dimensions results in an incomplete well-being assessment, which could lead to inaccurate conclusions and ineffective management.

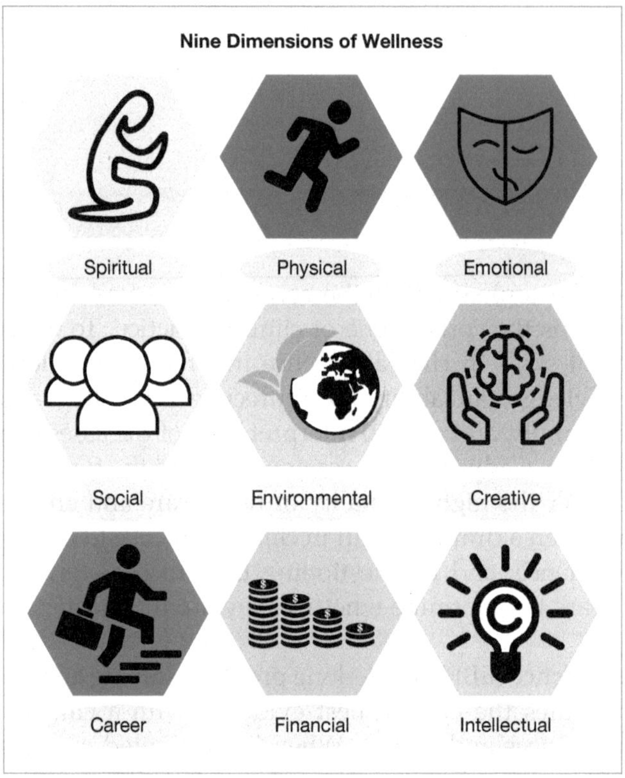


**Figure 2.1** Nine dimensions of wellness: physical, emotional, financial, intellectual, career, social, creative, environmental, and spiritual.

## HISTORY TAKING

History taking is the primary way a clinician obtains comprehensive information about the patient and is, often, the most important aspect of the patient visit for diagnostic decision making. The approach to history taking will change based on the reason for the patient visit. There are different types of health histories that are collected during a patient visit. This chapter discusses collecting a history for an episodic visit, a wellness exam, a chronic care management visit, and the various components of each. The scope and degree of detail in history taking will depend on the patient's purpose for the visit, their chief concern, the complexity of the patient's medical condition, and the clinician's goals for the visit. Regardless of the type of history, the goal during the interview is to be attentive to the patient and receptive to the patient's needs. Tailor communication, decision-making, and treatment based on the purpose of the visit and patient preferences.

## HISTORY TAKING FOR AN EPISODIC VISIT

The episodic visit, scheduled for a recent, bothersome, or acute health problem, accounts for the majority of clinician visits. Episodic visits focus on a specific concern voiced by the patient. The patient can be either an established patient or a new patient. For an episodic visit, the extent of the history collected is variable and based on the clinician's judgment and the patient's presenting symptoms. For new patients, a comprehensive health history should be conducted. For established patients, a more limited health history is collected, tailored to the chief concern. The following list provides the general framework for the elements of history taking during an episodic visit. To begin the visit, the clinician introduces themselves and washes their hands.

### CHIEF CONCERN OR REASON FOR SEEKING CARE

History taking begins with clarifying the patient's main reason for the visit. Clarifying an individual's chief concern (CC) is a priority. The CC is the description of the symptom, problem, condition, diagnosis, or reason for seeking care. Often, documentation of the CC is in the patient's own words, e.g., "my left ear hurts."

### HISTORY OF PRESENT ILLNESS

The history of present illness (HPI) provides key information required for developing differential diagnoses, determining a diagnosis, and guiding treatment. Often a diagnosis can be made from the history alone, so this step is crucial. In the HPI, the patient provides detailed reasons for the visit and describes how the illness has progressed. It is important for clinicians to allow the patient to tell the story in their own words about their concerns, including their perception of the illness or health problem. The history of the present illness contains eight core elements to assess, summarized with the mnemonic OLDCARTS:

- **Onset:** When did symptoms start? Are symptoms recent? How did symptoms begin?
- **Location:** Specific location of symptoms?
- **Duration:** Are symptoms persistent or transitory? Increasing or unchanged?
- **Characteristics:** How would you describe the symptoms? Is there itching, burning, drainage, pain, swelling, bruising, or redness? How does the symptom feel (i.e., sharp, dull, stabbing, burning, crushing, throbbing, nauseating, shooting, twisting, or stretching)?
- **Aggravating factors:** What actions or activities may have precipitated the symptoms or caused the symptoms to worsen?
- **Relieving factors:** What actions or activities decrease the symptoms? What medications has the individual taken to help with the symptoms? (Note that treatment may be listed as a distinct component of the HPI).
- **Temporal factors/timing:** How do symptoms respond to treatment, relieving factors, situations, or conditions? Are symptoms constant?
- **Severity:** How severe are the symptoms on a scale of 0 to 10? Do symptoms limit participation in activities at school/work/home?

## PAST MEDICAL HISTORY

Also referred to as history of illness, health history, or past medical and surgical history, the assessment of past medical history is important to obtain and review during all visits; even when established patients follow up with clinicians, their health history should be updated. Assessment of past medical history includes asking the patient about experiences with illnesses both acute and chronic (may include pertinent childhood illnesses), hospitalizations, surgeries, sexual/reproductive health issues, and hereditary conditions that could place the patient at risk. When asking health history questions, review all current medications, prescribed, over-the-counter, and/or herbal; when an individual shares history of allergies, ask specifics about their reaction to the allergens.

Components of past medical history:

- History of physical or mental health conditions
  - Ask if ever diagnosed with specific conditions (e.g., heart disease, elevated blood pressure, cancer, diabetes, depression, arthritis, asthma)
  - Clarify whether conditions are current or past health problems
- History of hospitalizations and surgeries
  - Clarify reason and dates
- Recent illness, accidents, injuries, or exposures
- History of emergency department or urgent care visits
- Immunization status, record of vaccines
- Gender identity and sexual orientation with age-appropriate considerations
  - **Women's health history:** Menstrual, gynecological, obstetric, and sexual health
  - **Men's health history:** Sexual and reproductive health
  - **Pediatric health history:** Birth history, growth, and development
- Medications
  - Prescribed medications including dose and frequency
  - Over-the-counter medications or supplements, including dose and frequency
- Allergies
  - Allergies to medications, including reaction
  - Seasonal, environmental, and/or food allergies, including reaction

## FAMILY HISTORY

The family history is a review of the immediate family members' history related to medical events, illnesses, and hereditary conditions that place the patient's current and future health at risk. Immediate family includes parents, grandparents, siblings, children, and grandchildren. As details are provided during the family history, inquire whether the relative is alive or deceased. If the person is deceased, ask about the age at death and the cause of death, especially for first-degree relatives.

Assess family history for:

- Chronic diseases
  - Hypertension, heart disease, obesity, diabetes, cancer, epilepsy, and asthma
- Acute or recent episodic illnesses
  - Infectious diseases, allergies, environmental exposures
- Mental health disorders
  - Anxiety, depression, bipolar disorder, or severe, persistent mental illness
  - Substance use disorder, alcoholism, addiction

- Intellectual disabilities, learning disorders, developmental delays
- Genetic or hereditary conditions

Obtaining a patient's family history provides valuable insight into health risks and supports recommendations for screening and/or referral for genetic counseling. Genetic conditions can be inherited in a variety of patterns, depending on the gene involved (e.g., autosomal dominant, autosomal recessive, X-linked dominant, X-linked recessive, Y-linked, codominant, mitochondrial, and polygenic.)

## SOCIAL HISTORY

An individual's social history provides information regarding their health beliefs and behaviors, support systems, and safety, and allows a clinician to identify risk factors that may impact well-being. Note that the influence of culture on health beliefs, behaviors, practices, perceptions, and approaches is vast; this component of history requires a sensitive and humble approach that respects cultural, family, community, and personal values and norms.

Components of social history:

- Substance use history
  - Tobacco use in any form (pipe, snuff, chewing tobacco, e-cigarettes, hookah, vaping, cigars, cigarettes)? If yes, assess smoking history, readiness to quit.
  - Alcohol use? If yes, screen for binge drinking, problematic use.
  - Other substances (e.g., medications not prescribed, illicit drugs)?
    - Ask if the individual has ever taken medications not specifically prescribed for them
    - Ask if the individual has ever taken substance for how it would make them feel
- Relationships, including marital status; living arrangements
  - Family dynamics
  - Friends and social support system
  - Strengths, including spiritual, religious, and ethnic/cultural support systems
  - History of trauma, victim of violence, and adverse childhood events
- Safety of home, work, and/or school environments
  - Exposure to hazards—fumes, radiation, chemicals, viruses
  - Risk or current exposure to violence, trauma, stressors
  - Behaviors involving risk-taking, risk of falls
  - Safe participation in sports and physical activities
  - Screen for use of seat belts, bicycle/motorcycle helmets
  - Screen for smoke detectors in home
  - Screen for access to guns in home, neighborhood, and at work
  - Assess social determinants of health (see Chapter 15, "Determinants of Health and Wellness," for more information)

## PREVENTIVE CARE CONSIDERATIONS

Assess an individual's participating in behaviors to prevent disease and illness:

- Healthy lifestyle behaviors, including diet/nutrition, physical activity/exercise, and sleep
- Management of stress, coping with stressors
- Recent/needed health screenings (e.g., blood pressure, anxiety, depression, mammogram, colonoscopy, cholesterol, lead, sexually transmitted infections [STIs], and vision/hearing)

## REVIEW OF SYSTEMS

A review of systems (ROS) collected during a patient visit is an inventory of symptoms that is obtained by a series of questions that are organized by body systems. The ROS offers essential information about current or potential disease processes or health problems that may otherwise go unnoticed. The history information provided by the ROS includes pertinent positive and negative findings. Important to note: the ROS is subjective information provided by the patient, not the clinician's observation or findings.

Clinicians choose the depth of the ROS based on the acuity of the individual who is presenting to them, whether the patient is established or new, and according to the level of diagnostic decision-making that is required during a visit. The ROS can be focused, extended, or complete.

Example ROS history questions:

- **General or constitutional**: Recent illness? Weight gain or loss? Fatigue? Changes in sleep pattern? Night sweats? Fever? Frequent infections?
- **Integumentary:** Lesions or rashes? Changes in skin, hair, nails? Itching? Eczema?
- **Head, neck:** Headache? Neck pain? Dizziness? Pain related to head injury?
- **Lymphatic/hematologic:** Swollen or tender lymph nodes? Abnormal bleeding? Bruising?
- **Ears, eyes, nose, throat (EENT):** Eye drainage or redness? Vision changes? Itchy eyes/ears/nose? Ear pain? Hearing loss? Rhinorrhea or congestion? Sore throat? Trouble chewing or swallowing? Bleeding gums? Dental pain?
- **Cardiovascular:** Chest pain? Palpitations? Exercise intolerance? Orthopnea? Edema?
- **Respiratory:** Cough? Dyspnea or shortness of breath? Wheezing? Hemoptysis?
- **Breast:** Tenderness? Palpable lumps or masses? Skin changes or discharge?
- **Gastrointestinal**: Pain? Change in bowel habits? Blood in the stool? Nausea? Vomiting? Heartburn? Change in appetite?
- **Genitourinary:** Urinary frequency? Pain with urination? Nocturia? Urgency? Hematuria? Unusual discharge or odor? Pelvic or groin pain? Dyspareunia?
- **Musculoskeletal**: Back pain? Muscle aches? Joint swelling? Limitations of function?
- **Neurologic:** Numbness or tingling? Syncope? Memory loss? Restlessness? Changing level of consciousness? Loss of coordination? Tremors?
- **Endocrine**: Increased thirst? Heat or cold intolerance?
- **Psychiatric/mental health:** Worry? Sadness, helplessness, hopelessness? Insomnia? Change in mood? Irritability? Difficulty coping with stress? Trouble concentrating?

## HISTORY TAKING FOR A WELLNESS EXAM

Wellness exams can be an important health promotion and disease prevention strategy, as the goals of the visit include early identification of health risks, and/or detection of health problems at an early stage when treatment is most likely to be effective. Sports physicals, well child exams, work physicals, and annual exams are examples of wellness exams; these clinician visits require age- and gender-appropriate history and physical exam.

Because the patient history taking during wellness exams is not problem-oriented, the history will not include a chief concern, although reason for the visit can be listed. In addition, there is not likely to be a need to collect HPI, or history of present illness. Rather, a wellness exam should include a comprehensive history and physical examination appropriate to the patient's age and gender, counseling and anticipatory guidance, risk reduction interventions, the ordering or administration of vaccine-appropriate immunizations, and the ordering of appropriate laboratory and/or diagnostic testing. The wellness exam differs from the episodic visit and chronic care management visit because the components of the wellness exam are based on age and risk factors, not a presenting problem.

### COMPONENTS OF WELLNESS EXAMS

- Comprehensive, culturally sensitive history and physical examination
- For infants and children, will include assessment of growth and development
- Anticipatory guidance regarding risks to health and well-being
- Recommendations for immunizations, screenings, diagnostic testing
- Anticipatory guidance and support regarding reaching health and wellness goals

## HISTORY TAKING AND CHRONIC CARE MANAGEMENT

More than half of all adults in the United States have a chronic condition; chronic diseases are among the leading causes of death and disability. Common chronic diseases include:

- Heart disease
- Cancer
- Chronic lung disease
- Stroke
- Alzheimer's disease
- Diabetes
- Chronic kidney disease
- Depression
- Anxiety
- Obesity

These chronic conditions place the patient at risk for adverse health events. Managing these conditions effectively requires face-to-face visits along with non–face-to-face visits. The focus of chronic care management is the patient's relationship with the healthcare team (not just the clinician); establishing and achieving individual health goals; coordination of community and social services; medical, functional, and psychosocial assessment; and preventive care.

History taking during a chronic care management visit includes all the components of an episodic visit, in addition to assessing and prioritizing the patient's ability to manage their chronic illness. Health behaviors play an important role in the risk for chronic disease. Tobacco use and exposure to secondhand smoke, poor nutrition, lack of physical activity, and excessive alcohol use have been found to be key contributors to increasing a patient's risk of acquiring a chronic disease. Assessment priorities for chronic care management include:

- Functional and psychosocial assessment, with disease-specific concerns
- Assessment of wellness, dimensions of wellness, and healthy lifestyle behaviors
- Individual health goals; motivation and readiness, confidence, and self-efficacy
- Problem list, treatment goals, expected outcomes, and collaborative management
- Self-management support; options for coaching, team-based care, and group visits

## THERAPEUTIC COMMUNICATION

Regardless of the type of patient visit, the goal during the history-taking is to be attentive to the patient and receptive to the individual's needs. Conducting the patient history requires patient-centered interviewing skills, which includes skillful use of therapeutic communication.

Therapeutic communication techniques include:

- **Open-ended questions:** The use of open-ended questions allows the patient to express their concerns.
- **Active listening:** Providing an opportunity for an individual to share their history and concerns without interruption and with full engagement communicates nonverbally that what is being said is being heard.
- **Reflection**: The use of reflection demonstrates active listening and acknowledges the patient's response.
- **Empathy:** The patient's emotions are central to effective decision-making. Affirming the patient's emotions demonstrates that the clinician appreciates how the patient is feeling.
- **Seeking clarification:** Asking follow-up questions to history statements is helpful in obtaining an accurate history, and with establishing trust with the patient.
- **Summary or restatement:** Summarizing patient statement to demonstrate an understanding of a patient's values and preferences allows the clinician to develop a partnership with the individual.

History questions are intended to be asked in a confidential and sensitive manner. In doing so, the clinician will encourage the patient to disclose their perspectives about health, wellness, and illness. Implementing evidence-based, patient-centered assessment requires sensitivity and openness to the patient's responses as specific details of their history and perspectives are shared.

## POPULATION HEALTH AND LIFE-SPAN CONSIDERATIONS

There are unique considerations when obtaining a history from children, parents, pregnant women, and older adults. These populations are covered in Chapter 16, "Pediatric and Adolescent Populations"; Chapter 17, "Pregnant Populations"; and Chapter 18, "Older Adult Populations."

# PHYSICAL EXAMINATION

## FUNDAMENTAL PHYSICAL EXAMINATION TECHNIQUES

The evidence-based physical examination has four fundamental practices that are typically utilized during each visit. These are the general survey, inspection, palpation, and auscultation. Some body systems also employ the use of percussion and select special tests.

The general survey is the initial impression of the patient as the clinician enters the room. The initial assessments of a general survey are completed to determine whether the individual being evaluated is in distress. Observing whether a patient is well or unwell is essential and can be completed quickly. Additionally, vital signs can offer information in this assessment.

Inspection is the close observation by the clinician of the patient using their eyes, ears, and nose. This is the process of observing the patient's appearance, behaviors, color, shape, symmetry, size, position, posture, facial expressions, body habitus, gait, respiratory rate, and odors.

Palpation is when the clinician uses the tactile pressure from their fingers and hands to assess an area of the body. This technique can be used to determine the temperature of the skin or the presence of pain, edema, elevation, size, texture, moisture, or contour on a body part or on a lesion.

Auscultation is a technique that involves using the bell and diaphragm of the stethoscope to listen to heart, lung, and circulatory sounds. This technique allows the clinician to detect normal and abnormal sounds within the body.

Percussion is the practice of striking a body surface in a quick, rapid motion to produce different sounds that provide information about the underlying body structures. This is typically done by using the third finger as the striking finger again the distal third finger of the opposite hand as it is placed firmly on the body surface. Dullness, tympany, and resonance can also be detected using this method.

Special tests are system dependent and are employed to provide additional evidence to support or refute a diagnosis. These tests vary in specificity and sensitivity.

## SEQUENCE OF PHYSICAL EXAMINATION

A physical examination can be focused or comprehensive based on the reason for the visit. Most clinicians prefer a head-to-toe approach. The head-to-toe approach generally follows the following sequence:

- General survey and vital signs
- Mental status
- Skin
- Head and neck
- Eyes, ears, nose, and throat
- Respiratory (chest and thorax)
- Heart and circulatory
- Abdomen
- Breasts

- Genitalia, anus, and rectum
- Musculoskeletal
- Neurological
- Mental health

Evidence-based assessment lays the foundation for building a comprehensive differential diagnoses or problem list, provides the strategies for triaging the acuity of the patient, and creates the groundwork for integration of wellness, health promotion, and disease prevention into the plan of care based on the best and latest evidence. Thorough history-taking and physical examination provides the clinician with key subjective information and tangible, objective information on which to base current and future decision making. Only with comprehensive, accurate, and evidence-based assessment can a clinician ensure patient safety, quality, and cost-effective care.

# KNOWLEDGE CHECK: EVIDENCE-BASED HISTORY AND PHYSICAL EXAM

1. Evidence-based practice is BEST described as a problem-solving approach to the delivery of care that incorporates:

   A. Patient preferences, clinician expertise, and best evidence from well-designed studies
   B. Practice findings based on how things have been done over long periods of time
   C. Research findings from published studies, and NOT clinician or patient preferences
   D. The values, beliefs, and the preferences of the patients and the providers

2. The clinician is reviewing several published research articles about measures to prevent transmission of the SARS-CoV-2 virus. Which type of study would offer the strongest level of evidence?

   A. Case–control studies
   B. Cohort studies
   C. Randomized trials
   D. Systematic reviews

3. A clinician assesses an individual who presents with ongoing fatigue. MATCH the patient findings with the components of an episodic exam.

   A. Lungs are clear to auscultation bilaterally
   B. History of depression as a teen, treated with antidepressant
   C. Fatigue began 3 months ago, with the loss of employment
   D. Shares pattern of drinking" two glasses of wine every evening
   E. Denies nausea, abdominal pain, weight loss, or weight gain

   1. History of present illness
   2. Past medical history
   3. Family, social, and cultural history
   4. Review of systems
   5. Physical exam

4. Which three red flags in the subjective history that indicate need for genetic counseling? (Select THREE.)

   A. Cancer diagnosed in paternal great-grandparent
   B. Cancer diagnoses in the family occur in every generation
   C. Early age of onset of cancer in a family member
   D. Ethnic predisposition to a genetic disorder
   E. Genetic predisposition to a genetic disorder is unknown

*(See answers next page.)*

**1. A) Patient preferences, clinician expertise, and best evidence from well-designed studies**

Evidence-based practice incorporates three considerations: patient preferences, clinician expertise, and best evidence. Clinical practices based on how things have always been done, or without consideration of patient preferences and clinician expertise, are not considered evidence-based practice.

**2. D) Systematic reviews**

Critical appraisal requires an understanding of the levels of evidence. Level I evidence (the strongest level) is from systematic review, or meta-analysis of all relevant randomized controlled trials. Level II evidence is obtained from at least one well-designed randomized control trial. Level III evidence is derived from well-designed research studies without randomization. Level IV evidence is derived from case–control or cohort studies.

**3. A) Physical exam, B) Past medical history, C) History of present illness, D) Family, social, and cultural history, and E) Review of systems**

An episodic visit helps to guide the clinician in completing a thorough patient assessment. (1) History of present illness assessment includes information about current symptoms, i.e., onset, location, duration, characteristics, aggravating factors, relieving factors, treatment tried, and severity. (2) Past health or medical history includes medical and surgical history, previous diagnoses, and medications. (3) Family, social, and cultural history includes a review of factors that increase/decrease risk of illnesses and wellness. (4) The review of systems is an inventory of findings that are pertinent to the present illness and support differential diagnoses. (5) Physical exam assessments are objective findings of the examiner.

**4. B, C, and D) Cancer diagnoses in the family occurs in every generation, early age of onset of cancer in a family member, ethnic predisposition to a genetic disorder**

Significant cancer history warrants a referral to genetic counseling, which includes: cancer in every generation, early onset, or condition in less-often affected gender (male with breast cancer). Genetic counseling is also necessary when ethnic predisposition exists (e.g., Ashkenazi Jewish ancestry). Cancer in a paternal great-grandparent and/or unknown predisposition does not indicate the need for counseling.

**5.** A young adult presents to the office for a wellness exam. The clinician assesses the individual's use of seat belts. Which component of the wellness exam is being addressed?

**A.** History of illness and health history
**B.** Health promotion and anticipatory guidance
**C.** Review of pertinent negatives and positives
**D.** Secondary and tertiary screenings

**6.** Implementing evidence-based practice (EBP) begins with having a spirit of inquiry and assessing the patient to determine a clinical problem or question. What are the subsequent steps of an evidence-based approach to assessment? Place the subsequent steps in order:

**A.** Critically appraise the evidence
**B.** Integrate evidence with clinician expertise and patient preferences
**C.** Ask a focused clinical question
**D.** Search for the best evidence to answer the question
**E.** Evaluate the outcomes of the practice decisions

**7.** In reviewing the evidence about the accuracy of a specific screening test, the clinician has found that the test has a sensitivity of 80%. Which interpretation of this finding is accurate?

**A.** The test correctly identifies 80% of individuals who do not have the disease (true negatives)
**B.** The test correctly identifies 80% of individuals who have the disease (true positives)
**C.** 80% of individuals without the disease are likely to test positive (false positives)
**D.** 80% of individuals with the disease are likely to test negative (false negatives)

**8.** Which statement is true about the use of the PHQ-2 and PHQ-9 screening tools to assess depression?

**A.** Screening tools should only be used when individuals present with symptoms
**B.** Screening tools should not be used for establishing the diagnosis of depression
**C.** These tools are recommended and evidence-based, and can be used during wellness exams
**D.** These tools are screenings that are accurate only before starting treatment for depression

*(See answers next page.)*

**5. B) Health promotion and anticipatory guidance**

All wellness exams should include anticipatory guidance to promote health by addressing risk factors. Assessing seatbelt use is not a cultural assessment, is not related to illness, is not routinely part of the review of systems, and would be primary screening, not secondary or tertiary.

**6. C, D, A, B, E) Ask a focused clinical question, search for the best evidence to answer the question, critically appraise the evidence, integrate evidence with clinician expertise and patient preferences, evaluate the outcomes of the practice decisions**

The steps of evidence-based practice begin by cultivating a spirit of inquiry, which allows the clinician to be aware of clinical problems. The subsequent steps of the process are 1) asking the clinical question in a focused PICOT format, 2) acquiring relevant evidence, 3) critically appraising the evidence, 4) integrating the best evidence with one's clinical expertise and patient/family preferences and values in making a practice decision or change and 5) evaluating outcomes of the practice decision or change based on evidence. The final step of the evidence-based practice process includes disseminating outcomes of an EBP decision or practice change.

**7. B) The test correctly identifies 80% of individuals who have the disease (true positives)**

Sensitivity is how likely the test will correctly identify individuals who have the condition for which the tool or test was designed; a screening test that is 80% sensitive will correctly identify 80% who have the disease, true positive, and will miss 20% of individuals who should test positive (false negatives). The specificity of a test refers to the likelihood that the test will correctly identify those without the condition for which the screening was designed. A highly specific test is one in which there are few false-positive results.

**8. C) These tools are recommended and evidence-based, and can be used during wellness exams**

Evidence-based screening tools like the PHQ-2 and PHQ-9 can be used to confirm the diagnosis of depression, note the severity of the symptoms, and monitor treatment outcomes. These depression screenings are evidence-based and recommended during wellness exams for the adolescent and adult population, including pregnant and postpartum women. These screenings are accurate for well individuals, for those with symptoms, and to monitor treatment.

9. An older adult presents to the office for a wellness exam. The clinician reviews all current medications that the individual takes on a regular basis and as needed. Which component of the wellness exam is being addressed?

   A. Cultural and family history
   B. History of illness and health history
   C. Health promotion and anticipatory guidance
   D. Review of pertinent negatives and positives
   E. Secondary and tertiary screenings

10. A clinician is reviewing a journal article based on a committee report that summarizes clinical recommendations for addressing flu vaccine hesitancy. Which level of evidence is the clinician appraising in review of this publication?

   A. Systematic reviews
   B. Randomized trials
   C. Cohort studies
   D. Expert opinion

*(See answers next page.)*

**9. B) History of illness and health history**

All wellness exams should include a review of medications prescribed and over-the-counter, noting the dose and frequency of each medication; this is a key component of the health history. Medication use and reconciliation is not a cultural assessment, is not routinely part of the review of systems, is not a secondary or tertiary screening, and is not specifically a component of anticipatory guidance. However, discussions of health promotion and anticipatory guidance may be based on pertinent health history.

**10. D) Expert opinion**

Critical appraisal requires an understanding of the levels of evidence. Level I evidence (the strongest level) is from systematic review, or meta-analysis of all relevant randomized controlled trial. Level II evidence is obtained from at least one well-designed randomized control trial. Level IV evidence is derived from case–control or cohort studies. Level VII evidence is based on expert opinion of authorities or committee reports.

# Part II
# Evidence-Based Assessment and Diagnosis

# Integumentary System

## KEY HISTORY CONSIDERATIONS

- Any changes or worsening of a rash/lesion (Table 3.1)
- Affected areas of the body
- Systemic symptoms or pain accompanying the rash/lesion
- Exposures (other people, environmental, occupational)
- Immunization(s) status
- History of any personal or family chronic diseases
- Previous treatments

**Table 3.1 Primary and Secondary Skin Lesions**

| Lesion | Description | Examples |
|---|---|---|
| **Primary Skin Lesions** | | |
| Bullae | Elevated, fluid-filled, round or oval; thin, translucent walls; >0.5 cm | Contact dermatitis, friction/fracture blister, large burn blister |
| Cyst | Elevated, encapsulated, fluid- or semisolid-filled, or solid; >1 cm | Sebaceous cyst, epidermoid cyst, acne |
| Macule | Flat, nonpalpable; <1 cm | Freckles, flat moles (nevi), petechiae* |
| Nodule | Elevated, solid, palpable mass; <2 cm | Small lipoma, squamous cell carcinoma, fibroma |
| Papule | Elevated, solid, palpable; <0.5 cm | Elevated moles, warts, insect bites |
| Patch | Flat, nonpalpable; >1 cm | Vitiligo, Mongolian spots, port-wine stains |
| Plaque | Groups or papules; >5 cm | Psoriasis, actinic keratosis, lichen planus |
| Pustule | Elevated, pus-filled; size varies | Acne, impetigo, carbuncles |
| Tumor | Elevated, solid, palpable, irregular borders; >2 cm | Carcinoma, hemangioma, benign tumor |
| Vesicle | Elevated, fluid-filled, round or oval; thin, translucent walls; >0.5 cm | Herpes simplex, poison ivy, small burn blister |
| Wheal | Elevated, often reddish area with irregular borders; size varies | Insect bites, hives (urticarial), allergic reaction |
| **Secondary Skin Lesions** | | |
| Atrophy | Thinning or wasting of skin due to loss of collagen and elastin | Striae, aged skin |
| Crust | Dried blood, serum, or pus from ruptured vesicles or pustules; slightly elevated; red, brown, orange, or yellow; size varies | Eczema, impetigo, herpes simplex |

(*continued*)

**Table 3.1 Primary and Secondary Skin Lesions (*continued*)**

| Lesion | Description | Examples |
|---|---|---|
| Excoriation | Absence of superficial epidermis, causing a moist, shallow depression | Scratch marks, abrasion, scabies |
| Fissure | Linear crack/break with sharp edges; moist or dry | Cracks at corner of mouth, fingers, or on feet (athlete's foot) |
| Keloid | Elevated area of excessive scar tissue that extends beyond the site of original injury (caused by excessive collagen formation during healing) | Keloid for ear piercing or following surgery |
| Lichenification | Rough, thickened, hardened area of the epidermis resulting from chronic irritation (e.g., scratching, rubbing) | Chronic dermatitis |
| Scale | Flakes of greasy keratinized skin tissue; white, gray, or silver; fine or thick texture; varies in size | Dry skin, dandruff, psoriasis |
| Scar | Elevated, irregular area, may be red or purple (new) or silvery or white (old) | Healed surgical wound or injury, healed acne |
| Ulcer | Irregularly shaped area, concave, depth varies | Stasis and decubiti ulcers, aphthous ulcers |

*Petechiae are unique in this list because they are nonblanching vascular lesions. They can be considered a subcategory of macules.

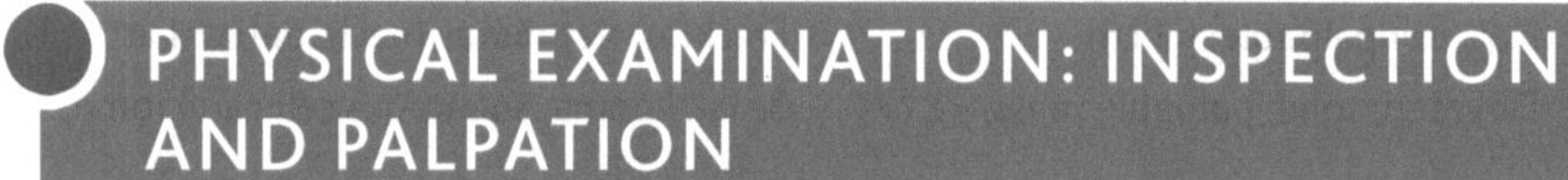

# PHYSICAL EXAMINATION: INSPECTION AND PALPATION

## INSPECTION

1. Inspect the skin in a head-to-toe sequence, ensuring the entire skin surface is systematically examined. Even if a rash/lesion is localized to one area of the body, it is good practice to look at all areas of the skin to ensure other areas are not affected.
2. Start with a general survey of the skin, including color, pigmentation, vascularity, bruising, lesions, color variations, and general hygiene.
3. With long hair, part the hair in a systematic and organized fashion to visualize the scalp. Look in and around the ears.
4. Use a tongue blade to look into the mouth and inspect the oral mucosa.
5. Look at the palms and soles of hands and feet and between fingers and toes.
6. The breast, buttock, and genitalia should be examined last and with the patient's permission.
7. Measure all skin lesions. Note the number, location, size, color, shape, morphology, distribution, and configuration.

8. Inspect the finger and toenails. Any nail polish should be removed. Inspect the color, texture, and shape.
9. Inspect the hair. Note the distribution, texture, and quantity of hair. Note any areas of hair loss or any abnormal hair growth.

## INSPECTION: ABNORMAL FINDINGS

- When a rash or lesion (Table 3.2) is present, the following should be noted:
  - Primary morphology
  - Size
  - Demarcation
  - Color
  - Secondary morphology
  - Distribution

**Table 3.2 Common Rash and Lesion Diagnoses**

| Condition | History and Physical Findings | Visual |
|---|---|---|
| **Acne**<br>Chronic inflammatory dermatosis affecting the pilosebaceous follicles of the skin | ■ Most common in adolescents<br>■ Pain, tenderness, and/or erythema in affected areas<br>■ History of PCOS<br>■ Character: closed/ open comedones (non-inflammatory); papules, pustules, nodules, cysts (inflammatory); post-inflammatory hyperpigmentation and/or atrophic scars (moderate-to-severe acne)<br>■ Location: face, chest, back, upper arms | |
| **Actinic Keratosis (Solar Keratosis)**<br>Premalignancy that forms from abnormal production of keratinocytes after excessive UV exposure | ■ Most common in adults aged >50 years with excessive sun exposure<br>■ History of sunburns, immunosuppression<br>■ Character: erythematous, hyperkeratotic scaly macules, papules, and plaques on sun-damaged skin; may be white, yellow, pink or red; rough on palpation; average 6–8 lesions<br>■ Location: Face, ears, scalp, neck, extremities<br>■ Without treatment, it can progress to squamous cell carcinoma | |

(*continued*)

**Table 3.2 Common Rash and Lesion Diagnoses (*continued*)**

| Condition | History and Physical Findings | Visual |
|---|---|---|
| **Basal Cell Carcinoma**<br>Malignancy that evolves from basal cells in the lower layer of the epidermis; most common malignancy in humans | ■ Most commonly develops on sun-exposed skin areas; fair-skinned patients disproportionately affected<br>■ History of sun damage<br>■ Character: Slow-growing, non-healing sore; friable and umbilicated; waxy papules with central depression, erosion, ulceration, or pearly; crusting; rolled border; translucent; surface telangiectasia<br>■ Bleeds with trauma<br>■ Usually does not metastasize | 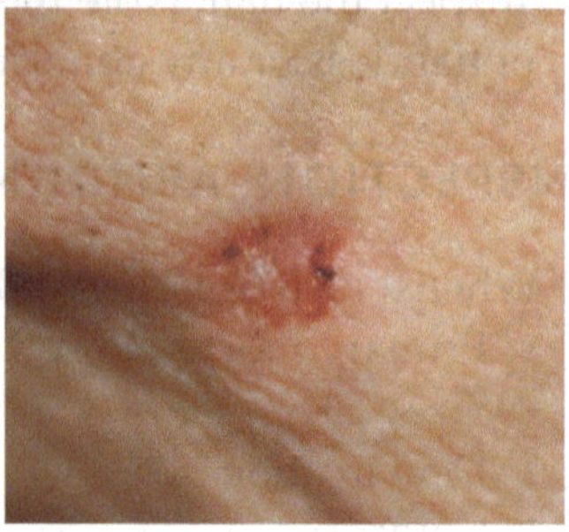 |
| **Cellulitis**<br>Bacterial infection of the deeper dermis and subcutaneous tissues; caused by group A streptococcus, *Staphylococcus aureus* (adults) and *Haemophilus influenzae* type B (children <3 years) | ■ Fever, leukocytosis, mildly elevated sedimentation rate<br>■ History of lymphedema, venous insufficiency, venous insufficiency, tinea pedis, obesity, previous history of cellulitis<br>■ Character: Trauma to the skin; erythema; calor; edema of the skin; pain; unilateral; indistinct borders<br>■ Location: Typically affects the lower legs but can occur on any skin surface area<br>■ Can quickly progress to fulminant sepsis with necrotizing fasciitis, especially in patient with comorbidities | 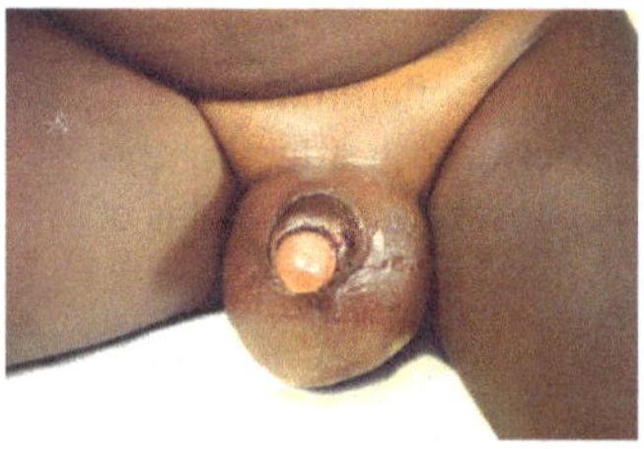 |

| Condition | History and Physical Findings | Visual |
|---|---|---|
| **Contact Dermatitis**<br>Eczematous inflammatory skin condition caused by contact with irritants (80% of cases) or allergens | ■ Painful, dry, and/or itchy skin; areas with thinner epidermis at increased risk<br>■ History of exposure to an allergen (e.g., jewelry metals, cosmetics, fragrances) or irritant (e.g., poison ivy, detergents, soaps)<br>■ Certain professions at higher risk (e.g., construction workers, hairstylists, landscapers, janitors)<br>■ Character: Pruritic papules, vesicles, and/or bullae with an erythematous base; crusting and oozing; lichenification, scaling, fissuring (chronic presentation)<br>■ Location: Can occur on any part of the body; areas with thinner epidermis at increased risk | 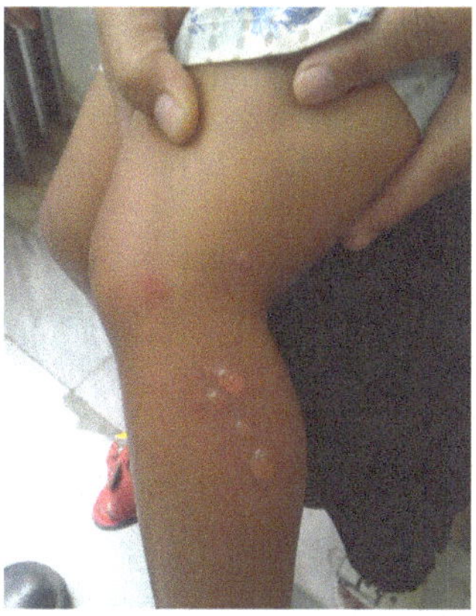 |
| **Eczema (Atopic Dermatitis)**<br>Inflammatory skin disorder with unknown etiology | ■ Most common in infants aged 3–6 months<br>■ Exacerbation/remission of dry, itchy, erythematous skin; scratching increases inflammation<br>■ History of asthma, allergic rhinitis, urticaria, acute allergic reactions to certain foods<br>■ Character: Pruritis; scaly, erythematous patches; xerosis; lichenification; excoriation;<br>■ Location: Can occur on any part of the body; commonly appear in elbow or knee creases, nape of neck | 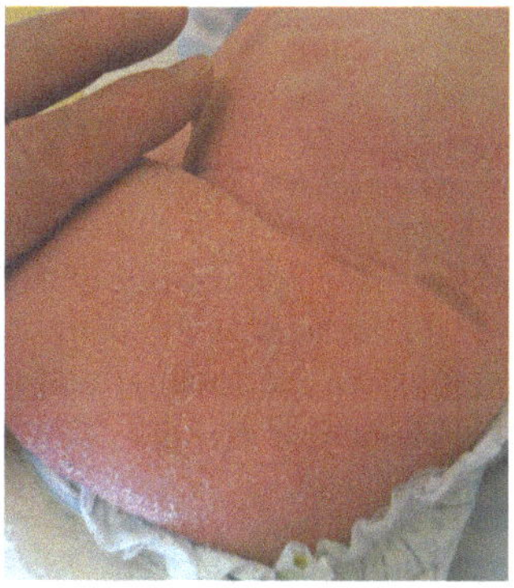 |

(*continued*)

**Table 3.2 Common Rash and Lesion Diagnoses (*continued*)**

| Condition | History and Physical Findings | Visual |
|---|---|---|
| **Erythema Migrans**<br>Bulls-eye rash associated with the first stage of most cases of Lyme disease; caused by *Borrelia burgdorferi* | ■ Rash; fever, myalgias, lymphadenopathy, fatigue, malaise<br>■ History of tick bite or being outdoors<br>■ Character: Distinct bulls-eye appearance; appears 3–30 days after bite (average 7 days); gradually expands in size up to 12 inches in diameter; mild calor; rarely itchy or painful<br>■ Location: Site of tick bite | 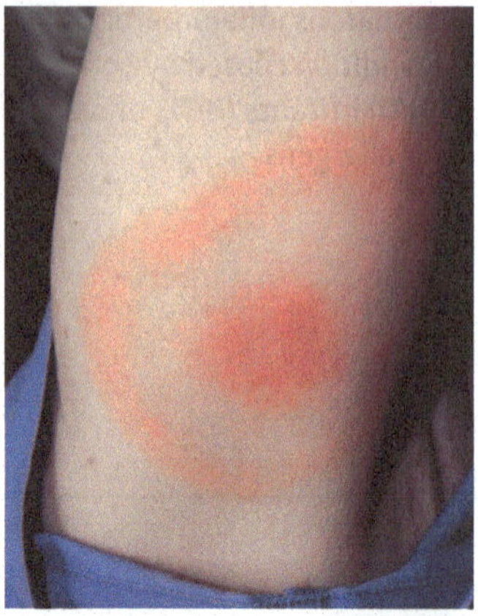 |
| **Fifth's Disease (Erythema Infectiosum)**<br>Rash caused by parvovirus B19; transmitted through respiratory secretions and blood | ■ Primary rash; fever, rhinorrhea, myalgias, headache<br>■ Secondary rash can appear a few days after primary; appears on chest, back, buttocks, arms, legs<br>■ Character: "Slapped cheek" appearance<br>■ Location: Face (primary); chest, back, buttocks, arms, legs (secondary) | 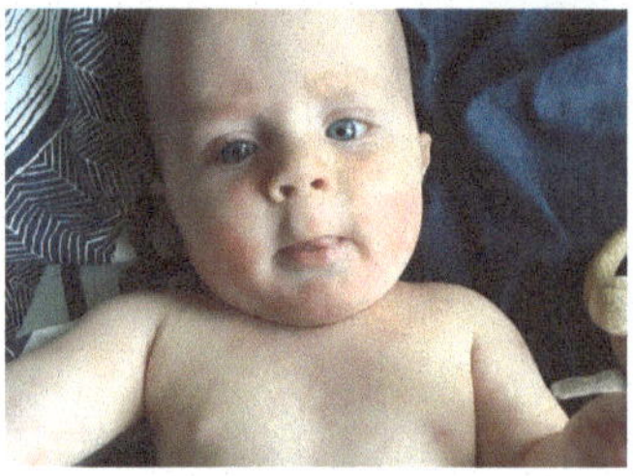 |
| **Hand, Foot, and Mouth Disease**<br>Rash caused by coxsackievirus A16; transmitted through respiratory secretions, fecal-oral route, or vesicle fluid | ■ Most common in children aged <5 years<br>■ Starts with fever, malaise, sore throat, and anorexia; followed by rash; typically occurs in summer and early fall<br>■ Character: Painful macular or vesicular lesions<br>■ Location: Mouth, palms of hands, soles of feet | 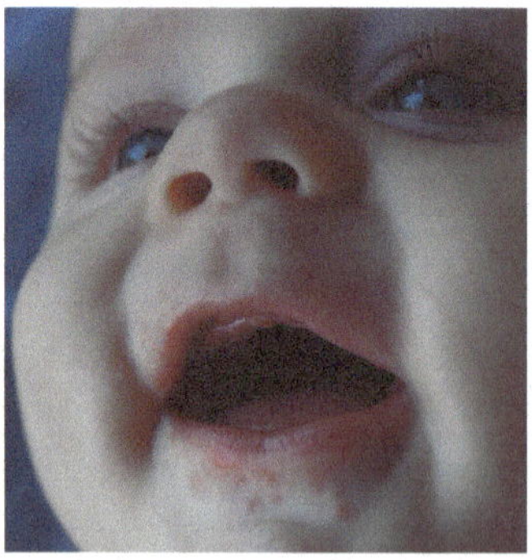 |

| Condition | History and Physical Findings | Visual |
|---|---|---|
| **Herpes Simplex**<br>Viral infection from exposure to herpes simplex virus types 1 and 2 | ■ Fever, especially with primary lesions; tingling and burning sensation prior to eruption<br>■ Stress and sun exposure may stimulate occurrence<br>■ Character: Erythematous plaque that progresses to grouped vesicles with clear to yellow fluid; erosion occurs with "punched out" appearance<br>■ Location: Mucocutaneous sites (e.g., perioral area, nose, distal fingers, genitalia) | 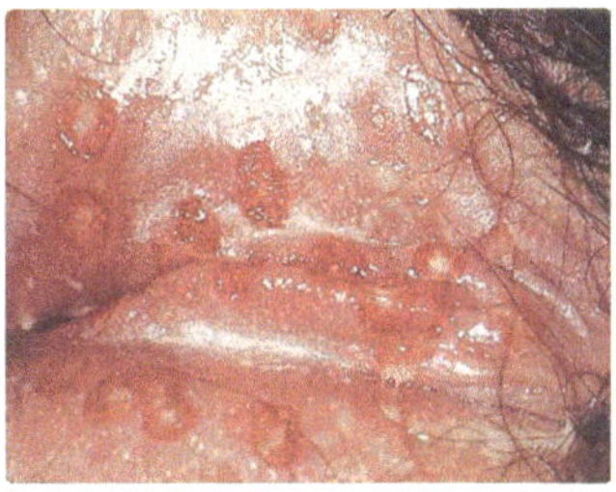 |
| **Herpes Zoster (Shingles)**<br>Viral infection caused by the reactivation of the varicella-zoster virus, the same virus that causes varicella | ■ Most common in older adults<br>■ Low-grade fever, fatigue, malaise, headache, regional lymphadenopathy<br>■ Tingling, pruritus in the area prior to the eruption of the rash<br>■ Burning, throbbing, or stabbing ("knife-like") pain in the dermatomal area<br>■ Character: Unilateral lesion eruption; initially erythematous and maculopapular, then becomes clusters of clear vesicles; crusts in 7–10 days<br>■ Location: Dermatomal; thoracic and lumbar areas most common | 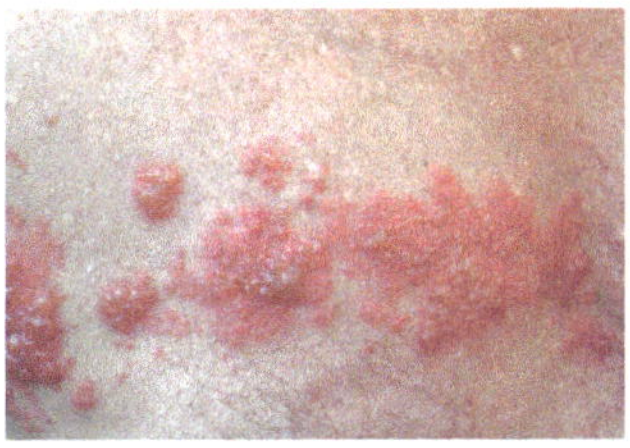 |
| **Impetigo**<br>Bacteria introduced through break in skin; caused by *Staphylococcus aureus* or *Streptococcus pyogenes;* three types: bullous, non-bullous, and ecthyma | ■ Most common in children aged 2–6 years<br>■ Mild itching and discomfort<br>■ Character: Vesicular lesions that burst develop honey-colored crusts (non-bullous); large blisters (bullous); deep, painful ulcers (ecthyma)<br>■ Location: It can occur anywhere; most common on face, nose, hands, feet; can spread by fingers, clothing, towels | 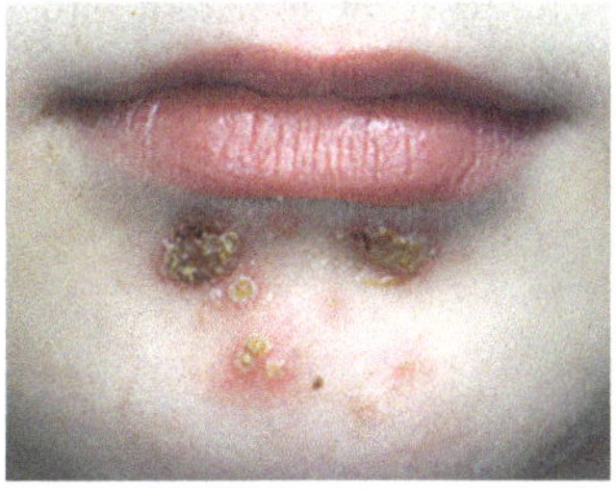 |

*(continued)*

Table 3.2 Common Rash and Lesion Diagnoses (*continued*)

| Condition | History and Physical Findings | Visual |
|---|---|---|
| **Melanoma**<br>Malignancy of the pigment-producing melanocytes in the basal layer of the epidermis; often diagnosed in later stages in Hispanics and African Americans, leading to poorer survival rates | ■ Spot or sore that burns, itches, stings, crusts, bleeds<br>■ A new mole or lesion in adulthood (aside from pregnancy); a mole that looks different from surrounding moles (ugly duckling)<br>■ Typically has one or more of following: **A**symmetry, **B**order irregularity, **C**olor variegation, **D**iameter >6 mm, **E**volution or timing of the lesion's growth (ABCDE acronym)<br>■ Character: Typically black or brown, but can be skin-colored, pink, red, purple, blue, white; spread of pigment from the border of spot into surrounding skin; satellite lesions that grow near an existing mole<br>■ Location: Most common in sun-exposed areas; in African Americans, Asians, Filipinos, Indonesians, and Native Hawaiians, 60–75% of lesions on palms, soles, mucous membranes, nails | 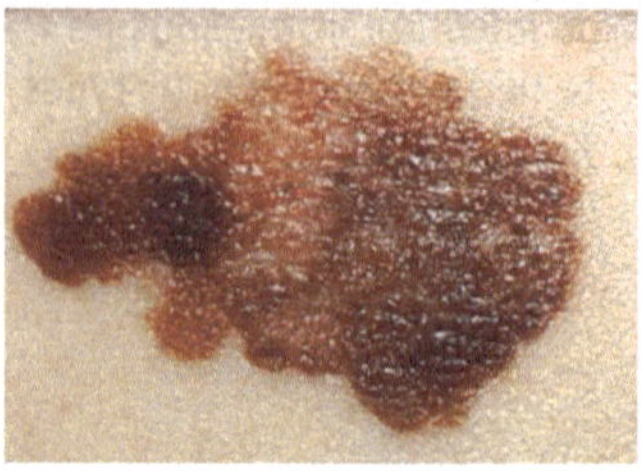 |
| **Onychomyocosis**<br>A disease of the nail(s) caused by yeast (*Candida*), dermatophytes, and nondermatophyte molds; microscopy consistent with fungus | ■ Most common in older adults<br>■ History of diabetes, HIV, immunosuppression, obesity, smoking, and older age<br>■ Can have an associated foul odor, pain, paresthesia<br>■ Character: Discoloration (whitish, yellow, brown); thickened and brittle; distortion of shape (ragged, crumbly); onycholysis<br>■ Location: Most common in toenails | 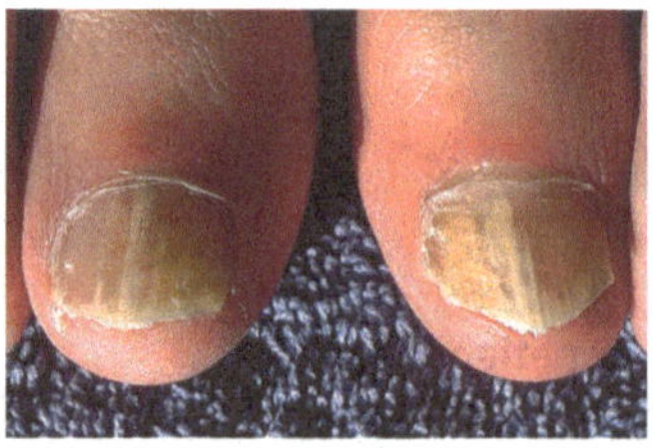 |

| Condition | History and Physical Findings | Visual |
|---|---|---|
| **Psoriasis**<br>Complex, inflammatory, multisystem disease characterized by hyperproliferation of the keratinocytes in the epidermis; most common type is plaque psoriasis | ■ Exacerbation/remission of pruritic skin lesions is often the most prominent and only recognized feature<br>■ Joint pain, conjunctivitis, blepharitis, Dystrophic nails<br>■ History of recent streptococcal throat infection, viral infection, immunization, trauma; family history of psoriasis<br>■ Character: Reddish-pink, well-demarcated macules, papules, and plaques with a silvery scale; Auspitz sign (pinpoint bleeding with removal of scales) is a hallmark sign; can be painful<br>■ Location: Can occur anywhere; typically scalp, elbows, knees, lower back | 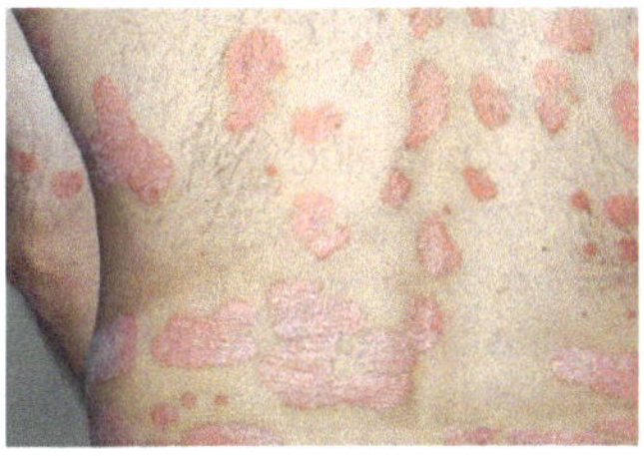 |
| **Rosacea (Acne Rosacea)**<br>Common, chronic, and relapsing inflammatory skin condition with unknown etiology | ■ Most common in fair-skinned women aged 30–50 years<br>■ History of facial flushing<br>■ Can be triggered by UV light (most common), stress, exercise, wind, heat, spicy foods, dairy, alcohol<br>■ Ocular involvement may be present<br>■ Character: Nontransient erythema; papulo-pustular lesions; telangiectasia; roughness of skin; thickening of skin of nose (rhinophyma); can resemble acne<br>■ Location: Face (most common), neck, upper chest | 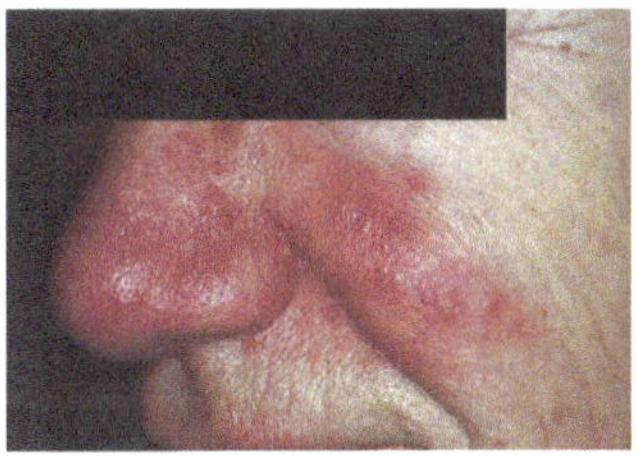 |

*(continued)*

**Table 3.2 Common Rash and Lesion Diagnoses (*continued*)**

| Condition | History and Physical Findings | Visual |
|---|---|---|
| **Scabies**<br>Highly contagious skin infestation caused by *Sarcoptes scabiei*, tiny parasites that burrow into the skin and lay eggs; spread by direct (skin-to-skin) and indirect (sharing articles) contact | ■ Intense, pruritic rash that worsens at night; can appear 2–6 weeks after exposure<br>■ Infants and young children may be irritable and not want to eat or sleep<br>■ Institutionalized individuals are higher risk<br>■ Character: Maculopapular rash; lesions can appear in linear patterns; can resemble pimples, eczema, insect bites<br>■ Location: Most common between fingers and toes, under jewelry or watches, in armpits, skin folds, genitalia; may appear on palms of hands, soles of feet, face, scalp, and neck in infants and young children | 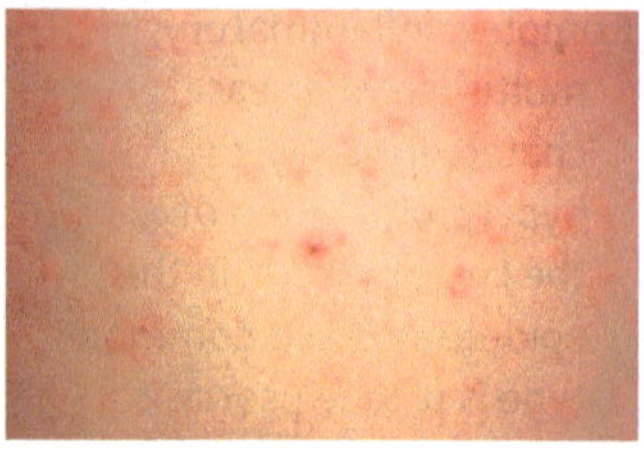 |
| **Scarlet Fever (Scarlatina)**<br>Rash caused by an erythrogenic exotoxin emitted by group A hemolytic streptococcus; commonly seen in conjunction with strep pharyngitis | ■ Most common in children aged 5–15 years<br>■ Typically starts with high fever and sore throat; rash appears after 1–2 days and fades in 4–5 days, followed by diffuse desquamation<br>■ Tongue may appear white with red, swollen papillae (white strawberry tongue); by day 4/5, it becomes bright red (red strawberry tongue)<br>■ Character: Maculopapular, exanthematous; looks like sunburn, feels like sandpaper; linear bright-red coloration of the creases in the axillary and inguinal folds (Pastia's sign)<br>■ Location: Initially appears neck and chest, then spreads over the body | 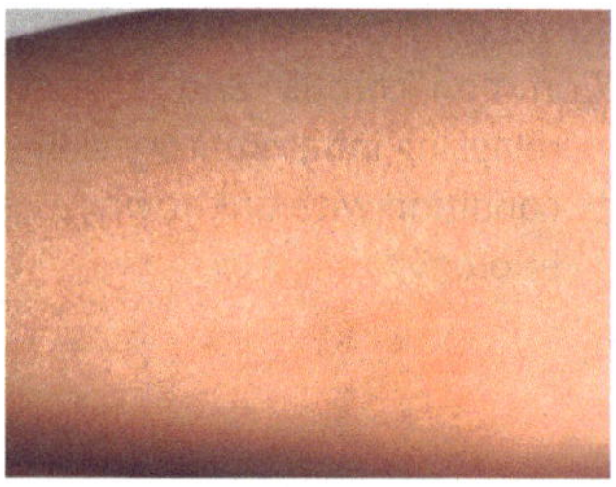 |

| Condition | History and Physical Findings | Visual |
| --- | --- | --- |
| **Squamous Cell Carcinoma**<br>Slow-growing malignancy that arises from the epidermal keratinocytes; poses substantial risk for morbidity and mortality | ■ Most common in the elderly and fair-skinned individuals<br>■ History of sun damage, actinic keratosis, radiation<br>■ Most common skin cancer in Blacks<br>■ Isolated or multiple lesions that itch or feel sore, tender, and/or numb<br>■ Character: Raised, firm, skin-colored/pink, hyperkeratotic papule or plaque; non-healing sore or patch of rough skin; firm, dome-shaped growth; tiny, rhinoceros-shaped horn; wart-like growth; black line under nail<br>■ Location: Most common on sun-exposed areas (head, upper extremities) | 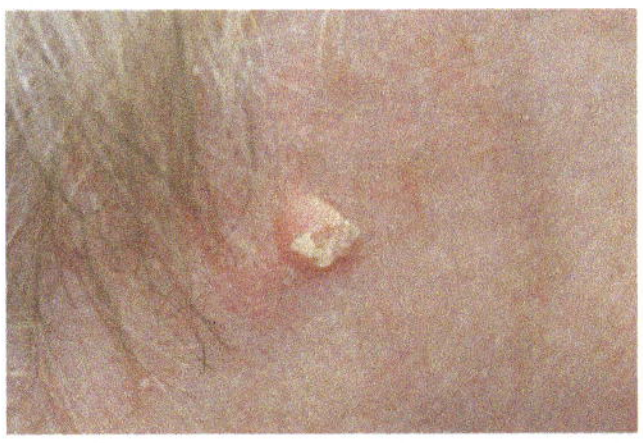 |
| **Tinea Corporis (Body)**<br>Highly contagious dermatophyte infection; microscopy consistent with fungal hyphae; an also occur on the head (tinea capitus), groin (tinea cruris), and feet (tinea pedis) | ■ Most common in children, especially those who play contact sports (e.g., wrestlers)<br>■ History of diabetes or obesity<br>■ Lives or visits tropical, humid areas<br>■ Lesions may be pruritic or asymptomatic, occasionally burn, and vary in number<br>■ Character: Red, scaly patch with distinct annular borders, central clearing; size typically 1–5 cm; inflammation, scale, crusts, papules, vesicles and bullae can develop at border | 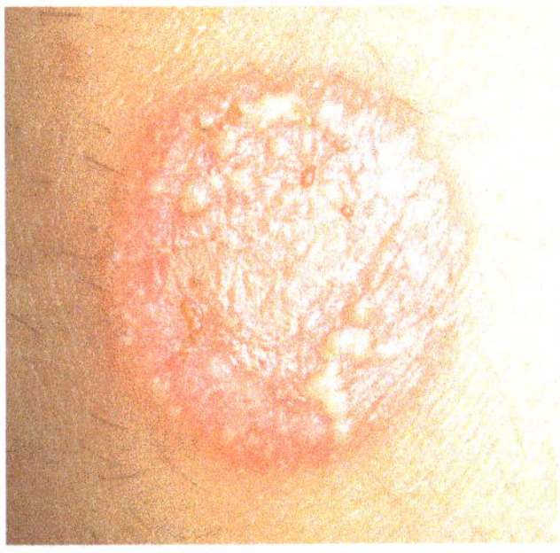 |
| **Tinea Versicolor**<br>Benign fungal infection caused by *Malassezia furfur;* microscopy consistent with fungal budding and hyphae | ■ Most common in adolescents and young adults<br>■ Most often occurs in summer<br>■ Character: Pruritic; multiple tan, brown, salmon, pink, or white scaling patches that may coalesce<br>■ Location: Trunk, neck, abdomen, face (occasionally) | 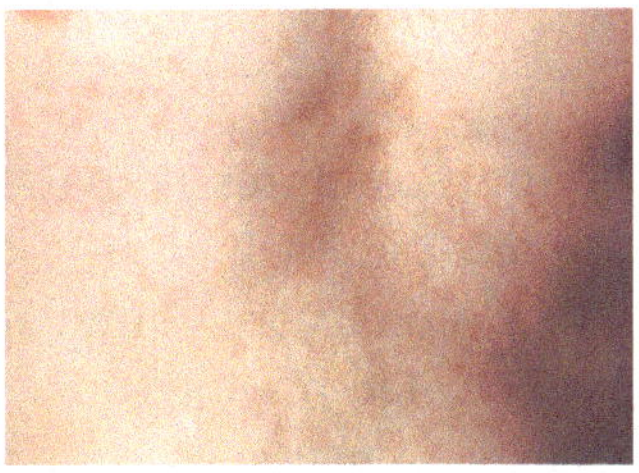 |

*(continued)*

**Table 3.2 Common Rash and Lesion Diagnoses (*continued*)**

| Condition | History and Physical Findings | Visual |
|---|---|---|
| **Urticaria (Hives)**<br>Acute or chronic infection caused by the release of histamine and other inflammatory mediators from mast cells and basophils in the dermis | ■ May cause significant pruritus and discomfort; usually resolves within 24 hours<br>■ Recurrence frequently associated with sun exposure, exercise, stress, water exposure<br>■ Character: Raised wheals that blanch with palpation; linear, annular (circular), or arcuate (serpiginous)<br>■ Location: Can occur anywhere | |

polycystic ovarian syndrome; UV, ultraviolet.

## PALPATION

1. Palpate the skin and note the temperature, texture, moisture, and turgor. Skin should be warm, dry, and intact without any erythema, edema, or drainage.
2. Palpate the fingernails and toenails for texture and note the capillary refill time. Normal capillary refill time is less than 2 seconds.
3. Palpate appropriate lesions, assessing the texture of the lesion, presence of tenderness or pain, temperature of the lesion and surrounding skin, fluidity, and blanching capacity.
4. Palpate any surrounding lymph nodes to check for enlargement or tenderness.

### PALPATION: ABNORMAL FINDINGS

- Skin that feels very warm or very cool is an abnormal finding, especially if it is localized to one particular area. For example, cellulitis will often feel warm in the area that is affected but surrounding tissue is unaffected. Vascular diseases can cause cool or cold skin.

## RED FLAGS IN HISTORY AND PHYSICAL EXAM

- Immunosuppressed patient
- Severe pain
- Very old or very young age
- Associated photophobia, fever, and headache
- Start of a new medication
- Toxic appearance
- Unstable vital signs
- Fever and a petechial/purpura or erythematous rash
- Scalded skin appearance

- Rash covering more than 90% of the body
- Non-blanching rash
- Mucosal lesions
- Rash or lesion that does not go away
- ABCDE for a mole (Box 3.1)

**Box 3.1 ABCDE of Melanoma**

A: Asymmetry
B: Border (irregular)
C: Color (multiple colors)
D: Diameter (greater than 6 mm or ¼ inch)
E: Evolving (changes in size, shape, or color over time)

# POPULATION HEALTH AND LIFE-SPAN CONSIDERATIONS

## INFANTS AND CHILDREN

- Approximately 50% of newborns experience physiologic jaundice, which is a normal phenomenon resulting from increased hemolysis of red blood cells following birth.
- Seborrheic dermatitis (cradle cap) may be present on the scalp of infants and appears as a scaly crust.
- There may be various harmless markings on newborns such as tiny, white facial papules (milia), vascular markings (salmon patches/stork bites), and Mongolian spots (congenital dermal melanocytosis).
- Bruising to lower legs may be present as the child becomes mobile.
- Bruising to the torso, ears, or neck for any child less than or equal to 4 years old or bruising in any location on an infant less than 4 months old should prompt the clinician to initiate a workup for physical abuse and also investigate for other occult injuries.
- Bruises in different stages of healing, bite marks, burns, signs of injury to other body systems, or skin markings that have a pattern (e.g., belt pattern) require further investigation for potential child mistreatment.
- There are a variety of different rashes that typically occur only in childhood but are rarely seen in adults. See Key Differentials in Children.
- Increased perspiration, oiliness, and acne are common in adolescents due to increased sebaceous activity.

## OLDER ADULTS

- Skin may appear pale and to hang from the frame.
- Normal older adult skin variations may include solar lentigo (liver spots), seborrheic keratosis, and acrochordon (skin tag).

- Skin tears may also be present due to the fragility of the skin.
- The hair may be thin, gray, and coarse with symmetric balding in men.
- The amount of body hair decreases (body, pubic, and axillary hair).
- Men have an increase in the amount and coarseness of nasal and eyebrow hair, and women may develop coarse facial hair.
- The clinician must be cognizant of signs of maltreatment in the older adult by assessing for bruising, lacerations, pressure ulcers, dehydration, and poor hygiene.

### OTHER CONSIDERATIONS

- Hispanics, Asians, American Indians (including Pacific Islanders), Africans, and Black Americans have unique skin presentations. A predisposition to scarring and pathogenesis of skin disorders are unique and common to these groups.
- There is a greater susceptibility to forming melasma, keloids, and dyschromia in races other than Caucasians. These benign lesions tend to be larger than the site of trauma and are often distressing to patients.
- Skin cancer occurs at a lower rate in skin colors other than white; however, the morbidity and mortality rate is significantly higher in persons of color due to late diagnosis.

## KEY DIFFERENTIALS FOR SKIN

### ADULTS

- Abuse
- Acne
- Actinic keratosis
- Basal cell carcinoma
- Bed bug bites
- Cellulitis
- Contact dermatitis
- Eczema
- Epidermoid cyst
- Erythema migrans
- Folliculitis
- Herpes zoster
- Melanoma
- Pityriasis rosea
- Psoriasis
- Rosacea
- Scabies
- Squamous cell carcinoma
- Tinea (barbae, capitis, corporis, cruris, faciei, pedis)
- Tinea versicolor
- Urticaria
- Verruca vulgaris

### CHILDREN

- Abuse
- Eczema
- Fifth disease
- Hand, foot, and mouth disease
- Impetigo
- Infantile seborrheic dermatitis
- Measles (rubeola)
- Milia
- Molluscum contagiosum
- Mongolian spots
- Mumps
- Roseola
- Rubella
- Salmon patches
- Scarlet fever
- Varicella

## KEY DIFFERENTIALS FOR NAILS

- Beau's lines
- Chronic hypoxia (clubbing)
- Leukonychia
- Koilonychia
- Onychomycosis
- Onycholysis
- Psoriatic nails
- Terry's nails

## KEY DIFFERENTIALS FOR HAIR

- Alopecia (traction, areata, scarring, totalis, universalis, ophiasis)
- B12 deficiency
- Tinea capitus
- Telogen effluvium
- Trichotillomania

# KNOWLEDGE CHECK: INTEGUMENTARY SYSTEM

1. Thickened white plaques on the tongue or oral mucosa that cannot be scraped off and may be premalignant are called:

   **A.** Crypts
   **B.** Koplik spots
   **C.** Leukoplakia
   **D.** Thrush

2. A child with suspected scarlet fever is likely to have a positive strep test and:

   **A.** Erythematous lesions that feel like sandpaper
   **B.** Maculopapular rash that evolved to vesicles
   **C.** Purpura that began on lower extremities
   **D.** Vesicular lesions on hands and feet

3. Which common primary skin lesions is BEST described as a circumscribed, elevated, fluid-filled lesion less than 0.5 cm in diameter?

   **A.** Bulla
   **B.** Papule
   **C.** Pustule
   **D.** Vesicle

4. An adult male is seeking care for a "red, raised, itchy rash" on his forearms that began 6 months ago when he began making furniture at home. He confirms that he wears a protective mask and gloves when using paint, wood stains, and varnish; however, he often gets these chemicals on his arms and is using cleaning agents to remove them. Which diagnosis is the MOST LIKELY?

   **A.** Atopic dermatitis
   **B.** Second-degree burns
   **C.** Contact dermatitis
   **D.** Cellulitis

5. A herald patch is a hallmark finding in which condition?

   **A.** Herpes zoster
   **B.** Pityriasis rosea
   **C.** Psoriasis
   **D.** Tinea corporis

*(See answers next page.)*

**1. C) Leukoplakia**

Oral leukoplakia, which presents as a white patch or plaque, is the most frequent potentially malignant lesion of the oral mucosa. Crypts are pits or spaces, most notably found within tonsils; large crypts in tonsils can collect debris and exudate. Koplik spots are small, bluish-white spots on the buccal mucosa that are associated with rubeola (measles). Thrush, or oral candidiasis, presents as a white patch that can be easily scraped off with gauze.

**2. A) Erythematous lesions that feel like sandpaper**

Scarlet fever is characterized by a positive strep test and "sandpaper rash;" typically, the small, bright, erythematous lesions begin on the trunk and spread all over the body. Maculopapular rashes more likely have viral causes in children. Varicella (chicken pox) begins as a maculopapular rash, and the lesions evolve to vesicles. Purpura is vascular and associated with sepsis. Vesicular lesions on the hands, feet, and in the perioral area are more indicative of hand, foot, and mouth disease (HFMD) caused by coxsackieviruses.

**3. D) Vesicle**

Vesicles are circumscribed, elevated, fluid-containing lesions that less than 0.5 cm in greatest diameter. They may be intra-epidermal or sub-epidermal in origin. Bullae are similarly defined, except that the lesions are more than 0.5 cm in diameter. Papules are solid, raised lesions up to 0.5 cm in greatest diameter. Pustules are circumscribed, elevated skin lesions containing purulent fluid.

**4. C) Contact dermatitis**

Contact dermatitis is an inflammatory skin condition provoked by exposure to an external irritant or allergen. Nearly 90% of occupational cutaneous conditions are contact dermatitis. While soaps and cleaners can exacerbate atopic dermatitis, the rash usually begins in early childhood and is persistent with exacerbations. Second-degree burns cause blistering and pain. Cellulitis, a bacterial skin infection, causes pain, inflammation, and tenderness; cases can worsen quickly to include fever and sepsis.

**5. B) Pityriasis rosea**

Pityriasis rosea begins with a single, circular erythematous lesion (a herald patch) that is followed by an eruption of smaller patches on the cleavage lines of the trunk in the configuration of a "Christmas tree." Herpes zoster begins with pain, itching, and or burning along a dermatome. Psoriasis presents with macules, papules, and plaques with silvery scales. The herald patch can be mistaken for the type of scaly lesion with a distinct border and central clearing associated with tinea corporis; however, lesions associated with tinea are pruritic, raised, and are not precursors to linear erythematous lesions.

6. A child presents with complaints of itching primarily at night, and their physical exam reveals papules and areas of excoriation on both hands and around the waist (as pictured in the image). Which diagnosis is MOST LIKELY?

   A. Fifth disease
   B. Impetigo
   C. Scabies
   D. Tinea corporis

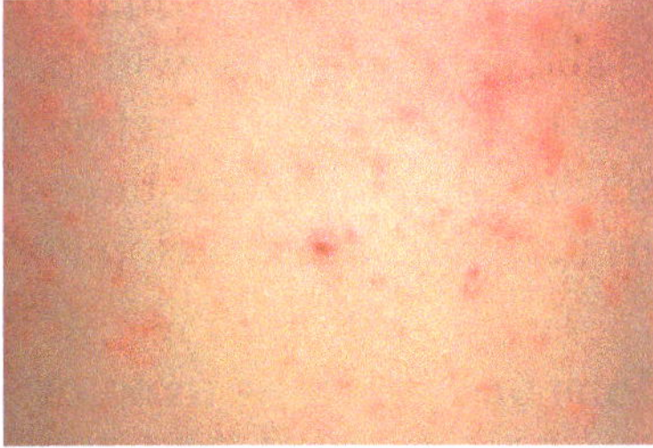

7. When assessing an older adult who has numerous moles, the clinician should be most concerned about lesions that have:

   A. A waxy, scaly, wart-like appearance
   B. Been intact since childhood
   C. Discolorations or variations in color
   D. Raised, well-defined borders

8. Which case scenario is LEAST LIKELY to suggest sepsis development?

   A. A 2-year-old child who developed a macular rash after resolution of a high fever
   B. A 5-year-old child with fever, peeling lips, petechial lesions, and loss of appetite
   C. A 65-year-old female with fever, tachypnea, and clammy skin with poor capillary refill
   D. An 89-year-old male with mottled skin and rapid mental status change over the past 2 days

9. Which three conditions are treated with antifungal medications? (Select THREE.)

   A. Eczema
   B. Impetigo
   C. Intertrigo
   D. Onychomycosis
   E. Tinea pedis

10. Early signs of Lyme disease include:

    A. Fever, fatigue, and erythema migrans
    B. Headaches and pruritic, painful rash
    C. Scaly, hypo-pigmented skin lesions
    D. Significant joint inflammation and pain

(*See answers next page.*)

**6. C) Scabies**

Scabies commonly presents as an intense, pruritic rash; the associated itching is worse at night. The maculopapular rash associated with scabies tends to occur between the fingers and toes, and at skin folds. While tinea corporis has pruritus associated, the lesions are circular and erythematous, with distinct borders and central clearing. The rash associated with Fifth disease, or erythema infectiosum, appears as a facial rash that has a "slapped cheek" appearance. Impetigo is common in children but presents as vesicular lesions that burst and develop honey-colored crusts.

**7. C) Discolorations or variations in color**

Lesions that have variations in color or are discolored are of concern for malignancy. Use the ABCD criteria (i.e., asymmetry, border irregularity, color variegation, and diameter of the skin lesion) to assess for melanoma. In older adults, benign seborrheic keratosis is more common, and can be waxy, scaly, velvety, smooth, or raised wart-like growths. Lesions that are raised, well-defined, or unchanged throughout the life span are more likely benign.

**8. A) A 2-year-old child who developed a macular rash after resolution of a high fever**

The appearance of a rash after resolution of a high fever in a pediatric patient is consistent with the diagnosis of roseola and is not an emergent condition. In the case of the 5-year-old, the peeling lips, petechiae, and malaise are suggestive of a toxicity in child; possible causes include meningococcemia and Kawasaki disease. In adults and older adults, symptoms of sepsis include fever, headache, changes in respiratory rate, cold, clammy, mottled, or pale skin with slow capillary refill, and changes in mental state, including confusion, disorientation, slurred speech, and loss of consciousness.

**9. C, D, E) Intertrigo, Onychomycosis, Tinea pedis**

Intertrigo, onychomycosis, and tinea pedis are all caused by fungal infections, and are responsive to treatment with oral or topical antifungal medications. Intertrigo is an inflammatory condition of skin folds, onychomycosis is a fungal infection of toenails or fingernails, and tinea pedis is commonly called "athlete's foot." Impetigo is a bacterial infection of the skin and requires antibiotic treatment. Causes of eczema include environmental irritants, allergens, and genetic predisposition; mainstays of treatment include corticosteroid creams and ointments, and barrier repair moisturizers.

**10. A) Fever, fatigue, and erythema migrans**

Lyme disease is a bacterial infection transmitted to humans through the bite of an infected tick. During the early stage of Lyme disease, a classic bulls-eye rash (erythema migrans) occurs, and individuals often have fever, lymphadenopathy, and fatigue. If untreated, Lyme disease can cause multiple systemic symptoms, including significant joint pain, severe headaches, facial palsy, neuralgias, and carditis. The rash associated with Lyme disease is not painful. The key to preventing systemic disease sequela is to diagnose and treat Lyme disease in the earliest stage.

4

# Head, Neck, and Lymphatics

## KEY HISTORY CONSIDERATIONS

- Headache (acute, chronic, recurring)
- History of injury or trauma to the head or neck
- Limited mobility of neck or jaw
- Neck pain
- Lymphadenopathy (acute or chronic)
- Symptoms of thyroid disorders
- Smoking history
- Human papillomavirus (HPV) vaccination
- Personal and family history of cancer, specifically lymphoma, neck, or thyroid cancers
- Family history of thyroid disorders
- Exposure to pollutants and/or environmental exposures

## PHYSICAL EXAMINATION: INSPECTION AND PALPATION

### INSPECTION

1. Note the position of the head and neck. They should appear midline and relaxed without deformities or tremors.
2. Inspect the cranium for symmetry; note the quality and condition of the skin of the scalp. Systematically parting the hair may be needed for a thorough assessment.
3. Observe the hair of the head for texture and distribution.
4. Note the facial features, including symmetry, shape, and facial expression.
5. Check cranial nerves V and VII. Ask the patient to clench their jaw and then test sharp, dull, and light touch with the patient's eyes closed. Ask individuals to raise their eyebrows, smile, frown, and puff their cheeks to observe symmetry in their facial movements. For more detailed information on the neurologic exam, refer to Chapter 8, "Nervous System."
6. Inspect the skin of the face and neck.
7. While an individual holds their head in a neutral position, inspect the neck anteriorly, posteriorly, and from each side. A thorough, complete physical exam includes assessing for limitation or pain with movement.
8. Have the patient tip their chin to their chest, turn their head to each side, and tip their head toward each shoulder. Patients should exhibit a full range of motion in their neck, and it should be completed without pain or discomfort.

## INSPECTION ABNORMAL FINDINGS

- **Head:** Observe for head tremor. A head tremor can indicate some type of movement disorder such as essential tremor or Parkinson's disease. Cerebellar, psychogenic, and metabolic-induced tremors can also occur. Tremor can also be a side effect of taking certain medications.
- **Position and symmetry of facial features:** An accurate assessment of symmetric alignment of the eyebrows, eyes, ears, nose, and mouth, and position of facial features relative to the face, including palpebral fissures and the nasolabial fold, can reveal genetic, endocrine, or neurologic disorders. Prominence or depression of the forehead, cheeks, and chin should be noted.
  - The facial features associated with fetal alcohol syndrome include epicanthal folds, a flat nasal bridge, small palpebral fissures, "railroad track ears," upturned nose, a smooth philtrum, and a thin upper lip.
  - Cleft lip and palate abnormalities occur when the lip and/or hard/soft palate do not completely form. Degree varies from mild notch to severe large opening extending to the nasal cavity.
  - Craniosynostosis occurs from early fusion of the bones of the skull. This results in increased intracranial pressure and/or skull abnormalities. This differs from plagiocephaly, which is a flat area on the head or side of the infant's head resulting from positioning (i.e., pressure from being repeatedly in a supine position can cause the back of the skull to flatten).
  - Down syndrome is a genetic disorder caused by an extra chromosome (trisomy 21). Associated craniofacial abnormalities include flattened nasal bridge, shortened neck, small low-set ears, slanted epicanthal folds.
  - Hemangioma is an abnormal collection of blood vessels in the skin that is faint at birth, then appears larger and darker in the first months after birth; also known as portwine stain, salmon patch, or strawberry hemangioma.
  - Treacher Collins syndrome (TCS) is a genetic disorder that causes maxillary hypoplasia and auricular deformities, in addition to a smaller skull or microcephaly.
  - Turner syndrome is a genetic disorder that affects development in females. The appearance can include a thickened neck, low hairline, prominent earlobes, and crowding of the teeth.
- **Facial movement:** Asymmetric facial movement can indicate a neurologic disorder, including a stroke or Bell's palsy.
- **Hair:** Hair that is abnormally coarse, thin, and/or has areas or patterns of hair loss are abnormal. This can be due to a variety of causes such as thyroid disorders, B12 deficiency, alopecia, or tinea capitus. See Chapter 3, "Integumentary System," for more information on hair abnormalities.
- **Skin:** Ecchymosis, particularly under the eyes or behind the ears, is a worrisome sign. Battle sign is the term used when there is ecchymosis over the mastoid process and typically means there is a fracture at the base of the skull. This is a medical emergency. Raccoon eyes, where ecchymoses develop under and around the eyes, typically mean there is a basal skull fracture. The head and neck are also common places for skin cancer to occur. Any new or changing lesions should raise suspicion for malignancy. See Chapter 3, "Integumentary System," for more information on skin abnormalities.

- **Signs of respiratory distress:** Signs of respiratory distress include skin color changes, tripoding, pursed lips, grunting, head bobbing, accessory muscle use, retractions, paradoxical respirations, and nasal flaring. For more information on respiratory distress, see Chapter 7, "Respiratory System."
- **Neck:** Complete range of motion of the neck and inspect for deformities, pulsations, areas of edema, and limitations in movement. With significant thyromegaly, the thyroid gland is often visible on the outside of the neck. If the patient has any limitations or pain while moving the neck, further investigation is needed. Cervical strain, torticollis, osteoarthritis, epidural abscess, whiplash, or cervical fracture are all possible causes. If the patient appears toxic with a headache and fever, meningitis should also be suspected. If a pulsation is noted, auscultation is necessary. Refer to Chapter 6, "Cardiovascular System," for more information.
- **Lymph nodes:** Lymph nodes should never be visible on inspection.

## PALPATION

1. Palpate the head for areas of edema, tenderness, including the mastoid processes.
2. Test sensation of light touch by asking the patient to close their eyes. Use a cotton swap to lightly touch the skin on forehead, cheeks, and chin. The patient should be able to identify when they are feeling the soft touch and what area of the face is being touched.
3. Palpate the jaw while the individual clenches their teeth, opens, and closes their mouth. The jaw should move smoothly and fluidly.
4. Palpate the submental, submandibular, retropharyngeal, tonsillar, pre-auricular, post-auricular, anterior, and posterior cervical lymph nodes.
5. Palpate the thyroid gland to assess for nodules and enlargement. Note the size, shape, and consistency of the gland. An anterior or posterior approach can be used for thyroid palpation (Figure 4.1).
   - **Posterior approach:** Ask the individual to tip their chin slightly forward; stand behind the individual and place fingers on the individual's neck just below the cricoid cartilage. Ask the individual to swallow while keeping fingers steady in this position and the thyroid isthmus can be felt rising under the pads of the fingers as the person swallows. To palpate the lobes of the thyroid, the clinician can ask the individual to tip their chin to their chest, displace the individual's trachea slightly and gently to the right with their left hand, and in this position, palpate the right thyroid lobes with their right hand. Repeat this technique on the other side, by displacing the trachea to the left with the right hand and palpating the left thyroid lobes.
   - **Anterior approach:** Ask the individual to tip their head back slightly and use the landmarks of the notched thyroid cartilage and the cricoid cartilage to locate the thyroid. Palpate the region below the cricoid cartilage to identify the contours of the thyroid. Simultaneously moving the sternocleidomastoid muscles further apart causes the skin to be taut over the thyroid gland and can enhance the anterior inspection and palpation techniques. To verify the location of the thyroid gland, ask the individual to swallow, and note movement of the thyroid isthmus. With palpation, the thyroid gland is normally soft, without distinctly palpable nodules.

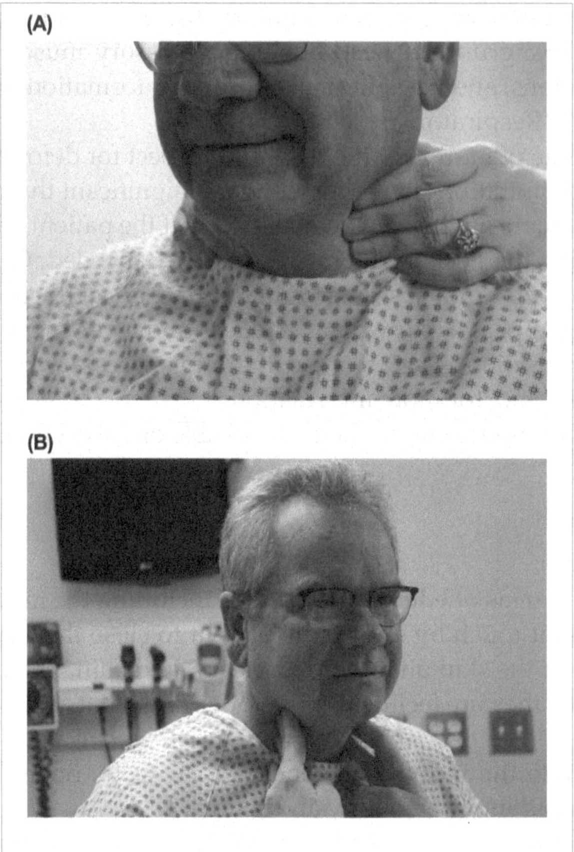


**Figure 4.1** Palpation of the thyroid. (A) Posterior approach; (B) anterior approach.

6. Palpate the lymph nodes in the head and neck. Ask the individual to remove all clothing from the regions of the head, neck, and upper shoulders. Have the patient tilt their head slightly down and relax the neck and shoulder muscles. Using both hands, palpate the occipital and posterior cervical lymph nodes. Have the patient return their neck to its upright position and ask the patient to raise their chin. Palpate the submental, submandibular, retropharyngeal, tonsillar, pre-auricular, post-auricular, and anterior cervical lymph nodes. Ask the patient to move their shoulders slightly forward and palpate the supraclavicular fossa for supraclavicular lymph nodes (Figure 4.2). Then palpate below the clavicles to feel for any infraclavicular lymph nodes. Palpation should be completed using a fluid, circular motion. Soft palpation should be followed by deeper palpation in order to feel for any hidden enlargement. Care should be taken to ensure the entire surface area of the lymphatic region is palpated. When palpating for the lymph nodes, it is important to remember what part of the body a particular lymph node drains so the examiner can also examine this particular area to look for local signs of infection or abnormality. It is also important to palpate the surrounding tissues since lymph nodes are often found in chains.

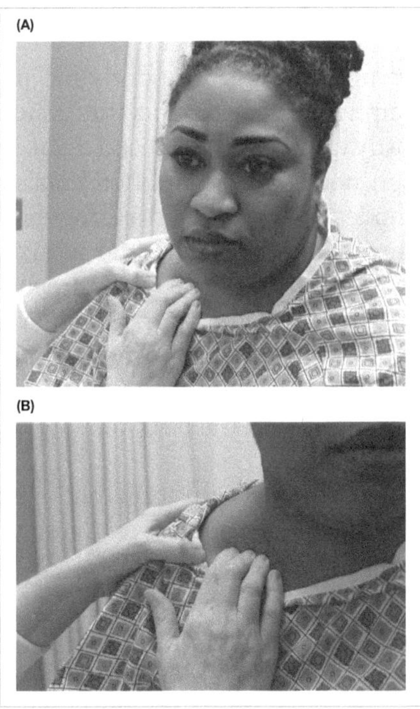


**Figure 4.2** Palpation of supraclavicular lymph nodes.

7. If a lymph node is palpated, the examiner should note the size, consistency, discreteness, mobility, tenderness, warmth, symmetry, and border edges of the lymph node.

## ABNORMAL FINDINGS OF THE HEAD AND NECK

- Edema and tenderness are common following trauma to the head/face/skull. Physical signs of a skull fracture include: a bump, bruise, depression, or soft point at the site of impact. Clear fluid or blood could be coming out of the ears or nose if there is a severe fracture. A visibly crooked or bent nose, bloody drainage from the nose, or difficulty breathing can indicate a broken nose.
- Tenderness to palpation of the frontal or maxillary sinuses can indicate sinusitis.
- Tenderness to palpation of mastoid processes can indicate a mastoiditis.
- Inability to identify sensation on the face indicates a neurologic disorder. See Chapter 8, "Nervous System," for more information.
- If the jaw has shifted from midline or has any associated popping, clicking, or grinding, this indicates temporomandibular joint dysfunction (TMJ).
- Thyromegaly is often seen in iodine deficiency, Graves' disease, and Hashimoto's thyroiditis. If the thyroid is tender on palpation, this can indicate a thyroiditis. If the thyroid is soft and nodular, Graves' disease should be suspected. If it is firm, Hashimoto's thyroiditis or malignancy should be considered.
- Thyroid nodules can sometimes be palpated on exam. These can be solid or fluid-filled. The majority of these do not cause symptoms and are not cause for concern. Nodules that are firm, hard, fixed, progressively growing, or associated with sudden pain are more concerning for malignancy. If the patient is younger than 14 or older than 70 and has a nodule, this is also more suspicious for malignancy.

### ABNORMAL FINDINGS OF THE LYMPHATIC SYSTEM

- Enlarged lymph nodes are often a sign of underlying infection and are common, especially in children. Lymph nodes are found throughout the body, but the palpable lymph nodes are mostly clustered in the head and cervical, axillary, and inguinal regions. Cervical lymph nodes are more often enlarged than other lymphatic regions. Enlarged lymph nodes are considered more worrisome when they exhibit the following qualities: hard, fixed, matted, >1cm in size, unilateral, generalized, located in the supraclavicular, iliac, popliteal, or epitrochlear regions, or do not go away. If a lymph node is palpated in the supraclavicular region, it is cancer until ruled out. Lymphadenopathy is also more concerning if it is accompanied by systemic symptoms such as weight loss, fever, or night sweats. Shotty lymph nodes are small, mobile palpable lymph nodes in the neck that are commonly associated with viral illnesses.
- When lymphadenopathy is generalized, multiple regions of the body are affected. HIV, cat scratch disease, lymphoma, mononucleosis, sarcoidosis, and toxoplasmosis are several diagnoses that should be considered.

## SPECIAL TESTS OF THE HEAD AND NECK EXAM

The cardiovascular, ENT, and neurological exams can also be included as part of the head and neck exam. Refer to Chapter 5, "Eyes, Ears, Nose, and Throat;" Chapter 6, "Cardiovascular System;" and Chapter 8, "Nervous System;" for more information on these exams.

# RED FLAGS IN HISTORY AND PHYSICAL EXAM

- Thunderclap headache
- Change in pattern, type, or frequency of headaches
- Neurologic symptoms associated with a headache
- Progressive decline in consciousness; profound confusion
- Persistent mental status changes, incoherent speech
- Loss of coordination, seizures
- Pupil dilation
- Mastoid ecchymosis (Battle sign)
- Bruising around orbits of the eyes (raccoon eyes)
- Clear fluid drainage from the eyes, ears, or nose
- Symptoms in children may include persistent crying, inability to be consoled, or unusual irritability.

# POPULATION HEALTH AND LIFE-SPAN CONSIDERATIONS

## INFANTS AND CHILDREN

- Inspect the head of a newborn, infant, or child to assess size, shape, and form, including presence of fontanels and suture ridges. An accurate head circumference measurement, using a non-stretchable measuring tape to measure above the eyebrows and ears, should be compared with expected size on the growth chart. Inspect for symmetry or asymmetry of an infant or child's head from above and from all angles. Confirm that the line of the eyes is horizontal and that the child's ears are in alignment, to confirm head symmetry.

- During the first days of life, expect that the newborn will have cranial molding. Inspect and palpate the head, noting overlapping suture ridges. A newborn's scalp is likely to be diffusely soft and swollen, a condition called *caput succedaneum.*
- Inspect and palpate the fontanels of infants and children under 2 years of age. The small posterior fontanel is located where the two parietal bones join the occipital bone; the larger anterior fontanel is palpable where the two frontal and two parietal bones join. While the posterior fontanel is often not palpable beyond 2 months of age, the anterior fontanel can be palpable up to 2 years of age. Fontanels should be flat, not depressed or bulging, when palpated. Begin the exam while the infant is calm. Palpate the fontanels while the child is held in both supine and upright positions. Palpation of the anterior fontanel in the upright position may reveal a normal, slight pulsation. If the anterior fontanel has closed prematurely, percuss the skull near the junction of the frontal, temporal, and parietal bones to assess for Macewen's sign, an unusually resonant "cracked-pot" sound that indicates increased intracranial pressure. Infants with an asymmetrical shape of the cranium that has resulted from positioning, a condition known as plagiocephaly, will have normal cranial suture lines and flat fontanels.
- Observe the infant or child's neck control, head movement, and position. Palpate the neck for masses and/or lymphadenopathy. To more easily assess the neck of a newborn, elevate the upper back of the infant to allow the head to extend slightly. Infants and children should have a full and easy range of motion of the neck. Nuchal rigidity, or resistance to flexion of the neck, is associated with meningeal irritation. Postural torticollis, twisting of the neck muscles, is relatively common in newborns related to positioning in utero; associated physical exam reveals a preference for tilting the head in one direction.
- Palpable lymph nodes in children are common.
- Roughly 50% of healthy children have palpable lymph nodes at any one time that are either benign or infectious in etiology, with up to 90% of children aged 4 to 8 years having palpable cervical lymph nodes.
- The lymphadenopathy is typically self-limiting and does not require further work-up or treatment.
- Similar to adults, large and supraclavicular lymph nodes in children need further investigation in addition to the presence of systemic symptoms.

## OLDER ADULTS

- The appearance of the face and neck typically changes with age.
- Loss of muscle tone and thinning skin gives the face a flabby or drooping appearance. In some people, sagging jowls may create the look of a double chin.
- The skin on the face dries out, and wrinkles appear.
- There can be bone loss in the lower jaw, giving the appearance of a prominent forehead, nose, and mouth.
- Noses and ears may get bigger.
- In elderly patients, malignant disease is the most common cause of persistent lymphadenopathy.

## KEY DIFFERENTIALS FOR THE HEAD AND NECK

- Cluster headache
- Craniofacial disorders
- Fetal alcohol syndrome
- Head injury and/or head trauma
- Parathyroid disorders
- Hypothyroidism
- Hyperthyroidism
- Migraine
- Stroke
- Skull fractures
- Tension headache
- Thyroid malignancy
- Torticollis

## KEY DIFFERENTIALS FOR THE LYMPHATIC SYSTEM

- Cat scratch disease
- HIV
- Hodgkin lymphoma
- Infection
- Lymphedema
- Mononucleosis
- Non-Hodgkin lymphoma
- Sarcoidosis
- Toxoplasmosis

# KNOWLEDGE CHECK: HEAD, NECK, AND LYMPHATICS

1. Which history statement about headache(s) MOST indicates the need for an imaging study as part of the diagnostic workup?

   **A.** Headaches triggered by lack of sleep
   **B.** Onset of migraines at 60 years of age
   **C.** Recurrent migraines for 3 to 5 years
   **D.** Sinus infection concurrent with migraine

2. When assessing the lymph nodes of an individual with a viral upper respiratory illness, which finding would be MOST expected?

   **A.** Anterior cervical lymph nodes tender and mobile
   **B.** Non-tender pre-auricular nodes are 2 cm in diameter
   **C.** Palpable infraclavicular node is small, fixed, and hard
   **D.** Several small iliac lymph nodes palpable unilaterally

3. A 6-month-old infant is brought to the clinic with new onset of vomiting. Which physical exam finding is MOST reassuring?

   **A.** Bulging anterior and posterior fontanels
   **B.** Closure of all fontanels with palpable suture lines
   **C.** Depressed anterior fontanel and open posterior fontanel
   **D.** Flat anterior fontanel and closed posterior fontanel

4. An athlete has sustained an acute head injury while playing football. Which assessment should prompt immediate transport for evaluation?

   **A.** Accurate but slowed mental processing
   **B.** Decreasing level of consciousness
   **C.** Headache and dizziness
   **D.** Inability to recall details of the injury

5. In older adults, one of the more common signs of hyperthyroidism is:

   **A.** Markedly increased appetite
   **B.** New onset of atrial fibrillation
   **C.** Palpable nontender mass in the neck
   **D.** Palpable tender lymphadenopathy

*(See answers next page.)*

**1. B) Onset of migraines at 60 years of age**

Red flags indicating secondary headache disorders include new onset of migraine-type headache in individuals over the age of 50, as this can indicate inflammatory, infectious, or neoplastic processes. Primary headache disorders, which include migraine- and tension-type headaches, may be recurrent or chronic, and are commonly triggered by stress, illness, environment, and/or sleep disturbances.

**2. A) Anterior cervical lymph nodes tender and mobile**

Tenderness of a lymph node is most indicative of an infectious etiology; the anterior, posterior, and deep cervical chain areas are the most likely regions to assess lymphadenopathy associated with upper respiratory illnesses. Hard, matted, fixed, non-tender, or irregular lymph node(s) are more suspicious for pathogenicity, especially if unilateral change is noted. Lymph nodes greater than 1cm in diameter are considered abnormal and uncommon. Any palpable supraclavicular, infraclavicular, iliac, epitrochlear, or popliteal lymph nodes should also be considered abnormal, regardless of size.

**3. D) Flat anterior fontanel and closed posterior fontanel**

The small posterior fontanel usually closes during the first 2 months of life. The larger anterior fontanel usually closes by 15 months. Fontanels should be flat, not depressed or bulging, when palpated; a bulging fontanel can indicate increased intracranial pressure, and a sunken fontanel can indicate dehydration. Early closure of fontanels is associated with craniosynostosis.

**4. B) Decreasing level of consciousness**

Some form of ongoing assessment and observation is recommended for at least 24 hours after a mild traumatic brain injury (TBI) because of the risk of intracranial complications. Follow-up imaging is indicated immediately for those who experience deterioration of mental status. Commonly reported symptoms include fatigue, drowsiness, neck pain, headache, emotionality, dizziness, difficulty concentrating, and difficulty remembering.

**5. B) New onset of atrial fibrillation**

Older adults and individuals with milder hyperthyroidism often have isolated symptoms that warrant evaluation, including unexplained weight loss, decreased appetite, weakness, and new onset of atrial fibrillation. Most individuals with overt hyperthyroidism have a dramatic constellation of symptoms, including increased perspiration and heat intolerance, thinning of hair, exophthalmos and periorbital edema, tachycardia, dysphagia, weight loss, nocturia, anxiety, and palpitations. Palpable thyroid nodules and/or lymphadenopathy are not associated with hyperthyroidism. The finding of thyroid nodules can be incidental; if associated with lymphadenopathy, an evaluation for malignancy is warranted.

6. Which two problems are associated with thyroid hypofunction? (Select TWO.)

   A. Carpal tunnel syndrome
   B. Exophthalmos
   C. Graves' disease
   D. Myxedema
   E. Thyroid storm

7. A 35-year-old male presents with extremely painful headaches that started this week. The headaches occur several times a day in brief attacks of severe stabbing pain, during which the patient notes that he has a very runny nose, tears from his eyes, and a drooping eyelid. He appears distressed; cranial nerves II–XII are intact. Which diagnosis is MOST LIKELY?

   A. Basilar migraine
   B. Cluster headache
   C. Migraine with aura
   D. Tension-type headache

8. An individual presents to the emergency department subsequent to sustaining a head injury in a motor vehicle accident. Which signs and symptoms are most concerning?

   A. Bruising behind the ears and around both eyes
   B. Disorientation and dizziness
   C. Emotionality despite no loss of consciousness
   D. Headache and nausea

9. When enlarged, which lymph nodes are MOST LIKELY to be a sign of malignancy?

   A. Occipital
   B. Posterior cervical
   C. Submandibular
   D. Supraclavicular

10. When an individual presents with swelling of epitrochlear nodes, which two assessments of patient history are most pertinent? (Select TWO.)

   A. Are you experiencing trouble swallowing?
   B. Are you having tooth pain?
   C. Do you have a sore throat?
   D. Have you been scratched by a cat?
   E. Have you noticed any skin changes?

*(See answers next page.)*

**6. A and D) Carpal tunnel syndrome and myxedema**

Key assessments indicating hypothyroidism include: fatigue, weakness, dyspnea on exertion, intolerance of cold temperatures, weight gain, constipation, cognitive dysfunction, bradycardia, carpal tunnel syndrome, coarse skin, hair loss, periorbital edema, enlargement of the tongue, non-pitting edema (myxedema), decreased hearing, hoarseness, and arthralgia. Graves' disease is an autoimmune disorder that causes overactivity of the thyroid gland; overproduction of thyroid hormone can lead to exophthalmos and thyroid storm.

**7. B) Cluster headache**

Cluster headaches are recurrent, short, painful attacks of severe burning or stabbing pain that occur one to eight times daily for weeks. Ipsilateral lacrimation, congestion, and ptosis are associated autonomic symptoms. Tension headaches have a much more gradual onset, with the predominant symptoms of band-like pressure. Migraine headaches are unilateral and have a more gradual onset; migraine pain is more likely to be throbbing, aggravated by light and sound. The aura or prodrome of a migraine are usually sensory disturbances. Symptoms of migraines with brainstem aura (basilar migraines) include vertigo, diplopia, tinnitus, and confusion.

**8. A) Bruising behind the ears and around both eyes**

Basal skull fractures characteristically cause bruising behind the ears, known as "Battle sign" (mastoid ecchymosis) and/or bruising around the eyes/orbits, known as "raccoon eyes." Bruising behind the ears and around the eyes are red flags for one of the most serious skull fractures. The other listed symptoms (disorientation, dizziness, emotional lability, headache, and nausea) are consistent with head injury and warrant observation.

**9. D) Supraclavicular**

Any palpable supraclavicular, infraclavicular, iliac, epitrochlear, or popliteal lymph nodes should be considered abnormal, regardless of size.

**10. D and E) Have you been scratched by a cat? And have you noticed any skin changes?**

Epitrochlear nodes are part of the superficial lymphatic system of the upper extremities and are not likely to be enlarged. Inflammatory and infectious causes include cat-scratch fever, abscesses, and metastatic lymphadenopathies (primarily from melanoma). Disorders of the head and neck are not likely to cause epitrochlear enlargement or tenderness. Appropriate assessment of epitrochlear lymphadenopathies should review for various causes of swelling involving the elbow and arm.

# Eyes, Ears, Nose, and Throat

5

## KEY HISTORY CONSIDERATIONS

- Upper respiratory infection symptoms (e.g., cough, fever, chills, rhinorrhea, sore throat, postnasal drip)
- Watery, itchy eyes
- Change in vision (e.g., sudden change or loss of vision, double vision, blurry vision, loss of peripheral or central vision, decreased ability to see at night, increased sensitivity to glare)
- Presence of flashing lights, halos, or floaters in visual field(s)
- Pain or drainage from the eye(s)
- Recent trauma, head injury, or traumatic noise exposure (blast/explosion)
- Pain, pressure, or drainage from the ear(s)
- History of hearing loss (complete, partial, or decreased, fluctuating)
- Tinnitus
- Facial pain or pressure
- Oral lesions
- Dysphagia or odynophagia
- Quality of voice (coarse voice, breathy voice, aphonia)
- Dental caries or dental pain
- Head and neck lymphadenopathy
- History of allergies, asthma, or eczema
- Prior surgeries on ears, nose, sinuses, tonsils, adenoids, or neck
- Alcohol, smoking, or intranasal drug use
- Occupational exposures
- Exposure or risk for human papillomavirus (HPV)

## PHYSICAL EXAMINATION: INSPECTION, PALPATION, AND SPECIAL TESTS

### INSPECTION AND PALPATION

#### HEAD AND NECK

1. Inspect the size and shape of the head and the scalp.
2. Inspect for symmetry, masses, and signs of trauma.

3. Note any difficulty with breathing or speech.
4. Palpate the head, face, and scalp.
5. Use a firm, circular motion to palpate the lymph nodes of the head and neck.
6. Refer to Chapter 4, "Head, Neck, and Lymphatics," for more detail on the head, neck, and lymphatics.

## EYES

1. Measure visual acuity with a Snellen chart. The patient should be 20 feet from the chart. Each eye should be measured independently, then both eyes together. If the patient wears glasses for myopia, they should not be removed for the exam. Ask the patient to read the line with the smallest characters that they can see. The numbers at the end of the line provide an indication of the patient's acuity compared with those who have normal vision. Normal visual acuity is 20/20. A person with 20/20 vision can see what an average person can see on an eye chart when they are standing 20 feet away.
2. Measure near visual acuity with a Rosenbaum or a Jaeger eye chart. Hold the test card 14 inches from the eyes in adequate lighting. Use a tape measure to verify the distance. Have the patient cover one eye and test each eye separately then together. Have the patient read the smallest block of text they are able to read without squinting and have them read that passage aloud. Have them continue reading successively smaller blocks of print until they reach a size that is not legible and record that value.
3. In patients with visual or focal neurological concerns, assess the visual fields. Refer to Chapter 8, "Nervous System," for an explanation of this technique.
4. Inspect the eyelids, lashes, bulbar and palpebral conjunctiva, sclera, cornea, anterior chamber, and iris. There should be no edema, erythema, or discharge.
5. Assess pupils by inspecting their size, shape, reactivity to light (direct and consensual), and accommodation. Pupils should be equal, even, and reactive to light. Perform the pupillary exam in a dimly lit room. Have the patient focus on an object across the room. Shine a light in each pupil and note the size, position, shape, equality of the pupils, and their response to bright light. The pupils should constrict to direct illumination. Shining a light in one pupil should also cause the other pupil to constrict (consensual response). Assess direct and consensual response for each eye; appropriate pupillary response reflects the integrity of cranial nerves (CN) III, IV, and VI. Accommodation is normal when the pupils change in size when shifting focus on near and far objects. To assess the accommodation reflex, have the patient focus on a distant object, then focus on a penlight and slowly move the penlight toward the patient's nose. Both eyes should turn inward (convergence), and both pupils should constrict (accommodation).
6. Confrontation visual field testing is used as a screening for integrity of the optic nerve (CN II), visual field defects, scotomas (blind spots), and early signs of serious ocular disorders. To test visual fields by confrontation, the clinician should sit (or stand) approximately two feet away from the patient; the clinician and patient should face one another. Both clinician and patient should cover one eye (as a mirror image) and maintain eye contact. The clinician should extend their arm and raise a finger. Starting from the periphery, slowly advance the finger into the patient's field of vision. Ask the patient to say "now" when the finger becomes visible. Assuming

the clinician has normal peripheral vision, the patient should be able to see the finger at the same time the clinician does. This should be repeated on both sides and can include all fields of vision. Because the visual fields of both eyes overlap, each eye should be tested independently.

7. With the ophthalmoscope, assess the red light reflex bilateral. The "red reflex" refers to the red or reddish-orange reflection of light from the fundus. This can commonly be seen in photographs as "red eye." Direct the light of the ophthalmoscope into the pupil at a medial angle and watch for the red reflex. Slowly move toward the patient while following the red reflex. If the red reflex is lost, start over. The red-light reflex should be symmetrical and identical in shape, color, and size in both eyes. Follow the red reflex all the way in until the vasculature is seen. This technique works best in a dimly lit room. The clinician may need to view different angles to elicit the reflex.
8. If there is an eye concern, the appropriate equipment is available, and the clinician is appropriately trained, complete a fundoscopic exam. If the appropriate equipment is not available and/or an adequately trained clinician is not available, the ophthalmic exam should not be completed. To perform the exam, darken the room and ask the patient to focus on an object far away to help dilate the pupil. The clinician should place the ophthalmoscope firmly against their own cheek. The clinician and ophthalmoscope should move as one unit. Use the right hand/eye to assess the patient's right eye. Use the left hand/eye to assess the patient's left eye. Look through the ophthalmoscope to determine if it is in focus and adjust the diopter setting if needed. Using the red reflex as a guide, follow the direction of the blood vessels until the optic disc is visualized. Inspect the optic cup and disc, retinal blood vessels, retinal background, and macula. Arteries are narrower than veins. Vessels emerge from the nasal side of the optic disc. The optic disc should have sharp margins, and the retinal background should have even color without hemorrhages or exudate. The cup-to-disc (C/D) ratio is based upon a relationship of the diameter of the "cup" portion of the disc in comparison with the total diameter of the optic disc. Think of a hole in a tire. The hole represents the cup, and the surrounding tire represents the disc. If the cup fills one-tenth (1/10) of the disc, the C/D ratio is 0.1. The average C/D ratio is about 0.4. The macula is an oval-shaped, pigmented area in the center of the retina. In the center of the macula is a slightly darker area called the "fovea."

## EARS

1. Inspect the auricle and mastoid. Skin color should be uniform without edema, lesions, ecchymosis, or erythema.
2. With the otoscope, examine the external auditory canals (EAC), tympanic membranes (TMs), and any middle ear structures visualized through the TMs. The EACs should be free from edema, erythema, and drainage. Cerumen is a normal finding. Cerumen should appear soft and yellow/orange in color. The TMs should be pearly grey and translucent with no bulging or retraction. The cone of light should be visible at 5 o'clock in right ear and 7 o'clock in left ear. The lateral process of the malleus, pars tensa, and pars flaccida should be visualized.
3. Assess hearing one ear at a time with light finger rubbing or the whisper test. To complete the finger rub test, stand in front of the patient. The clinician should then hold their hands to the side of the patient's head. Gently rub the fingers on one side

together, asking if the patient hears the sound. Repeat on the other side. Wait for the patient's response. Repeat again with both hands, asking if the patient hears them equally on both sides.

4. To complete the whisper test, tell the patient that three words will be whispered to them, and the patient should repeat those words back to the clinician. The patient will be asked to occlude one ear canal. If the patient cannot do this, the clinician can press on the tragus occluding the ear canal. The clinician should stand behind the patient or cover their mouth to ensure that the patient does not read the clinician's lips. Standing about one to two feet away, the clinician should exhale fully and whisper softly three words or numbers toward the unoccluded ear. The words or numbers should be equally accented syllables like baseball or ninety-nine. If the patient responds correctly, the hearing is considered normal. If the patient does not respond correctly, repeat using three different words or numbers. The patient is considered to pass if they repeat three out of six answers correctly.
5. If hearing is abnormal, perform the Weber and Rinne tests. To perform the Weber test, place a 512 Hz vibrating tuning fork on the top of the patient's head at midline. Ask the patient in which ear the sound is best heard. The sound should be heard equally well in each ear.
6. To perform the Rinne test, place the vibrating tuning fork on the mastoid process. It is then held just lateral to the ear testing conduction of sound through air. The patient is asked which position produces the loudest sound. This technique is used to test conduction of sound through bone. Normally, air conduction should be better than bone conduction.

## NOSE AND SINUSES

1. Examine the external nose, nares, septum, and nasal cavities. Inspect the inside of the nose with an otoscope and the largest ear speculum available. Have the patient tilt their head back and press the nasal tip up to open the nasal vestibule. Look posteriorly and superiorly to visualize the anterior septum, anterior inferior turbinate, and possibly the middle turbinate. Evaluate the septum for deviation, lesions, perforation, bleeding, and/or crusting. Assess the nasal cavity and mucosa for color, lesions, drainage, ulcerations, and polyps. Assess the turbinates for color, size, polyps, lesions, or ulcerations.
2. Assess for nasal patency. Press on one naris at a time, asking the patient to breathe in and out, assessing airflow through the nasal vestibules.
3. If you suspect sinusitis, palpate the paranasal sinuses in the following areas for tenderness: above the eyes (frontal) and over the malar eminences (maxillary).

## ORAL CAVITY

1. Inspect the lips, buccal mucosa, tongue, floor of mouth, palate, palatine tonsils, and posterior pharyngeal wall.
2. Inspect the teeth and gums for caries and periodontal disease.

3. In patients with risk factors for oral cancer or symptoms of oral infection, salivary duct stone(s), or malignancy, palpate the submandibular glands, salivary ducts, and base of tongue.
4. Palpate the parotid glands.
5. Palpate temporomandibular joints (TMJ). Listen for clicking, popping, or crepitus. Feel for any jaw deviation from midline.

## INSPECTION AND PALPATION: ABNORMAL FINDINGS

### HEAD AND NECK

Refer to Chapter 4, "Head, Neck, and Lymphatics," for more detail on abnormalities in the head, neck, and lymph nodes.

### EYES

- Any score less than 20/20 on the Snellen chart requires further evaluation for myopia or other underlying conditions.
- Patients who cannot see the smallest letters or numbers on the Rosenbaum or Jaeger charts also require a referral to an eye specialist to evaluate for presbyopia, hyperopia, and any other underlying eye conditions.
- Any edema, erythema, or discharge noted on eyelids, lashes, bulbar and palpebral conjunctiva is abnormal and could suggest such diagnoses as conjunctivitis or allergic rhinitis. Severe allergic rhinitis can also cause darkened skin around the inferior eyes, often termed "allergic shiners."
- Anisocoria may be a normal variant, termed physiologic anisocoria, and is present in up to 20% of the population. Other causes include pharmacological dilation, Horner's syndrome, and third cranial nerve palsy.
- In the confrontation visual field testing, the patient should be able to see the finger at the same time the clinician does. A delay in seeing the finger would indicate impaired peripheral vision. Common causes of peripheral vision include glaucoma, stroke, scotoma, or retinitis pigmentosa. It can also occur during migraines but is typically temporary.
- The red reflex test can reveal problems in the cornea, the lens, the vitreous, and the retina; it is particularly useful in young children who may develop eye diseases but who are too young to complain of not seeing. Absence or a color other than red reflecting back during the red-light reflex test is abnormal. Any asymmetry of the red reflex may indicate an abnormality such as strabismus, refractive error, or media opacity. White reflex (leukocoria) may indicate a corneal scar, cataract, retinal scar, or retinoblastoma. A white reflex is the hallmark of a retinoblastoma in the eye; and it is the light reflecting from the tumor's white surface that can be seen when light reflects from a certain angle. This is a rare finding. A black or absent reflex may indicate a corneal scar, cataracts, or hemorrhage.
- The larger the C/D ratio, the more suspicious the clinician should be for underlying pathology, specifically glaucoma. If the C/D ratio is 0.8 or higher, consider glaucoma until otherwise ruled out.

- Abnormal findings when inspecting the optic disc include optic cupping, optic edema, cotton wool spots, flame hemorrhages, papilledema, emboli, infarct, Roth spots, drusen, or arterio-venous (AV) nicking. These findings are associated with other, often chronic, underlying conditions such as diabetes, hypertension, or increased intercranial pressure.

## EARS

- Tenderness to the auricle and tragus often indicates otitis externa. Painless edema to the auricle can be an auricular pseudocyst or perichondritis.
- Foul-smelling drainage in the ear canal can indicate such diagnoses as otitis externa (including malignant otitis externa) or cholesteatoma. Ear canals should also be checked for a foreign body, especially in children.
- Abnormalities to the tympanic membrane include perforations, tympanosclerosis, retraction, or a red/bulging appearance. Fluid or bubbles can accumulate behind the tympanic membrane, which is termed an otitis media with effusion. In rare cases, blood can be visualized behind the tympanic membrane, called "hemotympanum." This can occur after blunt head trauma, barotrauma due to scuba diving, spontaneous epistaxis, otitis media, blood disorders, or anticoagulation therapy.
- During the Weber test, if the sound lateralizes to one ear, the test is considered abnormal. It can mean one of two things: there is sensorineural loss on the side with the decreased sound, or there is conductive hearing loss on the side with the increased sound.
- The Rinne test is considered abnormal for sensorineural hearing loss, if air conduction is better than bone conduction and for conductive hearing loss, if bone conduction is better than air conduction.

## NOSE AND SINUSES

- Erythema and edema of the nasal turbinates or nasal discharge are considered abnormal and may indicate allergic rhinitis, upper respiratory infection, or sinusitis. Boggy, pale turbinates can also occur with allergic rhinitis.
- In more severe allergic rhinitis, there can also be a nasal or allergic crease seen on the nose. This is a transverse line across the top of the nose that develops from habitually rubbing the nose in an upwards motion with the palm of the hand to try and relieve itching.
- Nasal polyps are soft, painless growths on the lining of the nasal passages that hang down like grapes. They are often due to chronic inflammation from conditions such as asthma, recurring infections, allergies, drug sensitivity, or certain immune disorders.
- The nose should appear midline, and nasal passages should be equal in size. Septal deviation is present if the nose appears crooked and/or the nasal passages are unequal in size and shape. Septal deviation can be genetic, inherited, or caused by trauma.
- A hole visualized through the septum of the nose is called a "septal perforation." It can be the result of cocaine use, previous nasal procedures, infection, prolonged use of nasal steroids or decongestants, certain autoimmune conditions (e.g., lupus), or trauma to the nose and/or face.
- If sinuses are tender to palpation, this can indicate sinus inflammation or infection.
- Anosmia can occur due to various etiologies but has more recently been associated with COVID-19.

## ORAL CAVITY

- Oral lesions or lesions on the lips or surrounding skin can be a number of conditions. Appearance of the lesions should determine potential differential diagnoses (Table 5.1).
- Dental caries are often seen as visible holes or pits in the teeth. Brown, black, or white staining on any surface of a tooth can also indicate dental decay.
- The appearance of periodontal disease can vary based on the extent and severity of disease. Signs of periodontal disease include swollen/puffy gums, bright red/dusky/purplish gums, tenderness to gums when touched, gums that bleed easily, gum receding, new spaces or pus developing between teeth, halitosis, or in later stages, loose teeth.
- Enlargement of the tonsils can be a normal variation or associated with pathology such as streptococcal pharyngitis or tonsillitis.
- Clicking, popping, crepitus, or deviation from the midline with movement of the TMJ is abnormal.

**Table 5.1 Common Oral and Lip Lesions**

| Lesion | Description | Notes |
|---|---|---|
| Aphthous ulcers (canker sores) | Round or oval lesion with a white or yellow center and a red border; form inside the mouth—on or under the tongue, inside the cheeks or lips, at the base of the gums, or on the soft palate; painful | Usually appear during an immunocompromised state |
| Angular cheilitis | Chronic inflammatory condition of the corners of the mouth; cracking and fissuring of the corners of the mouth with redness, ulceration, drainage of pus, and tissue softness/tenderness; slightly painful | Usually associated with a fungal (*Candidal*) or bacterial (*Staphylococcal*) infection |
| Basal cell carcinoma | Flat, firm, pale, or yellow areas, similar to a scar; raised reddish patches that might be itchy; small, pink or red, translucent, shiny, pearly bumps, which might have blue, brown, or black areas; pink growths with raised edges and a lower area in their center that might contain abnormal blood vessels spreading out like the spokes of a wheel; open sores (which may have oozing or crusted areas) that do not heal or heal and then come back | Often fragile and might bleed after shaving or after a minor injury |
| Leukoplakia | White patches or spots on the inside of the mouth that cannot be rubbed off; can develop into malignancies | Caused by chewing tobacco, heavy smoking, and alcohol use |

(*continued*)

**Table 5.1 Common Oral and Lip Lesions (*continued*)**

| Lesion | Description | Notes |
|---|---|---|
| Squamous cell carcinoma of the lip (SCC of lip) | Skin lesions may appear as crusted ulcer, plaques, and nodules that may ulcerate and bleed; in majority of the cases, condition is asymptomatic and does not present with any signs or symptoms (during the initial period) | Generally slow-growing tumors; an aggressive form of cancer |
| Oral candidiasis | White patches on the inner cheeks, tongue, roof of the mouth, and throat; cracking and redness at the corners of the mouth; cotton-like feeling in the mouth; loss of taste; pain while eating or swallowing | Caused by *Candida*, a yeast (a type of fungus) |
| Orofacial herpes ("cold sores") | Painful sores on the upper and lower lips, gums, tongue, roof of the mouth, inside cheeks or nose, and sometimes on face, chin, and neck; can cause symptoms such as lymphadenopathy, fever, and myalgias | Caused by herpes simplex virus; also termed *HSV-1, type 1 herpes simplex virus*, or *herpes labialis* |

## SPECIAL TESTS

Refer to Chapter 8, "Nervous System," for instructions on how to complete a cranial nerve exam. Sometimes completion of the cranial nerve exam is needed during the HEENT exam to access for certain conditions.

# RED FLAGS IN HISTORY AND PHYSICAL EXAM

## EYE

- Severe eye pain (especially with a sudden onset)
- Acute change in visual acuity, loss of vision
- Halos around lights, double vision
- Severe headache with photophobia, fever, and/or petechial rash
- Intense eye redness of conjunctiva, sclera, lens, cornea
- Severe, purulent discharge from eye(s)
- Lens opacities, hazy cornea
- Loss of vision, visual field defects, change in visual acuity
- Pupil dilation, or pupils unequal in size, shape
- Slow or absent pupil reaction to light

- Papilledema
- Periorbital or orbital erythema, edema, and tenderness
- Ptosis
- Painful or limited extraocular movements

### EAR AND NOSE

- Suspected foreign body in the ear or nose
- History of sudden or rapidly progressive hearing loss
- Unilateral hearing loss of sudden or recent onset
- ENT symptoms associated with unintentional weight loss or other systemic symptoms
- History of pain, active drainage, or bleeding from an ear
- Acute, chronic, or recurrent episodes of dizziness
- Evidence of congenital or traumatic deformity of the ear
- Unilateral or pulsatile tinnitus

### THROAT

- Severe edema
- Stridor
- Presence or suspicion of foreign body
- Oral lesions or a persisting lump or ulcer in the mouth
- Dysphagia
- Painless neck lump

## POPULATION HEALTH AND LIFE-SPAN CONSIDERATIONS

### INFANTS AND CHILDREN

- The American Academy of Pediatrics recommends that formal vision screening be performed at ages 4 and 5 years, and then every other year beginning at age 6 years (Hagan, Shaw & Duncan, 2017). Normal visual acuity in the newborn ranges from 20/100 to 20/400 and gradually develops to 20/20 by 5 to 6 years of age; this development of vision is known as emmetropization. The clinician should refer children to ophthalmology for an abnormal visual acuity for age, or more than a two-line difference between eyes, for example, right eye 20/20 and left eye 20/30.
- At each routine wellness visit, the following assessments should be performed on all children aged newborn to 3 years:
  - Vision assessment including visual fixation, tracking, visual interest, and attentiveness
  - Inspection of eyes including lids, eyelashes, conjunctiva, corneas, sclera, irises, pupils
  - Assessment of corneal light reflex and movement of the eyes (EOMs)
  - Pupillary function including reaction to light, accommodation, and convergence
  - Red reflex

- Normal findings will vary based on age. The pupillary light reflex is underdeveloped until 5 months of age, and transient nystagmus can be a normal finding in infants younger than 6 months. Extraocular muscle function is not well established in the first 6 months of age, therefore, intermittent phorias/strabismus may be observed. Phorias are the natural inward or outward eye posture. Poor muscle coordination and abnormal ocular alignment after 6 months of age may warrant referral and further evaluation.
- Test the red reflex after birth, at the age of 6 weeks, during routine consultations, or when parents are concerned about the child's vision or the appearance of their eyes. If this is abnormal, a referral to a specialist is necessary for pupil dilation and a complete eye exam.
- Corneal light reflex and observation are the primary methods for assessing eye alignment in infants. In young cooperative children, the cover test (sometimes also called the "cover-uncover test") can be used. To perform the cover test, have the child focus on an object straight ahead. Check for deviation in either eye. Using your hand or an eye occluder device, cover one of the patient's eyes for 3 seconds. The tested, uncovered eye is observed for movement out of (or back into) its original position. The untested eye is uncovered, while the tested eye is again observed for any deviation out of (or into) alignment. Repeat for the other eye. Deviation out of (or into) alignment is a positive test and indicates strabismus.
- Hearing evaluation in infants is a screening requirement implemented by the Early Hearing Detection and Intervention (EHDI) Act.
- In children under the age of 3, the angle of the ear canal is less acute, so the clinician will need to pull back and down on the posterior helix. This allows for proper placement of the speculum into the external ear canal. It is helpful to have a parent or assistant stabilize the head for you.
- Otitis media with effusion (OME) can also cause significant hearing problems in children, resulting in speech and learning delays. According to the 2016 revised American Academy of Otolaryngology's clinical practice guidelines on otitis media with effusion, clinicians should assess children between the ages of 2 and 12 who exhibit speech or learning problems. Subtle symptoms of poor balance, behavioral problems, school performance issues, or speech delay may also point to an underlying hearing problem.
- The pediatric population has heightened activity of the tonsil and adenoid tissue from the ages of 4 to 10. The most common bacterial infection that affects this area is Group A Beta-Hemolytic Streptococcus (GABHS), which causes tonsillitis.
- When examining children or someone who may not be able to stay still, the clinician should stabilize the otoscope by using the side of their hand against the patient's head. Hold the handle of the otoscope between the thumb and fingers with the handle facing upward. Place the side of the hand against the patient's cheek to stabilize the otoscope. This will help prevent jerky movements and prevent trauma from sudden patient head movements. In many cases, the parent or an assistant can help stabilize the child's head.
- It may be difficult to see the posterior pharynx in an infant. It is best visualized when the infant is crying. If you cannot get good visualization, listen to the quality of infant crying, as this can indicate if there is any obstruction or restriction of the airway.

### OLDER ADULTS

Changes associated with structures of the eye include:

- Eyelid laxity and deepening of the lines of expression
- Changes in corneal curvature and decreased corneal luster
- Increased resistance to the outflow of aqueous humor in the trabecular network
- Hardening (nuclear sclerosis) of the lens
- Less collagen causes liquefaction of vitreous humor
- Decline in visual function including function of the lens results in presbyopia, far-sightedness
- Decreased contrast sensitivity resulting in reduced depth perception
- Increased susceptibility to age-related diseases (e.g., macular degeneration)
- In adults aged 60 or older, several eye diseases may develop that can change vision permanently. The earlier these problems are detected and treated, the more likely the patient can retain good vision.
- According to the U.S. Preventive Services Task Force 2018 draft statement on hearing loss screening, adults over the age of 50 should be screened for hearing loss
- Significant pathology is much more likely in older adults who present with oral lesions
- Cancer of the tongue is common in the older male population, especially in tobacco users

### SPECIAL CONSIDERATIONS

- There are multiple different eye shapes, such as hooded eyes, downturned eyes, and upturned eyes. Vision and eye shape are usually independent of each other. However, certain eye shape variations may affect vision.
- The red-light reflex may appear gray or cream-colored in individuals with darker pigmented skin.
- The most associated concern early in preeclampsia is blurry vision. However, severe preeclampsia can lead to retinopathy, optic neuropathy, and retinal detachments; retinopathy associated with preeclampsia may be more severe with underlying diabetes, chronic hypertension, and renal disease.

## KEY DIFFERENTIALS

### EYE

- Cataracts
- Chalazion
- Corneal abrasion
- Conjunctivitis: allergic, bacterial, fungal, irritant, keratoconjunctivitis, neonatal, viral (Figure 5.1)
- Dacryostenosis
- Dacryocystitis

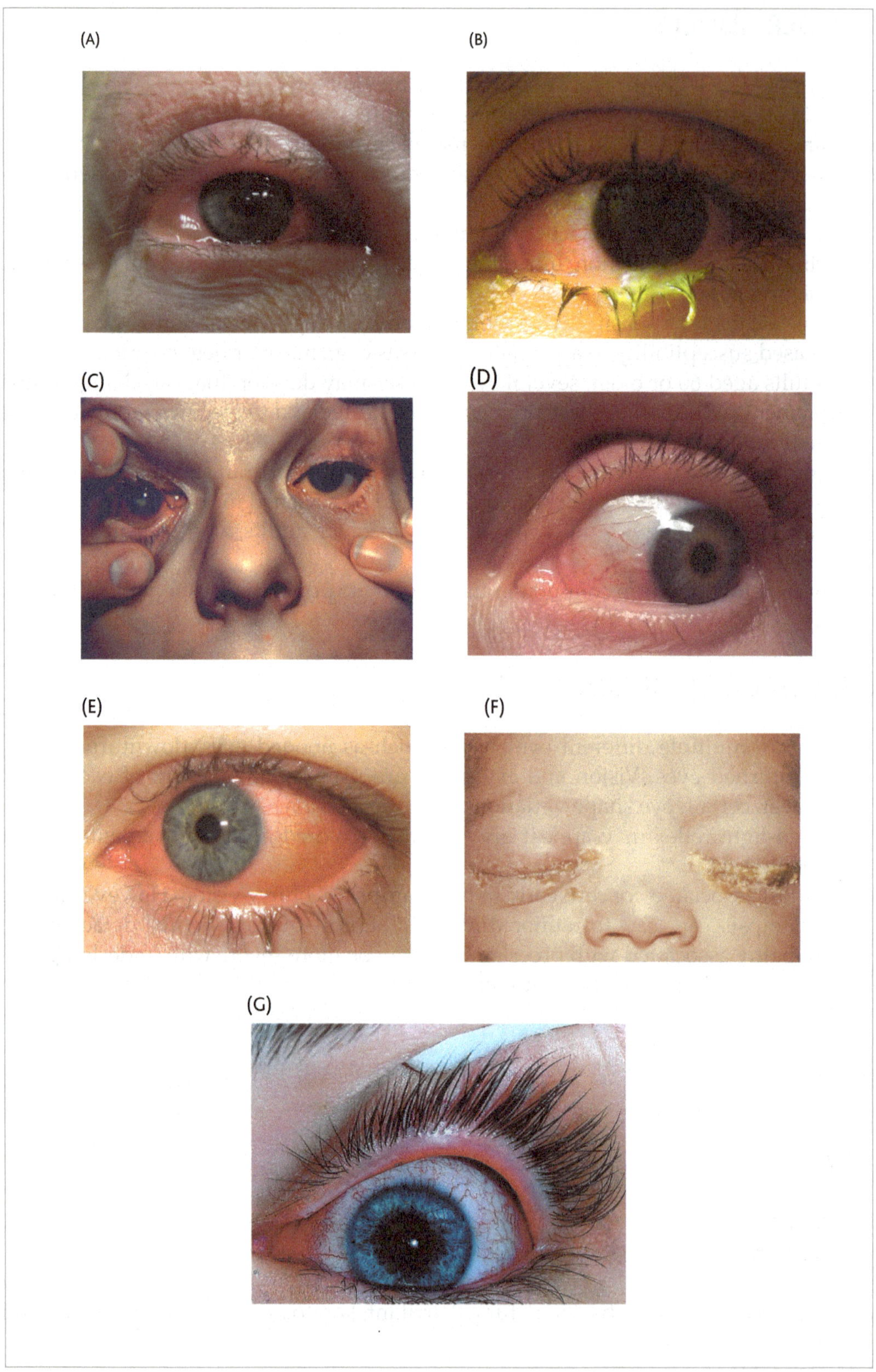


**Figure 5.1** (A) Allergic conjunctivitis. (B) Bacterial conjunctivitis. (C) Fungal conjunctivitis. (D) Irritant conjunctivitis. (E) Keratoconjunctivitis. (F) Neonatal conjunctivitis. (G) Viral conjunctivitis.

- Diabetic retinopathy (Figure 5.2)

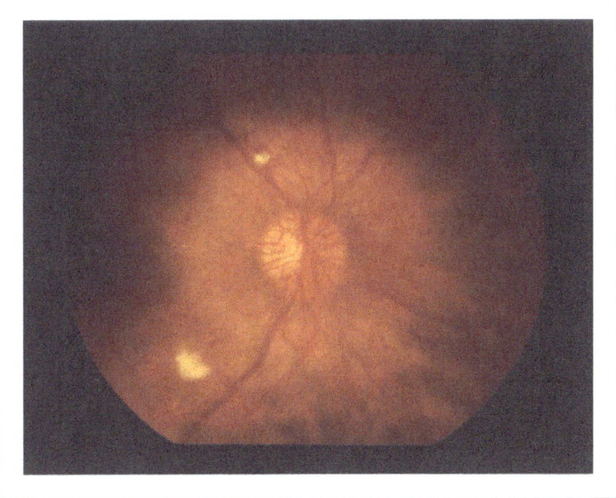

**Figure 5.2** Proliferative diabetic retinopathy.

- Dry eye
- Glaucoma
- Hordeolum
- Hyperopia
- Hypertensive retinopathy (Figure 5.3)
- Macular degeneration
- Myopia
- Optic (and retrobulbar) neuritis

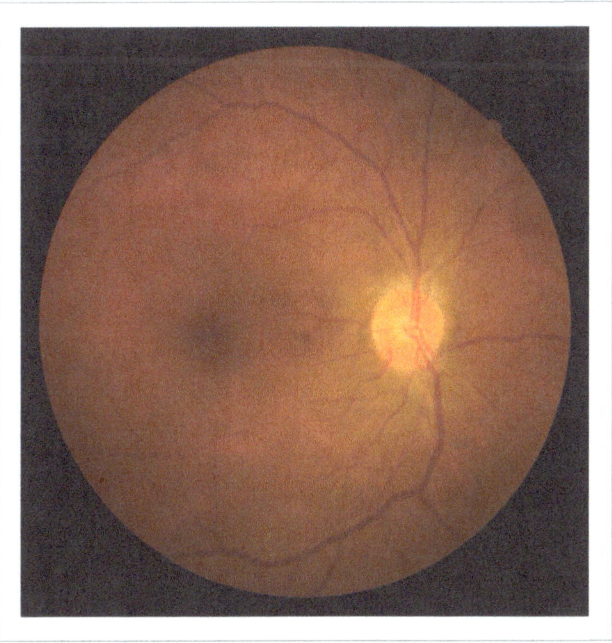

**Figure 5.3** Hypertensive retinopathy.

- Orbital (and periorbital) cellulitis
- Pingueculum
- Presbyopia
- Pterygium
- Retinal detachment
- Retinal tears
- Scleritis (and episcleritis)
- Strabismus
- Subconjunctival hemorrhage
- Uveitis

## EAR

- Anotia
- Cerumen impaction
- Cholesteatoma
- Eustachian tube dysfunction
- Malignant otitis externa
- Microtia
- Osteomas
- Otitis media (with and without effusion [Figure 5.4]
- Otitis externa
- Tinnitus

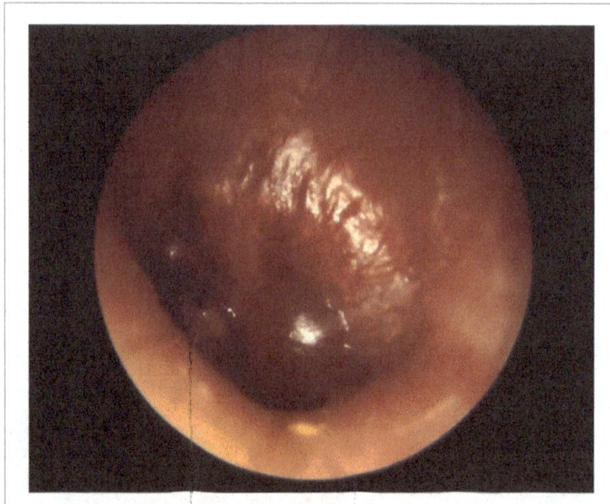

**Figure 5.4** Otitis media.

## NOSE AND SINUSES

- Allergic (and non-allergic) rhinitis
- Epistaxis
- Hearing loss
- Nasal polyp
- Septal deviation or perforation
- Sinusitis (acute and chronic)

## THROAT

- Angioedema
- Aphthous ulcers
- Herpangina
- Leukoplakia
- Oral cancer
- Oral candidiasis
- Streptococcal pharyngitis
- Tonsil cancer

# KNOWLEDGE CHECK: EYES, EARS, NOSE, AND THROAT

**1.** Cotton wool spots found on fundoscopic exam commonly indicate:

**A.** Eye trauma
**B.** Glaucoma
**C.** Hypertension
**D.** Normal aging processes

**2.** A preschool-aged child presents with unilateral, purulent, foul-smelling nasal drainage, and a history of epistaxis. Which physical exam finding would be consistent with the MOST LIKELY diagnosis?

**A.** Bulging tympanic membranes
**B.** Nasal foreign body
**C.** Nasal septum perforation
**D.** Scattered bruising

**3.** Which history is most consistent with the diagnosis of acute bacterial sinusitis?

**A.** Child with irritant cough triggered by exercise for 3 months
**B.** Adult with congestion and dental pain worsening after initial improvement
**C.** Adult with mild, persistent mid-facial fullness and tenderness for 3 days
**D.** Older adult with rhinitis triggered by foods and cold weather

**4.** An 18-year-old male presents with recent onset of "red eyes." He had nasal congestion and nonproductive cough for 2 days with no other symptoms until today. Now he has an oral temperature of 99.9°F. The conjunctivae of both eyes are diffusely red without itching and with minimal clear discharge. His ear exam reveals gray tympanic membranes. Pharynx is clear without lesions or exudate. The MOST LIKELY diagnosis is:

**A.** Allergic conjunctivitis
**B.** Bacterial conjunctivitis
**C.** Keratoconjunctivitis
**D.** Viral conjunctivitis

*(See answers next page.)*

**1. C) Hypertension**

Cotton wool spots are an abnormal finding on fundoscopic exam; the retinal background should be a deep red color, without exudate or hemorrhages. Damage to the retina caused by micro-infarctions associated with diabetes or hypertension may appear as cotton wool spots (i.e., fluffy white exudate). Trauma to the eye is likely to cause a corneal abrasion, not internal eye abnormalities, unless there is penetrating trauma (ruptured globe) evidenced by clear drainage of aqueous humor. Glaucoma is an optic neuropathy characterized by elevated intraocular pressure (IOP) from insufficient drainage, or over-production of aqueous humor, which damages the optic nerve, causing vision loss and blindness if untreated.

**2. B) Nasal foreign body**

Nasal foreign bodies (NFB) are commonly seen in the pediatric population; a high index of suspicion is required, especially in children ages 2 to 5. The usual presentation for NFB includes unilateral, foul-smelling purulent nasal drainage, with or without epistaxis. Septum perforation can co-occur but is not as common. Sinusitis, acute otitis media, and periorbital cellulitis are possible complications; nasal drainage as the presenting symptom decreases the likelihood of clotting disorders as the cause of epistaxis.

**3. B) Adult with congestion and dental pain worsening after initial improvement**

Most cases of sinusitis have a viral cause. Acute bacterial sinusitis is characterized by purulent nasal discharge, maxillary tooth, or facial pain (especially unilateral), unilateral maxillary sinus tenderness, and worsening symptoms after initial improvement. Viral symptoms mostly resolve in 7 days. Consider asthma for children who have a persistent irritant cough with activity or environmental triggers. Older adults are predisposed to vasomotor rhinitis, triggered by environmental irritants, changes in weather, hot or spicy foods, medications, or stress, predisposing them to chronic sinusitis.

**4. D) Viral conjunctivitis**

Viral conjunctivitis usually occurs concomitantly with a viral respiratory infection, which leads to symptoms of cough, nasal congestion, low-grade fever, reddened sclera, and watery eye drainage. Note in the case presented that the eye drainage is clear and minimal, without itching. The key differentiating symptom of allergic conjunctivitis is pruritus. Key symptoms of bacterial conjunctivitis are purulent eye discharge and the crusting and matting of lids and lashes. Keratoconjunctivitis is an inflammatory and/or infectious condition that affects both the conjunctiva and the cornea; key symptoms include a foreign body sensation, scleral erythema, photophobia, and/or mucopurulent discharge in association with corneal opacity.

5. Which signs and symptoms meet the diagnostic criteria for acute otitis media?

   A. Dull retracted tympanic membrane and flat tympanogram; child has decreased hearing
   B. Erythematous tympanic membrane; crying infant has a history of teething
   C. Erythematous bulging tympanic membrane with minimal mobility; infant has fever
   D. Tympanic membrane pearly gray with landmarks easily visualized; child pulling on ears

6. An adolescent has had 2 days of tragus pain, otorrhea, and otic itching. Which history statement is most significant as a risk factor for the likely diagnosis?

   A. Acne treated by a dermatologist
   B. Athlete on the swim team
   C. History of acute otitis media as a toddler
   D. Recently air travel to visit family

7. A 5-year-old presents with persistent bilateral rhinorrhea; his nasal turbinates are pale and boggy. His mother is concerned because the child always looks like he has circles under his eyes. The MOST LIKELY cause is:

   A. Environmental or seasonal allergies
   B. Inadequate sleep hygiene
   C. Influenza or other respiratory virus
   D. Untreated bacterial infection

8. A young adult female presents with abrupt onset of fever (highest 102°F), progressively worsening sore throat, and difficulty swallowing. Her speech is muffled and sounds similar to a person speaking with a hot potato in their mouth. On exam, her right tonsil is swollen to twice the size of the left tonsil, and her uvula is displaced. Which diagnosis is MOST LIKELY?

   A. Dental abscess
   B. Peritonsillar abscess
   C. Mumps
   D. Tonsillar stone

*(See answers next page.)*

**5. C) Erythematous bulging tympanic membrane with minimal mobility; infant has fever**

Diagnostic criteria for acute otitis media include rapid onset of symptoms, bulging tympanic membrane, limited or absent mobility of the membrane, and erythema of the tympanic membrane or ear pain affecting sleep or normal activity. Fever is often present. A dull or retracted tympanic membrane with a flat tympanogram, obvious fluid bubbles, and decreased hearing are signs of effusion. Erythema of the tympanic membrane can occur with crying and is not solely diagnostic. Children may pull at their ears when they discover them, so this behavior is not always an indicator of ear pain. The presence of cold symptoms or teething is not diagnostic for otitis. A normal tympanic membrane is pearly gray with landmarks easily visualized.

**6. B) Athlete on the swim team**

Common presenting symptoms of otitis externa include otalgia (ear discomfort) and otorrhea (discharge from the external auditory canal); the discomfort can range from itching to pain exacerbated by motion of the ear, including tragus palpation and/or chewing. Otitis externa is referred to as "swimmer's ear" because repeated exposure to water increases the ear canal's vulnerability to infection and inflammation. Previous episodes of acute otitis media, acne treatment, or air travel would not predispose someone to otitis externa. Air travel can exacerbate eustachian tube dysfunction, however, which can cause ear pain.

**7. A) Environmental or seasonal allergies**

Signs and symptoms of allergies in children include nasal symptoms—e.g., runny nose (rhinorrhea), congestion, postnasal drip, and pale, boggy nasal turbinates. Children may also have itchy, watery, red eyes. These symptoms lead to allergic shiners, or dark circles under the eyes. While bacterial or viral infections can also cause nasal and sinus symptoms, infections most often cause erythema and edema of nasal turbinates and are not likely to create periorbital hyperpigmentation. Inadequate sleep would not cause rhinorrhea, although it could cause a child to appear fatigued.

**8. B) Peritonsillar abscess**

Individuals with peritonsillar abscess appear ill and report fever, worsening throat pain, dysphagia, and trismus, leading to a muffled or "hot potato" voice. Inspection of the oropharynx reveals swelling and erythema of the infected tonsil with uvular displacement. Complications of this condition can include life-threatening airway obstruction and hemorrhage. The physical exam in this case rules out dental abscess (which causes tooth/gum swelling), mumps (which affects salivary glands), or tonsillar stone (a hard white or yellow formation in the tonsil).

9. Which statement about pharyngitis is TRUE?

   A. Allergies predispose patients to chronic bacterial pharyngitis
   B. Most cases of acute pharyngitis are caused by bacterial infections
   C. Most cases of acute pharyngitis are caused by viral infections
   D. Tonsils that are 2+ or greater usually indicate strep pharyngitis

10. A 5-year-old child presents with congestion, rhinorrhea, and low-grade fever. His tympanic membrane is pictured below. The MOST accurate diagnosis is:

    A. Acute otitis media
    B. Bullous otitis media
    C. Otitis externa
    D. Otitis media with effusion

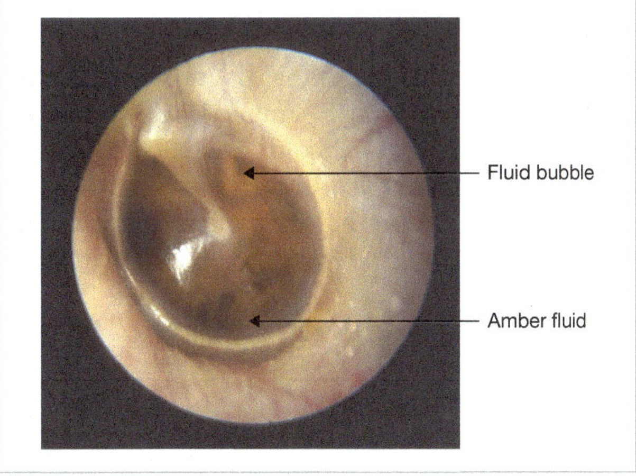


(*See answers next page.*)

**9. C) Most cases of acute pharyngitis are caused by viral infections**

Approximately 50% to 80% of pharyngitis cases are caused by viral infections, predominantly rhinovirus, influenza, adenovirus, coronavirus, and parainfluenza. The most common bacterial infection is Group A beta-hemolytic streptococci, which causes 5% to 30% of cases of acute pharyngitis. Centor criteria for GABHS diagnosis include tonsillar exudate, tender anterior cervical lymphadenopathy, history of fever, and absence of cough (not tonsillar enlargement). Environmental allergies and chemical exposures may also cause acute pharyngitis but do not lead to chronic bacterial infections.

**10. D) Otitis media with effusion**

Otitis media with effusion is diagnosed based on the visible fluid bubble, as well as the change of the color to amber. Children are more susceptible to effusions because they have more frequent colds and shorter eustachian tubes. In acute otitis media, the tympanic membrane is bulging and erythematous. In bullous otitis media, bullae or vesicles are noted on the tympanic membrane; moderate-to-severe pain is a common expected symptom. Otitis externa is associated with inflammation of the ear canal.

# Cardiovascular System

## KEY HISTORY CONSIDERATIONS

- Chest pain
- Left arm, jaw, or neck pain
- Unusual or extreme fatigue
- Shortness of breath
- Palpitations
- Lower extremity edema
- Hypertension
- Hyperlipidemia
- Calf pain
- Blood clots (including pulmonary embolus)
- Exercise (type, frequency, duration)
- Personal history of hypertension, hyperlipidemia, COVID-19, bleeding/clotting disorders, diabetes, sleep apnea, thyroid disorder
- History of stress tests, echocardiograms, EKGs, Holter monitors
- Family history of early myocardial infarction, stroke, or coronary artery disease
- Family history of congenital heart disease, sudden cardiac death, bleeding/clotting disorders, or long QT syndrome
- Tobacco use (past or present)
- Stress level (acute or chronic)
- Home monitoring of blood pressure and/or daily weight

## PHYSICAL EXAMINATION: INSPECTION, PALPATION, AND AUSCULTATION

### INSPECTION

1. Complete a general survey and observe the patient's overall appearance. Does the patient appear comfortable and calm or anxious and in distress?
2. Observe skin color, respiratory effort, and mental status.
3. Inspect the chest surface. Note the color of the skin and any movements of the chest. The chest should be free from rashes, scars, or pulsations.
4. The apical impulse is visualized at the same anatomic location where the Point of Maximal Impulse (PMI) is palpated. In normal-sized hearts, this normal pulsation is observed in the left fifth intercostal space (ICS) at or just medial to the mid-clavicular line (MCL).

5. Visual inspection of the chest should be completed with the patient in both the supine and seated positions. Lower the head of the bed so that the patient's head and chest are at a 30° to 45° angle. Young patients and healthy patients with no known or suspected cardiopulmonary disease may be examined lying flat.

## INSPECTION: ABNORMAL FINDINGS

- Those presenting with chest pain or shortness of breath should be closely observed for an urgent or emergent situation. Patients having an acute myocardial infarction often have clammy skin, diaphoresis, and shortness of breath. They may report having fatigue, dizziness, nausea, anxiety, or feelings of impending doom. Abnormalities in the skin color, respiratory effort, and mental status may indicate cardiovascular (CV) compromise.
- The skin should be inspected for any rashes, ecchymosis, scars, apparent heaves, lifts, or abnormal pulsations. Herpes zoster follows a unilateral dermatomal pattern. Patients typically have pain prior to the eruption of the rash, making diagnosis difficult. Ecchymosis can occur following trauma to the chest and can indicate underlying conditions such as broken ribs, internal bleeding, or a minor injury. Scars on the chest may provide evidence of prior surgeries or an implanted cardiac pacemaker or defibrillator. Heaves and lifts are abnormal outward thrusting or focal movement of the chest wall during the cardiac cycle that may indicate enlarged heart chambers, aneurysm, or an underlying valvular disorder.
- If the point of maximal impulse (PMI) is displaced, typically below the fifth intercoastal space, lateral to the midclavicular line (MCL), this is typically an indication of cardiomegaly. Other possible diagnoses for this include right pleural effusion, right tension pneumothorax, and/or left-sided pulmonary fibrosis. If there is a double impulse present over the apical region, hypertrophic cardiomyopathy should be considered. Epigastric and subxiphoid movements are typically seen with right ventricular hypertrophy, right ventricular dilation, or an abdominal aortic aneurysm.
- Note any chest abnormalities. Some common variations include pectus excavatum, pectus carinatum, or flail chest. These chest abnormalities are described in Chapter 7, "Respiratory System."

# PALPATION

1. Start by palpating the chest, costal cartilage, and ribs.
2. Palpate for the apical pulse with the palm of the hand and then the pad(s) of the finger(s). It should be less than 2.5 cm in diameter, approximately the size of a quarter. Note the location, size, amplitude (upstroke), intensity (strength/force), and duration of the pulse. The apical pulse represents the brief contraction of the left ventricle (LV) and, as such, is located at the apex of the heart, approximately fifth intercostal space (ICS) MCL. The apical impulse is the PMI in patients with normal-sized hearts and surrounding anatomy. PMI locates the left border of the heart and is typically in the fifth ICS, 7 to 9 cm lateral to the mid-sternal line (MSL). As noted above, palpation of the apical impulse and PMI provides information about the size of the heart. The apical impulse is palpated with the patient in the supine position but can also be performed in the left lateral position if there is difficulty identifying it while the patient is supine.
3. Next, palpate over the heart region to determine any thrills, lifts, or heaves. A thrill is a palpable murmur, and any grade 4/6 murmur or louder will have an accompanying palpable thrill.

## PALPATION: ABNORMAL FINDINGS

- Any tenderness, depressions, masses, deformities, or crepitus discovered during palpation of the chest is abnormal. Crepitus is the presence of air in the subcutaneous tissues, which can occur after a chest injury, invasive procedures, or surgery; crepitus can be both felt and heard as crinkling, a sensation often associated with "bubble wrap." Note that chest wall tenderness may be associated with inflamed pleura or costochondritis. Costochondritis is an inflammation of the costal cartilage (connective tissue where the ribs attach to the sternum) and can be distinguished from other etiologies when there is focal tenderness in the area of the costal cartilage. Focal tenderness on a rib(s) can indicate fracture.
- Deviation of the apical impulse from a brief, single impulse located at the fifth ICS MCL line suggests underlying pathology.
  - A forceful and hyperdynamic impulse can be palpated during states that increase the work of the heart such as seen during exercise; in hypermetabolic states such as anemia, hyperthyroid, or high-cardiac output states; or with mitral/aortic regurgitation or a ventricular septal defect.
  - A sustained impulse can also be seen in cardiac heart failure with a reduced ejection fraction.
  - A double apical impulse results from a forceful left atrial contraction against a highly noncompliant left ventricle and occurs in states of elevated end-diastolic pressure such as left ventricular hypertrophy, myocardial disease/cardiomyopathy, or a non compliant heart due to ischemia.
- A systolic thrill is strongly suggestive of significant underlying valvular disease.
- If a left lower parasternal heave is palpated, this may be normal in children or small/thin adults. If present, it can be palpated near the left parasternal intercostal spaces three and four. If it is present throughout systole, it is likely pathologic and suggestive of right ventricular hypertrophy.
- Other precordial pulsations that are significant include:
  - Right second intercostal pulsation may indicate an aneurysm of ascending aorta.
  - Left second (or third) intercostal pulsation, although less common, may indicate a dilated pulmonary artery.

# AUSCULTATION

1. Auscultate the apical pulse, noting the heart rate and rhythm. The rhythm should be regular, and the rate should be between 60 and 100 impulses/minute. Ideal heart rate is between 50 and 70 beats per minute.
2. Assess the radial pulse in conjunction with auscultation of the apical pulse.
3. Identify S1 and S2. These heart sounds will allow the clinician to identify systole and diastole and assist in identifying the timing of abnormal heart sounds. S1 indicates the beginning of systole and is heard as a "lub." S1 also coincides with the carotid artery pulse.
4. Auscultate the apical pulse while gently palpating the carotid artery to ensure the sound is S1. S1 is heard with each pulsation of the carotid artery. Refer to carotid pulse palpation later in this chapter for correct carotid palpation technique.
5. S2 indicates diastole, follows S1, and is heard as "dub." S1, representative of the closure of the mitral and tricuspid valves (atrioventricular [AV] valves), is heard best at the apex and is louder than S2 at this location. S2, indicating the closure of the aortic and pulmonic (semilunar) valves, is heard best at the base and is louder than S1 here.

6. Listen to the two sounds individually, denoting systole from diastole. A split in the S1 sound (heard best along the left sternal border [LSB]) and a physiological S2 split (heard best at the left second and third ICS) are normal.
7. The auscultatory exam may start at the apex or the base of the heart—either is appropriate. Regardless of the approach used, follow a "Z" pattern inching along the path, listening throughout systole and diastole at each site. Starting at the base of the heart, from the second right ICS move the stethoscope in turn to the second left ICS, the right sternal border, and the apex in the fifth ICS near the MCL. The order is reversed if starting at the apex. Listen with the bell first, then repeat the pattern listening with the diaphragm (Figure 6.1).

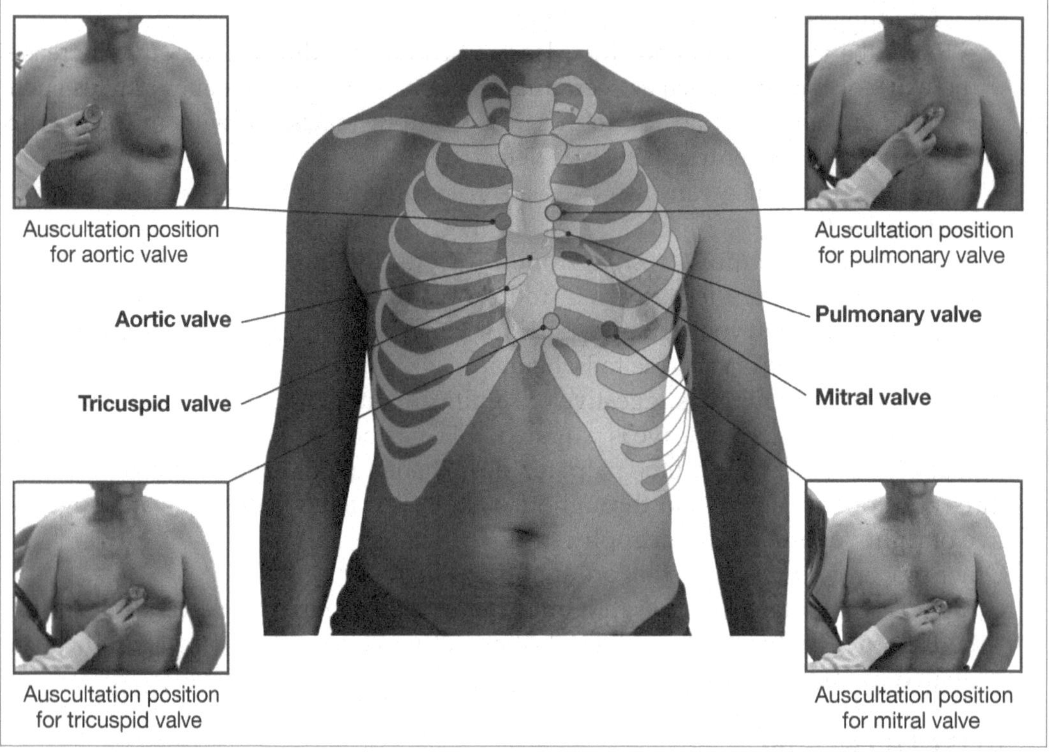


**Figure 6.1** Auscultatory sites for heart sounds. Positioning for the aortic valve, pulmonary valve, tricuspid valve, and mitral valve.

8. Before completing the seated portion of the cardiac exam, the patient is asked to lean forward and hold the breath after full exhalation while the clinician uses the diaphragm to listen along the left LSB. This position brings the left ventricular outflow tract closer to the chest wall and enhances the high-pitched sounds of the semilunar valves.
9. At each precordial site, listen first for systole and then diastole relative to S1 and S2.
10. Auscultation of the heart with the patient in the supine position is identical to the exam completed in the seated position, listening over all auscultatory sites with both the bell and the diaphragm. In addition, the patient is asked to turn to the left lateral position, and the clinician auscultates over the apex of the heart, left fifth ICS MCL, with the bell. In this position, the LV is closer to the chest wall accentuating S3, S4, and mitral murmurs, specifically mitral valve stenosis, if they are present.
11. The clinician will also auscultate the patient in the squatting and standing positions in certain circumstances.

## AUSCULTATION: ABNORMAL FINDINGS

- Tachycardia (elevated heart rate, typically considered >100 beats/minute): This can be a normal or abnormal finding. Tachycardia is a normal finding during exercise and can also occur during stressful situations. Abnormal tachycardia can originate in either the atria or ventricles. When the tachycardia is originating in the atria, the underlying cause can be atrial fibrillation, atrial flutter, supraventricular tachycardia, or Wolff–Parkinson–White syndrome. When the tachycardia is originating in the ventricles, ventricular tachycardia, ventricular fibrillation, or long QT syndrome can be the cause.
- Bradycardia (decreased heart rate, typically considered <60 beats/minute): This can also be a normal or abnormal finding. Bradycardia can be a normal finding in individuals who are very physically fit and/or at times, during sleep. Sick sinus syndrome, conduction blocks, or medication-induced bradycardias can also occur.
- For any irregular rhythm, note whether there is a regular or irregular pattern.
- Any difference between the apical rate and the radial pulse rate is noted as a pulse deficit and may indicate an abnormal cardiac rhythm.
- Persistent S2 splitting may indicate underlying conduction or valvular disorder. A fixed S2 split with no variation with respiration is concerning for an atrial septal defect (ASD) or a ventricular septal defect (VSD).
- Listen carefully for abnormal or extra heart sounds, such as the third (S3) and fourth (S4) heart sounds or murmurs. S3 and S4 can be normal or abnormal. S3 is auscultated in early diastole and S4 in late diastole. A pathological S3 is also referred to as a ventricular gallop and indicates decreased compliance of the ventricle and volume overload, as might occur in heart failure (HF) or high cardiac output states. Although not often detected in the outpatient setting, evidence strongly supports the utility of an S3 in the diagnosis of HF. S4, occurring immediately before S1, is a soft sound with low pitch. It is heard best with the bell of the stethoscope when the patient is in the left lateral position. A pathological S4, or atrial gallop, may occur because of decreased compliance of the ventricle and increased afterload. See Figure 6.2.

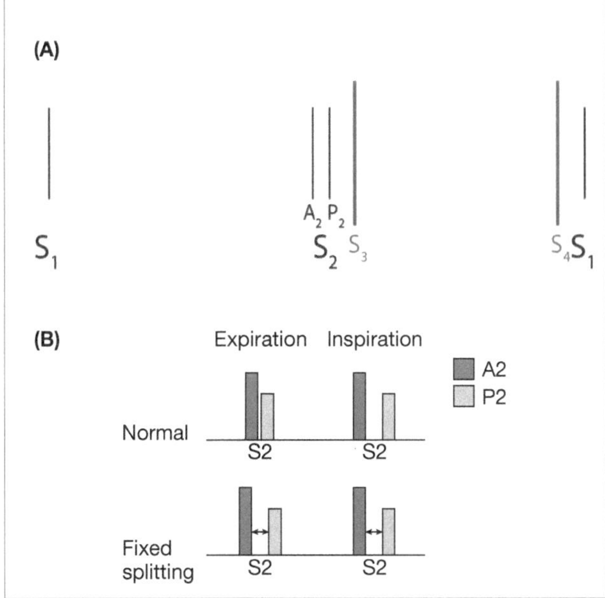


**Figure 6.2** (A) Physiological and pathological heart sounds. (B) Splitting of the S2 heart sound during the cardiac cycle.

- A variety of abnormal heart sounds may be auscultated over the precordium. These can include a variety of murmurs and pericardial friction rubs. Murmurs may be heard as a whooshing, clicking, snapping, vibrating, rumbling, or blowing sound. Murmurs can be benign (physiological) or pathological, related to congenital or acquired abnormalities, such as valvular disease and coronary heart disease. Murmurs are described according to eight characteristics: timing, loudness, pitch, pattern, quality, location, radiation, and posture. Types of heart murmurs are outlined in Table 6.1.
- Patients in whom a systolic murmur has been identified should be examined in additional positions to further delineate the origin of the murmur. Examining a patient in the squatting and standing positions can help to distinguish between the systolic murmurs of AS and hypertrophic cardiomyopathy (HCM). AS is best heard in the second right ICS while the murmur of HCM is best heard in the third to fourth left ICS. With the patient in the standing position, and preferably using the exam table for balance, the clinician stands next to the patient and places the stethoscope on the chest. The clinician asks the patient to squat and then stand while auscultating the heart. The patient is asked to momentarily pause while in the squatting position, then rise. The murmur of AS intensifies while the murmur of HCM decreases in intensity during the squatting phase as a result of increased arterial blood pressure, stroke volume, and left ventricular volume. The standing phase decreases arterial blood pressure, stroke volume, and left ventricular volume, thus decreasing the intensity of the AS murmur and intensifying the murmur of HCM. Patients may also be asked to perform the Valsalva maneuver (bear down like when having a bowel movement) while supine. The murmur of HCM intensifies during the Valsalva maneuver.

## INSPECTION OF THE PERIPHERAL VASCULAR SYSTEM

### JUGULAR VENOUS PRESSURE

1. Identify the jugular vein to be used for measurement of jugular venous pressure (JVP). The internal jugular vein lies deep in the sternomastoid muscle and can be difficult to see. Its pulsation is best visualized in the sternal notch. The top of the external jugular vein is visualized where it overlies the sternomastoid muscle.
2. Raise the head of the bed (HOB) 30° to 45° for visualization of the jugular vein and measurement of JVP. The angle may be more or less depending on at what elevation or height the jugular column (venous meniscus) is visualized. For patients suspected of hypovolemia, the HOB may need to be lowered for visualization of the jugular pulsation. For those suspected of fluid overload, the HOB may need to be raised higher.
3. Use a folded pillow or blanket behind the patient's head to elevate the head off the mattress while maintaining the shoulders on the mattress. Turn the patient's head away and elevate the jaw slightly. Traditionally, the right internal jugular vein has been used for this measurement; however, it can be difficult to locate. Studies affirm that using either the right or left internal jugular or right or left external jugular vein provides accurate results. Shine a tangential light across the neck to help visualize the venous motion. Place a ruler vertically on the sternal angle (the bony prominence on the sternum below the sternal notch). Use another straight edge as the horizontal reference line. Place the straight edge perpendicular to the ruler across

**Table 6.1 Characteristics of Heart Murmurs**

| Type of Murmur | Precordial Location | Timing in Cardiac Cycle | Radiation | Pitch | Sound Quality | Special Maneuvers |
|---|---|---|---|---|---|---|
| Aortic stenosis | Right second and third intercostal spaces | Mid-systolic | Toward carotid arteries | Crescendo–decrescendo; medium | Harsh | Best heard with patient sitting and leaning forward |
| Mitral stenosis | Apex | Diastole | None | Decrescendo; low | Rumbling | Use bell of stethoscope at PMI; best heard with patient in left lateral decubitus position |
| Aortic regurgitation | Left second to fourth intercostal spaces | Diastole | Toward apex | High | Blowing | Best heard with patient sitting and leaning forward with breath held following exhalation |
| Mitral regurgitation | Apex | Holosystolic | Toward left axilla | Medium/high | Harsh | Murmur should not vary with respiration |
| Tricuspid regurgitation | Lower left sternal border | Holosystolic | Toward xiphoid process | Medium | Blowing | Murmur will increase with inspiration |
| Pulmonic stenosis | Left second and third intercostal spaces | Mid-systolic | May radiate to left shoulder | Crescendo–decrescendo; medium | Harsh | None |

PMI, point of maximal impulse.

the highest point of the internal jugular pulsation or the point just above where the external jugular appears to collapse. Measure the vertical distance above the sternal angle where the horizontal and vertical points cross. If the measurement is above the sternal angle by no more than three cm, this is considered a normal finding.

4. Round the identified measurement to the nearest centimeter. If a jugular pulsation is not noted, it may lie below the level of the sternum, and, as such, the venous pressure is not elevated.
5. If venous pulsations are not visualized in the neck, JVP is likely normal. Lower the HOB until a pulsation is visualized to ensure that the pressure is not so high that it cannot be visualized.
6. If JVP is elevated, perform the hepatojugular reflux (HJR), also known as the "abdominojugular reflux." With the patient supine, the clinician places their right hand over the mid-abdomen below the right costal margin and pushes firmly for 10 to 15 seconds, observing the right jugular. If the jugular rises for a few seconds and then returns to baseline, the CVP is considered normal.

## ABDOMEN AND EXTREMITIES

1. With the shirt removed, inspect the abdomen and look for any pulsations and/or any masses.
2. Inspect the extremities. Note the skin color (keeping in mind the patient's race/ethnicity).
3. Assess the color and shape of the nails, noting any cyanosis or clubbing.
4. Check for capillary refill and nail angle. For more information on the capillary refill assessment and nail angle, refer to Chapter 7, "Respiratory System."
5. Examine the lower extremities for skin color, hair distribution, lesions, and edema. Arms and legs should be symmetric in size.

## INSPECTION OF THE PERIPHERAL VASCULAR SYSTEM: ABNORMAL FINDINGS

- A measurement of >3 cm above the sternal angle indicates an elevated JVP. An elevated JVP, and thus elevated right heart pressure, is a sign of congestive heart failure. Sustained elevation of the jugular is consistent with elevated CVP. In conjunction with an elevated JVP, positive HJR increases the likelihood (LR+ 8.0) of elevated venous pressure.
- Any visible pulsation on the abdomen should be noted. This may be a normal finding in very thin patients. If the patient has significant risk factors or does not have a thin frame, any pulsation, especially an abdominal pulsating mass, would be considered an abnormal finding, and an abdominal aortic aneurysm should be considered.
- Decreased hair distribution, cool skin, skin ulcerations, pale legs on elevation, and dusky red skin of the lower extremities in the dependent position may be signs of peripheral arterial disease (PAD). Brown pigmentation or petechiae of the skin, cyanosis with leg dependency, stasis dermatitis (dry, scaling, hyperpigmented skin), and ulcerations of the lower extremities may indicate venous insufficiency. Note any varicosities (engorged veins) of the legs. Note edema of the lower extremities as this may indicate poor venous return (as in venous insufficiency) or fluid retention, as occurs in HF. Table 6.2 reviews further signs and symptoms to help one delineate signs and symptoms of chronic venous insufficiency versus peripheral artery disease.

**Table 6.2 Chronic Venous Insufficiency Versus Peripheral Artery Disease: Signs and Symptoms**

| Sign/Symptom | Chronic Venous Insufficiency | Peripheral Artery Disease |
|---|---|---|
| Edema | Common | Uncommon |
| Ulcer location | Medial or lateral ankle | Toes or feet |
| Moisture | Common | Uncommon |
| Pain | Less common | More common |
| Other findings | Hyperpigmentation, lipodermatosclerosis | Absent pulses |

*Sources:* Grey, J. E., Harding, K. G., & Enoch, S. (2006). Venous and arterial leg ulcers. *BMJ, 332*(7537), 347–350. doi:10.1136/bmj.332.7537.347; Spentzouris, G., & Labropoulos, N. (2009). The evaluation of lower extremity ulcers. *Seminars in Interventional Radiology, 26*(4), 286–295. doi:10.1055/s-0029-1242204

## PALPATION OF THE PERIPHERAL VASCULAR SYSTEM

1. Palpate the right and left carotid arteries one by one. The patient should be in the supine position with the HOB elevated to 30° to 45°. The carotid arteries are located just medial to the sternomastoid muscle. Do not apply firm pressure or palpate both carotids at the same time, as this can compromise blood flow to the brain, causing syncope. Using several fingers, palpate the artery at the level of the cricoid cartilage. Use the right fingers to palpate the left carotid pulse and the left fingers to palpate the right carotid pulse. Avoid palpating near the top of the thyroid cartilage, the location of the carotid sinus, as pressure on this may cause slowing of the heart rate. Note the symmetry, rhythm, rate, amplitude (or upstroke), and intensity (or strength, force) of the pulse. The pulse should be smooth and symmetric with a brisk upstroke.
2. Palpation of the carotid artery may be done in conjunction with cardiac auscultation during identification of S1 and S2.
3. Palpate the arms and legs for skin temperature, texture, turgor, and edema.
4. Note the symmetry, rate, rhythm, amplitude (or upstroke), and intensity (strength or force) of the peripheral pulses. See Box 6.1 to see the three-point grading scale. The peripheral pulses include the radial, brachial, femoral, popliteal, posterior tibial (PT), and dorsalis pedis (DP). Light pressure on the pulse is important as firm pressure may obliterate the pulsation. In some adults, this pulse may be absent bilaterally.

**Box 6.1 Grading Scale For Pulses**

Pulses are graded on a 3-point scale according to the strength or force of the pulse:

- 3+: Bounding
- 2+: Normal
- 1+: Weak
- 0: Absent

## PALPATION OF THE PERIPHERAL VASCULAR SYSTEM: ABNORMAL FINDINGS

- Palpation of the carotid and femoral arterial pulses simultaneously is done for suspected coarctation of the aorta. With this condition, there is delayed transmission and amplitude of the femoral pulse as compared with the carotid.
- Lower-extremity edema is identified as either pitting or non-pitting, with pitting edema graded 1 to 4. Press firmly and gently with the thumb over the dorsum of the foot and pretibial area of the lower leg (shin). Hold the pressure for 5 seconds. Pitting is present if an indentation remains in the tissue after the thumb is removed. Grade the pitting and note the extent to which the edema ascends the extremity. See Box 6.2 for information on grading and documenting edema.

### Box 6.2 Documenting Edema

The following scale is used to grade pitting edema:
- 1+: Mild pitting with only slight indentation and no appreciable extremity edema
- 2+: Moderate pitting; thumb indentation resolves rapidly
- 3+: Deep pitting; indentation remains for a brief period of time and appreciable extremity edema present
- 4+: Severe pitting; indentation remains for a long time, and the extremity is obviously swollen

Nonpitting edema is graded according to severity:
- Mild
- Moderate
- Severe

Documentation also includes the extent to which the edema ascends the extremity (e.g., moderate nonpitting edema of the feet, ankles, and halfway up the calf).

- If unilateral edema is present, use a tape measure to document the difference between the two extremities. Measure at the smallest and largest difference of the calf and the circumference of the mid-thigh (if edema is present here). While there is a slight difference in the measurement of extremities, right to left, a difference of more than 1 to 2 cm is considered abnormal. Unilateral edema may be due to an injury, a venous thrombosis, lymphatic obstruction, or impaired venous return from a proximal obstruction.

## AUSCULTATION OF THE PERIPHERAL VASCULAR SYSTEM

1. Carotid artery auscultation is completed after palpation, when there is an indication of neurologic signs or symptoms consistent with decreased cerebral blood flow, as occurs with carotid artery stenosis, or when a palpable bruit is identified. To auscultate the carotid arteries, place the bell of the stethoscope over the identified carotid artery. Ask the patient to take a breath, exhale, and hold the breath. Holding the breath helps to avoid interpreting tracheal sounds as turbulent blood flow. This technique also avoids contraction of the levator scapulae muscle in the neck from dampening the sound.
2. The abdomen should be auscultated with the bell of the stethoscope over the aorta, iliac, renal, and femoral arteries.

### AUSCULTATION OF THE PERIPHERAL VASCULAR SYSTEM: ABNORMAL FINDINGS

- When listening over the carotid arteries, note any blowing or swishing sounds. This is a carotid bruit. Cardiac murmurs may be transmitted from the heart to the carotids. To avoid interpreting a heart murmur for a bruit, perform a complete precordial exam.
- Abdominal bruits (during systole) heard in the epigastric region of the abdomen are likely a normal finding in a healthy person; however, continuous bruits (across systole and diastole) or a bruit heard away from the midline are more concerning and deserve a more focused assessment.

## ADDITIONAL TESTING AND IMAGING

There are many other modalities for providing diagnostic information about the cardiovascular system. These modalities should be used in addition to a comprehensive history and physical exam when additional information is needed to make a diagnosis. The most common tests are described below, but additional advanced testing is available, including but not limited to coronary computed tomography angiography and coronary calcium scoring, coronary angiography, cardiovascular magnetic resonance imaging, cardiac computed tomography, and single-photon emission computed tomography.

### ELECTROCARDIOGRAM (ECG)

An ECG is a noninvasive test that measures the electrical activity of the heart. It uses electrodes placed on the skin of the patient's chest to measure voltage changes as the heart beats. By measuring the voltage across several vectors, an ECG can evaluate a variety of aspects of cardiac structure and function, the status of the conduction system, and identify signs of ischemia. It can be used to detect structural change(s) in the heart, such as chamber hypertrophy and enlargement, valve disease, and pericarditis. ECG is often ordered for the initial evaluation of patients with cardiovascular concerns.

### CHEST RADIOGRAPH

A chest radiograph or x-ray is a fast, relatively inexpensive test that can provide helpful clues to guide decision-making when faced with a patient with symptoms suspected to involve the heart. The x-ray beams that pass through the chest are picked up by a detector, and an image is created. A chest x-ray provides information about cardiac anatomy via the size and shape of its silhouette, but if combined with other findings, it can be diagnostic for various pathologies.

### ECHOCARDIOGRAM

#### *Transthoracic Echocardiogram*

A transthoracic echocardiogram (TTE) uses ultrasound (US) waves to create 2D and 3D pictures of the heart by detecting the reflection of the sound waves as they encounter tissue and blood. The speed and direction of blood flow can also be determined using Doppler imaging. This test is a useful way of determining the size and strength of the cardiac chambers and obtaining information about the structure and function of heart valves. It can also evaluate portions of the aorta, pulmonary arteries, and central veins.

#### *Transesophageal Echocardiogram*

A transesophageal echocardiogram (TEE) is similar to a TTE in its ability to obtain 2D, 3D, and Doppler images of the heart, but with one important difference: greater image quality. A TEE is performed by inserting a flexible probe that is tipped with a transducer into the esophagus and stomach. This positions the transducer directly behind the heart with very little tissue in between, so the image quality is much higher and allows for identification and measurement of small structures that may not be detected by TTE, such as valvular vegetations, thrombi, congenital defects, and aortic dissections, and can better define valvular function when TTE images are inadequate. Transesophageal echocardiograms require sedation as well as local anesthetic to the posterior pharynx to avoid stimulating the patient's gag reflex while the probe is inserted.

## STRESS TESTING

Stress testing refers to the process of evaluating the cardiovascular response to exercise. This can be done to look for evidence of cardiac pathology such as atherosclerotic cardiovascular disease (ASCVD), or to evaluate other parameters such as blood pressure response to exercise or the presence of arrhythmias, which may be induced by exercise. All stress testing involves inducing cardiovascular stress either with exercise or by pharmacological methods. Stress testing is most often performed to unmask cardiac ischemia in response to a reported patient symptom such as chest pain or pressure. A stress test is also frequently performed before surgery to determine whether underlying cardiac disease is present and stratify the risk of major adverse cardiac events.

#### *Treadmill Stress Electrocardiogram*

A treadmill stress ECG is a diagnostic test in which an ECG is performed during exercise. During the test, patients walk on a treadmill, and the intensity of exercise is gradually increased by adjusting the speed and incline of the treadmill at specified intervals. Heart rhythm, rate, and blood pressure are measured at regular intervals before, during, and after the test. During exercise, changes in the ECG such as T-wave inversions, ST-segment depression or elevation, or frequent premature ventricular contractions may be provoked, which indicate underlying myocardial ischemia.

#### *Stress Echocardiogram*

Stress echocardiography (echo) is another method of evaluating the cardiovascular response to stress. Stress echocardiograms are useful when a treadmill ECG is not sufficient to evaluate for ischemia because the patient cannot exercise, has a left bundle branch block, or the ECG is indeterminate and there is ongoing suspicion for ischemia. Exercise is performed on a treadmill, and once peak exertion is achieved, the patient is instructed to move to a table where a limited echocardiogram is performed. If a segment of the myocardium shows a reduced or absent ability to contract with exercise, this suggests that blood supply to that area of the heart is limited by an atherosclerotic plaque. If a patient is unable to exercise, external pacing or drugs such as dobutamine, dipyridamole, and adenosine can be infused to simulate stress. This test has high sensitivity (88%) and specificity (83%) for detection of coronary artery stenosis of greater than 50% of the luminal diameter.

## RED FLAGS IN HISTORY AND PHYSICAL EXAM

- Family history of premature ASCVD, sudden death, or bleeding disorders
- Chest pain suggestive of cardiac origin
- Unstable angina
- Calf pain or edema with a high likelihood of deep vein thrombosis (DVT)
- Sudden severe headache
- Dyspnea
- Hemoptysis
- Trauma to the chest, abdomen, or extremities
- Diaphoresis with reported chest pain, nausea/vomiting, left jaw/neck/arm pain
- Bleeding
- Tachycardia
- Bradycardia
- Pulselessness
- Sudden confusion
- Change in mental status
- Unilateral weakness
- Facial drooping
- Slurred speech
- Sudden trouble walking or seeing
- An extremity with color changes and a cool/cold temperature

## POPULATION HEALTH AND LIFE-SPAN CONSIDERATIONS

### INFANTS AND CHILDREN

- Many aspects of the physical exam in infants and children are the same as adults.
- Auscultation of heart sounds may indicate different disease processes in the pediatric population; however, they occur at the same landmarks and are described and classified in the same fashion.
- General appearance of the infant or child (happy or cranky), as well as nutritional and respiratory status, is very important in infants and children. Subtle changes in these systems can signal warning signs for congenital heart defects (CHD).
- Palpation of pulses is another very important exam technique in infants and children as differences in pulses between extremities can be indicative of a coarctation of the aorta, while bounding pulses may be indicative of a shunt lesion.
- Blood pressure evaluation in children is just as important as it is in adults and can help screen for heart diseases. Clinicians should be familiar with appropriate techniques for obtaining blood pressure as well as normative blood pressure ranges for infants and children by age.
- See Table 6.3 for an explanation of congenital fetal heart defects and common signs and symptoms found with these conditions.

**Table 6.3 Congenital Heart Defects**

| Congenital Heart Defect | Description | Exam Findings |
|---|---|---|
| Atrial septal defect | Opening between the right atrium and the left atrium, or the upper two chambers of the heart | ■ Young infants and children are often asymptomatic; infant with isolated ASD may present as symptomatic with signs of CHF<br>■ Older children may present with mild fatigue or dyspnea<br>■ Wide fixed split S2: hallmark finding<br>■ Systolic ejection murmur at the left parasternal area (midway between sternal border and midclavicular line); murmurs may be very soft in early childhood<br>■ Those with long-standing left to right shunting: left precordial bulge, and prominent RV impulse<br>■ Significant findings on chest x-ray, ECG, and TEE |
| Coarctation of the aorta | Defect of the aortic arch involving a narrowing of the arch; characterized as an obstructive lesion in which blood flow is diminished or nonexistent past the area of the obstruction; can present in varying degrees depending on the amount of narrowing | ■ Infants with critical obstruction to blood flow will present with acute symptoms of shock, metabolic acidosis, renal failure, and necrotizing enterocolitis; tachypnea and tachycardia; skin mottling, delayed capillary refill, and peripheral cyanosis<br>■ Older children or adults may present with systemic HTN and a systolic ejection murmur along the left sternal border.<br>■ Gallop rhythm common<br>■ Weak or absent femoral pulses<br>■ A delay between upper extremity and lower-extremity pulses will be appreciated<br>■ Significant findings on chest x-ray, ECG, and echo |
| Tetralogy of Fallot | Comprises four different defects: VSD, overriding aorta, PS, and RV hypertrophy; typically identified in utero | ■ "Tet spells": Deep blue skin, nails, and lips after crying or feeding<br>■ Murmur: Systolic ejection murmur at left lower sternal border with a single S2<br>■ Cyanosis: Varying degrees<br>■ Significant findings on chest x-ray, ECG, and echo |
| Ventricular septal defect | Opening between the right ventricle and the left ventricle; significance of defect depends on the size, location, and the amount of pulmonary and systemic vascular resistance encountered | Murmur is dependent on the size of defect:<br>● **Large defect:** May not have a significant murmur or may have a short systolic ejection murmur<br>● **Small defect:** Loud holosystolic murmur often recognized in early infancy<br>■ Significant findings on chest x-ray, ECG, and echo |

ASD, atrial septal defect; ECG, electrocardiogram; HTN, hypertension; PS, pulmonary stenosis; RV, right ventricle; TEE, transesophageal echocardiogram; VSD, ventricular septal defect

## OLDER ADULTS

- Arterial walls thicken and stiffen due to atherosclerotic changes, predisposing the older adults to isolated systolic HTN and widening pulse pressure.
- The myocardium loses elasticity and the walls of the atria and ventricles hypertrophy, decreasing cardiac reserve and ability to respond to stress and activity.
- Heart valves thicken, sclerose, and valve leaflets do not close efficiently. Resulting turbulent blood flow may produce murmurs, many benign.
- Age-related changes in the electrical system, including a decrease in pacemaker cells in the SA node, predisposing older adults to dysrhythmias.
- Clinically, cardiovascular disease may be difficult to detect and diagnose because it may be asymptomatic or present with vague, atypical symptoms in the older adult population.

## OTHER CONSIDERATIONS

### WOMEN

- Heart disease is the leading cause of death in women but typically develops 7–10 years later in women than in men.
- Women have smaller hearts and narrower blood vessels than their male counterparts which can lead to different pathophysiology and atypical symptoms of cardiac disease.
- Women are more likely to have cholesterol buildup in the heart's smallest blood vessels.
- The menopause transition is associated with a worsening cardiovascular risk profile.
- Women with a history of hypertension, gestational diabetes, pre-eclampsia, or eclampsia in pregnancy are at an increased risk for hypertension and premature atherosclerotic cardiovascular disease (ASCVD) in later life.
- Risk factors that are specific to cardiovascular disease in women include: endometriosis, high testosterone levels prior to menopause, increasing hypertension during menopause, autoimmune disease, stress/depression, and low-risk factor awareness.
- Women have more atypical heart attack symptoms including indigestion, shortness of breath, nausea, vomiting, diaphoresis, and/or pain in the neck, jaw, throat, back, or abdomen, sometimes in the absence of obvious chest discomfort.
- Under-recognition of heart disease in women leads to treatment delays and less aggressive preventive interventions.

### RACIAL/ETHNIC POPULATIONS

- Black Americans have the highest rates of cardiovascular disease with about 47% affected.
- Black Americans experience a nearly 30% higher death rate from cardiovascular disease and a 45% higher death rate from stroke compared with non-Hispanic White Americans.
- An earlier age of onset of obesity, hypertension, and diabetes mellitus is likely to contribute to the higher prevalence of cardiovascular disease (CVD) morbidity and mortality and to the lower life expectancy for Black Americans versus White Americans.

- Hypertension, in particular, is highly prevalent among Black Americans and contributes directly to the notable disparities in stroke, heart failure, and peripheral artery disease among Black Americans.
- Hispanic American adults are less likely to have ASCVD than non-Hispanic White American adults despite having higher rates of cardiovascular risk factors including obesity and diabetes mellitus. They also are less likely to die from heart disease than non-Hispanic White American adults.
- South Asian Americans have higher proportional mortality rates from ASCVD compared with other Asian American groups and non-Hispanic White Americans. This is in contrast to the finding that Asian Americans (Asian Indian, Chinese, Filipino, Japanese, Korean, and Vietnamese) as a group are at lower risk of ASCVD, largely because of the lower risk observed in East Asian populations.
- Acculturation, or the process by which foreign-born persons adopt the values, customs, and behaviors of their new environment, has generally been associated with the development of cardiovascular disease and unfavorable changes in cardiovascular risk factors and has been specifically noted among Chinese and Japanese Americans.
- Significant racial differences were seen in cardiac biomarkers, including lipids, adipokines, and biomarkers of endothelial function, inflammation, myocyte injury, and neurohormonal stress, which may contribute to racial differences in the development and complications of cardiovascular disease.

### GEOGRAPHICAL CONSIDERATIONS

- The stroke belt is described as an 11-state region with high stroke mortality across the southeastern United States. Stroke dead rates are 10% higher in Alabama, Arkansas, Georgia, Indiana, Kentucky, Louisiana, Mississippi, North Carolina, South Carolina, Tennessee, and Virginia than in other states.

## KEY DIFFERENTIALS

- Acute myocardial infarction
- Aortic regurgitation
- Aortic stenosis
- Arterial insufficiency
- Atherosclerotic cardiovascular disease
- Atrial fibrillation
- Atrial flutter
- Bundle branch block
- Cerebrovascular event
- Conduction block
- Congenital heart defects
- Congestive heart failure
- Deep vein thrombosis
- Hypertension
- Hypertrophic cardiomyopathy
- Intermittent claudication
- Long QT syndrome
- Mitral valve prolapse
- Mitral valve stenosis
- Pericarditis
- Pericardial tamponade
- Pulmonary emboli
- Sick sinus syndrome
- Supraventricular tachycardia
- Varicose veins
- Venous insufficiency
- Ventricular fibrillation
- Ventricular tachycardia
- Wolff–Parkinson–White syndrome

## KNOWLEDGE CHECK: CARDIOVASCULAR SYSTEM

1. Identify three of the leading modifiable risk factors for cardiovascular disease. (Select THREE.)

   **A.** Family history
   **B.** Hypertension
   **C.** Menopause
   **D.** Smoking
   **E.** Obesity

2. The most common arrhythmia resulting from valvular heart disease, as noted with the arrow in the following electrocardiogram, is:

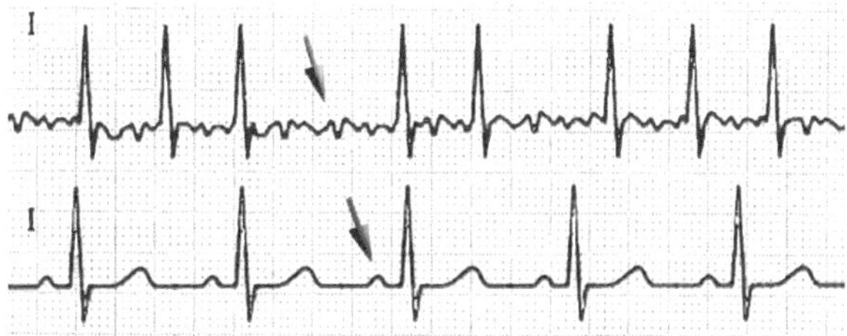


   **A.** Atrial fibrillation
   **B.** Paroxysmal supraventricular tachycardia
   **C.** Premature ventricular contractions
   **D.** Ventricular fibrillation

3. The QRS complex of the electrocardiogram represents:

   **A.** Atrial depolarization
   **B.** Atrial repolarization
   **C.** Ventricular depolarization
   **D.** Ventricular repolarization

4. Which murmurs are classified as systolic? (Select all that apply.)

   **A.** Aortic stenosis
   **B.** Aortic regurgitation
   **C.** Mitral valve prolapse
   **D.** Pulmonary stenosis

5. The diagnosis of heart failure is determined by:

   **A.** Cardiac catheterization
   **B.** Constellation of symptoms and signs
   **C.** Echocardiogram
   **D.** Edema and jugular venous distention

*(See answers next page.)*

**1. B, D, E) Hypertension; Smoking; Obesity**

Modifiable risk factors for cardiovascular disease include hypertension, diabetes, elevated cholesterol levels, smoking, and obesity. Non-modifiable risk factors include age, gender, family history, and race.

**2. A) Atrial fibrillation**

Atrial fibrillation is a rhythm in which the organized atrial activity is lost, causing the atria to quiver rather than contract; the ventricular rhythm becomes irregular and can at times become very fast. The correlation between atrial fibrillation and valvular heart disease is important to recognize, as these individuals require anticoagulation to prevent stroke. Paroxysmal supraventricular tachycardia is an arrhythmia that results in regular but rapid heart rate that starts and stops abruptly. Premature ventricular contractions can be related to structural heart disease, primarily heart failure and left ventricular hypertrophy. Ventricular fibrillation is an abnormal heart rhythm in which the ventricles quiver; the EKG depicts disorganized electrical activity.

**3. C) Ventricular depolarization**

The QRS complex represents the electrical impulse as it spreads through the ventricles and indicates ventricular depolarization; the QRS complex starts just before ventricular contraction. The T wave follows the QRS complex and indicates ventricular repolarization. Prior to the QRS complex, the P wave represents depolarization of the left and right atrium; the atria contract a split second after the P wave begins. Because it is so small, atrial repolarization is usually not visible on ECG.

**4. A, C, D) Aortic stenosis; mitral valve prolapse; pulmonary stenosis**

Timing of a murmur is key to accurate diagnosis. Stenosis of aortic or pulmonic valves results in a systolic murmur as blood is ejected through the narrowed orifice. Conversely, regurgitation of the same valves results in a diastolic murmur as blood flows backward through the diseased valve when ventricular pressures drop during relaxation. Regarding the mitral and tricuspid valves, stenosis results in a diastolic murmur and regurgitation and prolapse a systolic murmur.

**5. B) Constellation of symptoms and signs**

Heart failure is a clinical syndrome characterized by symptoms including dyspnea, orthopnea, and edema, and signs including elevated jugular venous pressure, pulmonary congestion, and reduced cardiac output. While labs and imaging are used to understand the functional classification of heart failure, no single lab, imaging, history, or physical exam finding is diagnostic. The constellation of signs and symptoms associated with heart failure guides classification and treatment.

6. A 70-year-old female presents to the clinic with heaviness in her lower legs. Her exam reveals 3+ pitting edema bilaterally; obesity; hyperpigmented, thickened skin; and healed ulcerations. Which additional finding would be consistent with her current assessment?

   **A.** Absent femoral pulses
   **B.** Dilated varicosities
   **C.** Limb-length discrepancies
   **D.** Stabbing pain with palpation

7. Adults who present for evaluation of elevated blood pressure MOST commonly presents with:

   **A.** Blurry vision
   **B.** Chronic headaches
   **C.** Fatigue
   **D.** No symptoms

8. The carotid pulse coincides with which of the following heart sounds?

   **A.** S1
   **B.** S2
   **C.** S3
   **D.** S4

9. Which term refers to a sound caused by turbulent blood flow?

   **A.** Bruit
   **B.** Thrill
   **C.** Friction rub
   **D.** Heave

10. Which statement is true regarding congenital heart disease?

    **A.** Acyanotic heart defects include hypoplastic left heart syndrome
    **B.** Defects like coarctation of the aorta may be present at birth but not be detected until adulthood
    **C.** Congenital heart defects always require surgery within the first year of life
    **D.** Nearly all congenital heart defects resolve spontaneously within the first few weeks of life

*(See answers next page.)*

**6. B) Dilated varicosities**

This presentation is consistent with chronic, venous insufficiency. Inspection and palpation would reveal evidence of venous disorders and prominent, dilated superficial venous abnormalities, such as telangiectasis and varicose veins. Absent femoral pulses are more likely to be assessed with arterial deficiencies or cardiac disorders. Sharp pain with palpation suggests neuralgia. Limb-length discrepancy is associated with degenerative and/or neoplastic disorders.

**7. D) No symptoms**

The vast majority of individuals with hypertension are asymptomatic, which often complicates timely diagnosis and treatment. Individuals with severe or uncontrolled hypertension may have headaches, dizziness, epistaxis, or palpitations; symptoms are often related to comorbidities or end-organ damage.

**8. A) S1**

S1 indicates the beginning of systole, is heard as a "lub," and can be auscultated with each pulsation of the carotid artery. S1, representative of the closure of the mitral and tricuspid valves (atrioventricular valves), is heard best at the apex. S2 indicates diastole, follows S1, and is heard as "dub." S2, indicating the closure of the aortic and pulmonic (semi-lunar) valves, is heard best at the base. S3 and S4 are abnormal or extra heart sounds heard in diastole. S2, S3, and S4 are auscultated after the carotid pulsation.

**9. A) Bruit**

A bruit is a vascular sound caused by turbulent blood flow and auscultated as a continuous murmur. These auscultatory sounds may be normal, innocent findings (e.g., a venous hum in a child) or may result from underlying pathology (e.g., a carotid artery bruit caused by atherosclerotic stenosis in an adult). A thrill is a vibratory sensation felt on the skin overlying an area of turbulent blood flow. Lifts or heaves are observable movements of the chest wall caused by forceful cardiac contractions; heaves can be slight or vigorous. Friction rubs are auscultated when two inflamed or roughened surfaces move against one another; pericardial friction rubs are auscultated with pericarditis, and pleural friction rubs are indicative of pleurisy.

**10. B) Defects like coarctation of the aorta may be present at birth but not be detected until adulthood**

Common acyanotic congenital heart defects may not be detected until adulthood. The most common symptom in adults is hypertension. Acyanotic heart defects include coarctation of the aorta, ventral and atrial septal defects, pulmonary and aortic stenosis, and patent ductus arteriosus. Cyanotic defects, on the other hand, cause hypoxia; these defects require surgery or some type of cardiac procedure within the first year of life. Hypoplastic left heart syndrome is one of the most severe, complex, and rare cyanotic heart defects.

# Respiratory System

## KEY HISTORY CONSIDERATIONS

- Acute versus chronic respiratory symptoms
- Sudden vs. insidious onset of respiratory symptoms
- Ability of the patient to speak in complete sentences
- Difficulty or decreased feeding in an infant/child
- Vaccination status
- Frequency of rescue inhaler use
- History of malignancy, immobility, surgery, emergency department visits
- History of allergic rhinitis and/or eczema
- Recent signs/symptoms or exposure to COVID-19
- Family history of pulmonary diseases or lung cancer
- Smoking history
- History of exposure to secondhand smoke
- Exposure to pollutants and/or environmental exposures

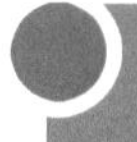

## PHYSICAL EXAMINATION: INSPECTION, PALPATION, PERCUSSION, AND AUSCULTATION

### INSPECTION

1. Observe the patient's overall appearance, posture, and position
2. Observe respiratory rate and effort, noting any signs of respiratory distress (Table 7.1)
3. Listen for audible wheezing or breath sounds (Table 7.2)
4. Inspect the face, neck, chest, and nails

**Table 7.1 Reference Ranges for Pediatric Respiratory Rate Based on Age**

| Age | Respirations per Minute |
|---|---|
| Infant (birth–1 year) | 30–60 |
| 1–3 years | 24–40 |
| 4–6 years | 22–34 |
| 6–12 years | 18–30 |
| 13–18 years | 12–16 |
| 18+ years | 12–20 |

*Source:* Data from Kleinman ME, Chameides L, Schexnayder SM, Samson RA, Hazinski MF, Atkins DL, Berg MD, de Caen AR, Fink EL, Freid EB, Hickey RW, Marino BS, Nadkarni VM, Proctor LT, Qureshi FA, Sartorelli K, Topjian A, van de Jagt EW, Zaritsky AL. Part 14: Pediatric Advanced Life Support: 2010 American Heart Association Guidelines for Cardiopulmonary Resuscitation and Emergency Cardiovascular Care. Circulation. 2010 Nov 2; 122(18 Suppl 3):S876–908.

**Table 7.2 Normal Breath Sounds**

| Breath Sound | Description | Inspiratory:Expiratory Ratio | Depiction |
|---|---|---|---|
| **Tracheal** | Tracheal breath sounds are the loudest and high pitched, usually heard over the upper aspect of the trachea and best heard on the anterior aspect of the neck | The duration of inspiration almost equals expiratory duration with an inspiratory:expiratory (I:E) ratio of 1:1 | Λ |
| **Bronchial** | Bronchial breath sounds are louder and higher in pitch and are usually heard over the lower aspect of the trachea and best heard over the manubrium | The duration of inspiration is shorter than expiration with an I:E ratio of 1:2 or 1:3 | ⌃ |
| **Bronchovesicular** | Bronchovesicular breath sounds are of intermediate intensity and pitch, and are usually heard over the major bronchi in the mid-chest area anteriorly or between the scapulae posteriorly | The duration of inspiration almost equals expiration with an I:E ratio of 1:1 | ^ |
| **Vesicular** | Vesicular breath sounds are of soft intensity, low pitched, with a rustling quality during inspiration and softer with expiration. They are usually heard bilaterally over most of the peripheral fields | The duration of inspiration is longer than expiration with an I:E ratio or 3:1 | ⌃ |

From Gawlik, K., Melnyk, B.& Teall, A. (2020). *Evidence-Based Physical Examination: Best Practices for Health and Well-being Assessment.* (1st Ed.). Springer Publishing LLC: New York, NY. ISBN: 978-0-8261-6453-7.

## INSPECTION: ABNORMAL FINDINGS

- **Color changes:** Skin may appear gray or pale if the patient is not getting enough oxygen. A bluish discoloration around the mouth or pallor on the inside of the lips or on the fingernails also indicate lack of sufficient oxygenation and/or respiratory distress.
- **Tripoding:** A body position when a patient is sitting or standing while leaning forward and supporting the upper body with the hands on the knees.
- **Pursed lips:** Lips flare out during expiration. This is a technique used to release trapped air in the lungs, keep the airways open longer, relieve shortness of breath, and prolong exhalation to slow the rate of breathing. This is a learned mechanism when the patient is experiencing increased expiratory effort.
- **Accessory muscle use:** Contraction of muscles other than the diaphragm during inspiration, usually the sternocleidomastoid and scalene muscles.
- **Nasal flaring:** Enlargement of the nasal openings during inspiration. This is more common in children than adults.

- **Grunting:** Short, repetitive grunt-like sounds expelled with each breath. This mechanism increases lung volume and alveolar pressure and slows expiratory flow. It is typically a sign of moderate to severe respiratory distress.
- **Paradoxical respiration (seesaw breathing):** Inward movement of the abdominal muscles during inspiration. Normally, the abdomen moves outward during inspiration as the diaphragm contracts and descends. If the diaphragm is weak or fatigued, it is pulled into the chest in inspiration and pulls the abdomen in with it.
- **Retractions:** The pulling or sucking in of soft tissue during inhalation, signifying that the individual is working hard to breathe due to increased airway resistance that is caused by slow filling of the lungs. The negative pleural pressure generated in inspiration pulls the soft tissue or intercostal muscles inward.
  - **Supraclavicular:** Occurs above the clavicles or above the sternal notch.
  - **Intercostal:** Occurs in the intercostal muscles, seen between each rib.
  - **Suprasternal:** Occurs above the sternum.
  - **Subcostal:** Occurs at or below the costal margins.
- **Head bobbing:** Extension of the head and neck during inspiration and falling forward of the head during exhalation, appearance that the head is moving up and down.
- **Chest/abdominal expansion:** Asymmetrical or no chest movement
- **$O_2$ saturation:** Less than 94% on room air or less than 90% at any time would be concerning.
- **Clubbed fingernails:** Characterized by enlarged fingertips and a loss of the normal angle at the nail bed due to chronically tissue hypoxia.
- **Audible breath sounds:** Crepitus, stridor, or wheezing noted while breathing is abnormal. Expiratory stridor alone suggests obstruction of a lower airway, as with an aspirated foreign body.
- **Chest movement with breathing:** Asymmetrical movement or any unilateral/bilateral bulging would be abnormal.
- **Chest abnormalities:** The presence of any skin lesions, masses, or discolorations; bruising may be noted over a fractured rib. Some common variations are as follows:
  - **Barrel chest:** The thoracic cage is described as a barrel chest when the anteroposterior (AP) diameter is equal to or greater than the lateral (transverse) diameter, or 1:1. Some rounding of the rib cage can be noted in aging adults or those with arthritis. However, hyperinflation of the lungs and an increasing stiffness of the respiratory muscles associated with chronic obstructive pulmonary disease leads to the barrel chest appearance.
  - **Pectus excavatum:** When the anterior chest wall is depressed with a low-lying sternum, it is called "pectus excavatum" or "sunken/funnel chest." The depression may be more noticeable on inspiration. This defect is usually congenital and asymptomatic. If the depression of the sternum is significant, then the reduction in lung volume and compression of the heart and great vessels may cause murmurs, palpitations, decreased exercise tolerance, and/or fatigue.
  - **Pectus carinatum:** When the sternum is displaced anteriorly and protrudes outward abnormally, it is called "pigeon's chest" or "pectus carinatum." With this less common chest wall deformity, the AP diameter will be increased. Individuals with pectus carinatum may have associated scoliosis, asthma, mitral valve prolapse, and connective tissue disorders affecting heart valves.

- **Flail chest:** When three or more ribs fracture in multiple places and a segment of the fractured ribs gets detached from the rest of the thoracic cage, the condition is known as "flail chest." A late sign of this life-threatening condition is when the detached segment is in paradoxical motion with the rest of the thoracic cage; a segment is in paradoxical motion when the segment is pulled into the thoracic cage with inspiration and pushed out during expiration, which is the opposite of normal thoracic cage mechanics. Patients with flail chest experience chest pain and shortness of breath.

- Variations of the vertebral column include scoliosis, kyphosis, and lordosis.
  - **Scoliosis:** Abnormal lateral curvature of the vertebral column.
  - **Kyphosis**: Excessive curvature of the upper thoracic vertebral column resulting in an exaggerated rounding of the back.
  - **Lordosis**: Excessive curvature of the lumbar vertebral column.
- Abnormal patterns of breathing (Table 7.3)

**Table 7.3 Abnormal Patterns of Breathing**

| Variation | Description | Depiction |
|---|---|---|
| Tachypnea | Abnormally increased respiratory rate associated with shallow breaths. Patient may describe sensations of shortness of breath. Typically noted in patients with hypoxemia, hypercapnia, and fever in whom the body is compensating to maintain homeostasis. Pathological causes include pneumonia, heart failure, central nervous system abnormalities such as tumors, and salicylate intoxication | 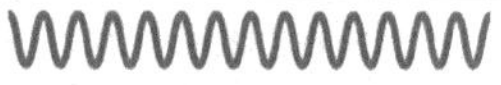 |
| Hyperpnea | An increased rate and depth of breathing that is commonly associated with an increase in metabolic demand resulting from exercise, high altitude, or anemia. Also noted in patients with severe metabolic acidosis related to diabetic ketoacidosis or renal failure. The hyperpnea associated with diabetic ketoacidosis is called "Kussmaul's respiration" | 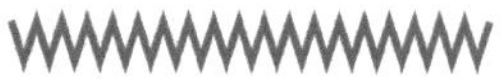 |
| Bradypnea | Abnormally slow respiratory rate that might affect alveolar ventilation. Etiology includes drug-induced respiratory depression, hypothyroidism, and neurologic conditions such as increased intracranial pressure or neuromuscular diseases such as Guillain-Barré syndrome or amyotrophic lateral sclerosis. In the United States, opioids are the primary cause of drug-induced respiratory depression and needs to be considered during history taking | 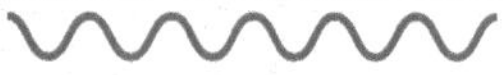 |
| Sighing Respiration | Normal reaction to mild emotional states or fatigue and typically nonpathological. Respiratory rate will be normal, but certain breaths will be deeper, leading to hyperventilation during those breaths | 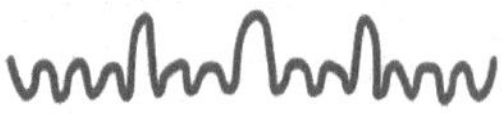 |
| Cheyne-Stokes Breathing | Abnormal breathing pattern where there are periods of progressively deeper breaths (crescendo–decrescendo) followed by periods of no breathing. Cheyne-Stokes breathing is commonly seen in patients who are in the final stages of dying. It can also be seen in patients with congestive heart failure, traumatic brain injury, carbon monoxide poisoning, hyponatremia, and medication overdoses (morphine) | 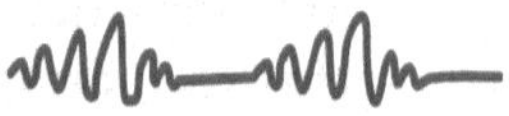 |

| Variation | Description | Depiction |
|---|---|---|
| Biot's Breathing | Regular deep respirations alternating with periods of no breathing due to damage to the pons caused by cerebrovascular accident, trauma, meningitis, or brain herniation | |
| Agonal | Occasional reflex-driven gasps, associated with anoxia, cardiac arrest, cerebral ischemia, or hypoxia | |
| Apnea | Absence of breathing that signals a life-threatening situation resulting in death if no intervention is carried out immediately | |

## PALPATION

1. Using the palmar surface of the hands, palpate the posterior and anterior chest wall.
2. Palpate for the position of the trachea. Using the index finger and thumb, palpate along the upper edges of each clavicle and up to the inner borders of the sternocleidomastoid muscles, above the suprasternal notch. It should be positioned in the midline, but a small deviation to the right side is considered a normal finding.
3. Palpate the spine, ribs, and costochondral cartilage.
   a. **Thoracic expansion or chest excursion:** Palpate the posterior thorax for symmetric chest expansion during respiration. With the patient sitting upright or standing with arms at the sides, place hands on the posterior chest wall, one on each side of the thorax near the level of the diaphragm, palms facing anteriorly with thumbs touching at the midline. Ask the patient to take a deep breath in, and then exhale. During inspiration, thumbs should separate, and each hand should rotate away from the midline equally.
   b. **Tactile fremitus:** Place either the ulnar surface of the hands or the palmar surface of the hands on posterior chest wall. This should be repeated on the anterior chest wall. Tactile fremitus should be symmetric.

### PALPATION: ABNORMAL FINDINGS

- Any tenderness, depressions, masses, deformities, or crepitus discovered during palpation of the chest is abnormal. Crepitus is the presence of air in the subcutaneous tissues, which can occur after chest injury, invasive procedures, or surgery; crepitus can be both felt and heard as crinkling, a sensation often associated with "bubble wrap." Note that chest wall tenderness may be associated with inflamed pleura or costochondritis.
- Focal tenderness or bruising over the spine is abnormal.
- **Tracheal deviation:** Trachea is significantly deviated from the midline. This can occur due to tumors/masses, pneumothorax, pleural effusion, pneumonectomy, pleural fibrosis, atelectasis, or kyphoscoliosis.
- **Decreased excursion of the chest:** Asymmetric and/or limited chest excursion is abnormal. Limited movement is associated with poor diaphragmatic excursion and hyperinflation, changes that occur with chronic obstructive pulmonary disease or neuromuscular disease. Asymmetric chest wall expansion is suggestive of unilateral lung pathology such as chronic fibrosis, lobar pneumonia, consolidation, or bronchial obstruction. Asymmetry can also be caused by pleural pathology or paralysis of one side of the diaphragm.

- **Decreased tactile fremitus:** Occurs due to respiratory system pathology that causes trapping of air in the lungs, which decreases the transmission of vocal and tactile fremitus; common causes include pneumothorax, emphysema, and asthma. Decreased fremitus can also be caused by thickened or scarred pleura, significant pleural edema or pleural effusion, or a tumor causing bronchial obstruction.
- Increased fremitus occurs with compression or consolidation of lung tissue and occurs only when the bronchus is patent and substantial consolidation extends towards the lung surfaces; examples include the presence of a tumor or pneumonia, as these conditions increase tissue density.
- Increased or decreased tactile fremitus is a finding that is understood to be a component of a constellation of signs and symptoms indicating respiratory disorders and is not solely diagnostic of pathology, as its sensitivity and specificity are limited.

## PERCUSSION

1. Percuss the chest posteriorly, comparing the right and left side from the apices to the interscapular areas to the bases. The technique of indirect percussion is done by placing the pleximeter (nonstriking) finger of the non-dominant hand on the chest wall firmly, while the remaining fingers are lifted slightly off the chest wall to avoid dampening the sound. The clinician then uses a quick, sharp wrist motion to strike the pressed finger at the midpoint between the proximal and distal interphalangeal joints with a plexor finger of the dominant hand to produce a sound.
2. Percuss the spine and the costovertebral angles, observing for focal tenderness.

### PERCUSSION: ABNORMAL FINDINGS

Resultant percussion sounds can be resonant, hyperresonant, dull, flat, or tympanic:

- Resonance is the hollow sound typically heard over normal lung tissue that is filled with air. This percussion sound is considered to be relatively loud with a low pitch.
- Hyperresonance is a very loud sound, lower in pitch and longer in duration than resonance. This sound is normally heard when percussing the chest wall of children or very thin adult patients. Hyperresonance also occurs when lungs are overinflated with air because of asthma or chronic obstructive pulmonary disease.
- Dullness is the sound heard when percussing over a dense area or solid organ, such as the heart or liver. The sound is of medium intensity, pitch, and duration. Dullness over lung tissue is an abnormal finding related to fluid or consolidation associated with pneumonia, masses or tumors, pleural effusions, hemothorax, or empyema.
- Flatness is lower than normal percussion sounds, soft in intensity but high in pitch and of short duration. Flatness is percussed normally over solid areas such as bones. Fluid in the pleural space from an effusion would result in flatness when percussed.
- Tympany is a loud and high-pitched drum-like sound that can be heard for a longer duration. Tympanic sounds are normal when percussed across the abdomen, and abnormal with percussion of the chest wall. Tympanic sounds can result from excessive air in the chest caused by a pneumothorax (collapsed lung).

# AUSCULTATION

1. Auscultate the chest using the diaphragm of the stethoscope placed firmly on bare skin, comparing left to right at each level (Figure 7.1):
   a. Posteriorly, from the apex to the interscapular area to the base
   b. Laterally, in the midaxillary line
   c. Anteriorly, over the upper lobes and right middle lobe

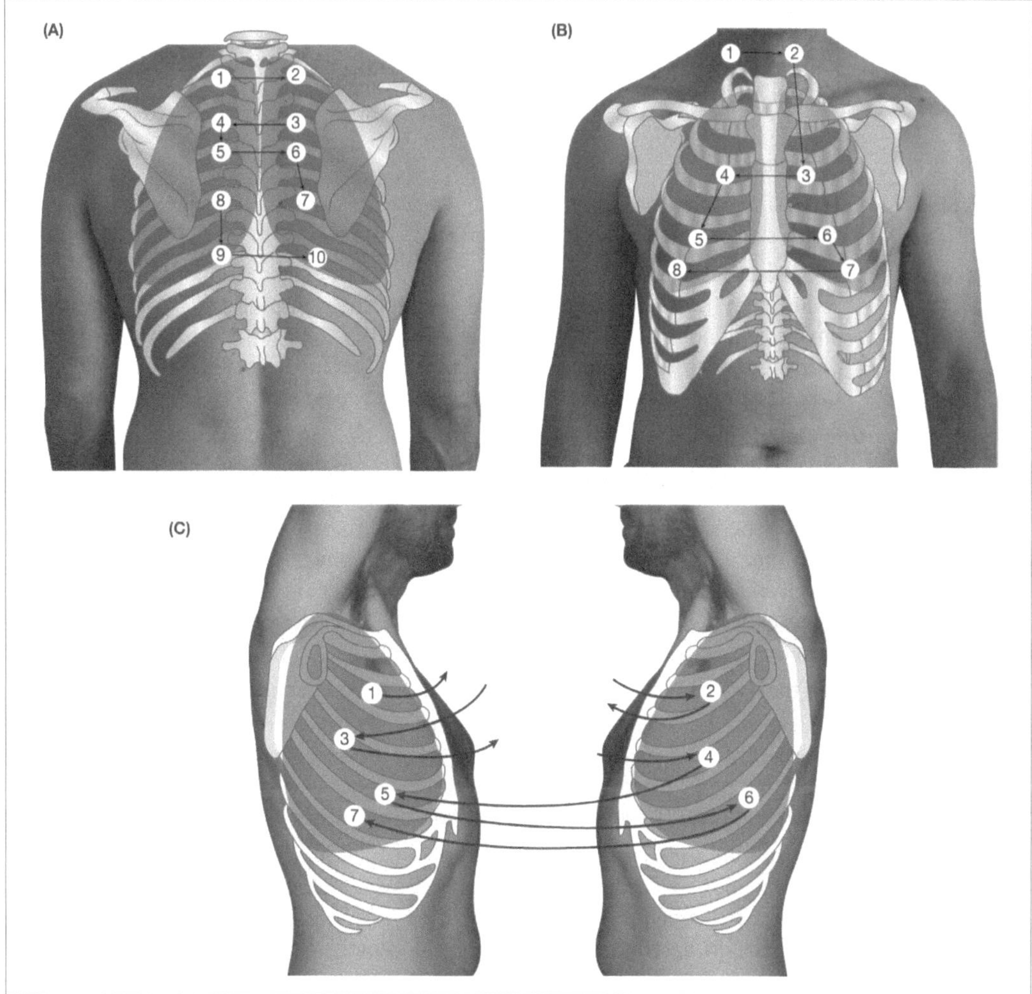


**Figure 7.1** Landmarks for auscultation of lung fields: (A) Anterior. (B) Posterior. (C) Lateral.

## SPECIAL TESTS DURING AUSCULTATION

- **Bronchophony:** Ask the patient to say "ninety-nine" while listening with the stethoscope. Normally, the sound of "ninety-nine" will sound very faint and muffled. If the voice sounds become clear and distinct, bronchophony is present. This occurs because sound transmits better through dense consolidation than through air.
- **Egophony:** Ask the patient to repeatedly say the sound "ee" while listening with the stethoscope. Normally, it will sound muffled but unchanged. If the sound changes to "aaay" while the patient is saying "ee," then egophony is present. This indicates the

presence of consolidation or fluid in the lungs. The "aaay" sound will also be louder in the presence of consolidated tissue.

- **Whispered pectoriloquy:** For the whispered pectoriloquy test, ask the patient to whisper a few numbers or a short phrase and continue to repeat it. For example, "1, 2, 3, 1, 2, 3, 1, 2, 3..." Auscultate while the patient is whispering. Normally, the whispered voice will be distant, muffled, and not intelligible. If there is consolidation in an area of the lung, the whispered voice will sound unusually clear and loud.

## AUSCULTATION: ABNORMAL FINDINGS (TABLE 7.4)

**Table 7.4 Abnormal Breath Sounds**

| Breath Sound | Description |
|---|---|
| **Bronchial** | Bronchial breath sounds are a normal finding unless they are heard peripherally, which suggests underlying consolidation. |
| **Crackles** | Crackles are classified as fine or coarse. Fine crackles are discontinuous high-pitched sounds that have a popping quality; these are usually inspiratory. Coarse crackles are discontinuous LOW pitched louder and longer. Crackles indicate abnormalities of the lungs or airways, such as pneumonia, congestive heart failure, or bronchitis. Crackles are heard as air is passing through fluid-filled airways. |
| **Wheezes** | Wheezes are continuous musical sounds that can be high or low pitched. Wheezing is usually heard during expiration but may be heard during both inspiration and expiration. High-pitched wheezes sound squeaky while low-pitched wheezes have a moaning quality. Wheezes are heard due to narrowing of the airways due to asthma, COPD, or bronchitis. The tone of the wheeze varies depending on which area of the airways are affected. If the smaller airways are narrow, then the wheezes are musical in nature (polyphonic) and if the larger airways are narrow, then the wheeze sounds hoarse (monophonic). |
| **Rhonchi** | When the larger airways are obstructed with secretions, continuous low-pitched rattling sounds, called "rhonchi," are heard. The rattling sounds may mimic snoring. The unique feature of rhonchi is that it clears with coughing or suctioning. Rhonchi is heard when pulmonary processes produce increased secretions, e.g., pneumonia, COPD, bronchiectasis, chronic bronchitis, or cystic fibrosis. |
| **Stridor** | Stridor is a loud and high-pitched sound caused by disrupted airflow. These abnormal breath sounds are produced typically during inspiration and associated with upper airway obstruction (above the thoracic cavity). When air cannot flow through the larynx, the disrupted airway creates the loud sounds. Upper airway obstruction can be caused by swelling-associated infection (croup, epiglottitis), chemical irritation (aspiration), or trauma (mechanical ventilation). Expiratory stridor may be present if the upper airway is blocked and air cannot escape through the trachea or upper airways. In rare situation, biphasic stridor may be heard when air cannot enter or leave the upper airways as subglottic stenosis due to granulation tissue. Stridor may indicate impending respiratory distress and/or failure. |
| **Pleural Rubs** | A pleural rub sound is the creaking or grating sound that can be heard during both inspiration and expiration as result of friction (lack of lubrication or irritation) between the pleura. The sounds can be described to that of two pieces of leather rubbing together. Pleurisy, an inflammation of the pleura, can cause pleural rubs. The pleural rub sound may not stop with coughing but will stop when the patient holds his/her breath. If the friction rub does not stop when the patient holds the breath, the etiology of the rub is more likely pericardial in nature. |

**Table 7.4 Abnormal Breath Sounds (*continued*)**

| Breath Sound | Description |
|---|---|
| **Diminished** | Diminished vesicular breath sounds may be heard in patients who are frail or elderly, and having shallow breathing. They might also be diminished in individuals who are obese or very muscular in whom the tissues impede the quality of the breath sounds. Obstruction related to a foreign body or thick secretions can generally decrease breath sounds, which are different than absent breath sounds. When minimal air is moving in or out of either lung, this is a worrisome sign, known as "silent chest," which signals the likelihood of severe hypoxia, respiratory distress, and/or respiratory failure. Absent breath sounds occurring on only one side of the chest can indicate pneumothorax, or a collapsed lung, which is also an emergency situation. |

From Gawlik, K., Melnyk, B.& Teall, A. (2020). *Evidence-Based Physical Examination: Best Practices for Health and Well-being Assessment.* (1st Ed.). Springer Publishing LLC: New York, NY. ISBN: 978-0-8261-6453-7.

## PULMONARY FUNCTION TESTS (SPIROMETRY)

- Spirometry is testing designed to detect the volume and capacity of the lungs to determine overall functioning of the respiratory system. Spirometry, or pulmonary function tests, identify lung volumes by direct measurement. Lung capacities are calculated using two or more measures of volume. The key volumes and capacities include:
  - **Tidal Volume:** Amount of air displaced at rest between normal inhalation and exhalation.
  - **Residual Volume:** Amount of air that remains in the lungs after a full exhalation.
  - **Inspiratory Reserve Volume:** Amount of air that can be inhaled after a normal inhalation.
  - **Expiratory Reserve Volume:** Amount of air that can be exhaled after a normal exhalation.
  - **Inspiratory Capacity:** Amount of air that can be inhaled after a normal exhalation. Inspiratory capacity is the sum of tidal volume and inspiratory reserve volume.
  - **Functional Residual Capacity:** Amount of additional air that can be exhaled after a normal exhalation. Functional residual capacity is the sum of expiratory reserve volume and the residual volume.
  - **Vital Capacity:** Maximum amount of air that can be inhaled or exhaled during one respiratory cycle. Vital capacity is the sum of tidal volume, inspiratory reserve volume and expiratory reserve volume.
  - **Total Lung Capacity:** Total amount of air that remains in the lungs after a maximal inhalation (Molnar and Gair, 2015).
- Additional measures taken during spirometry include the forced expiratory volume (FEV), which assesses how much air can be forced out of the lungs over a specific period, usually one second (FEV1), and the forced vital capacity (FVC), which is the total amount of air that can be forcibly exhaled (Molnar and Gair, 2015). These measures are significant because the ratio of these values (FEV1/FVC) is used to diagnose lung diseases including asthma and chronic obstructive pulmonary disease. If the FEV1/FVC ratio is high, this indicates that an individual was able to exhale most of their lung volume and/or that their forced capacity was low, which happens in pulmonary fibrotic disorders or restrictive diseases that create noncompliant lung tissue.

Conversely, when the FEV1/FVC ratio is low, there is resistance in the lung that is characteristic of obstructive diseases which cause individuals to have difficulty moving air out of their lungs; this is reflected in less exhalation volume in one second, and a much longer time needed to reach the maximal exhalation volume (Molnar and Gair, 2015).

- The air flow measurements taken during pulmonary function tests/spirometry are depicted in flow volume loops or spirograms as illustrated in Figure 7.2; the

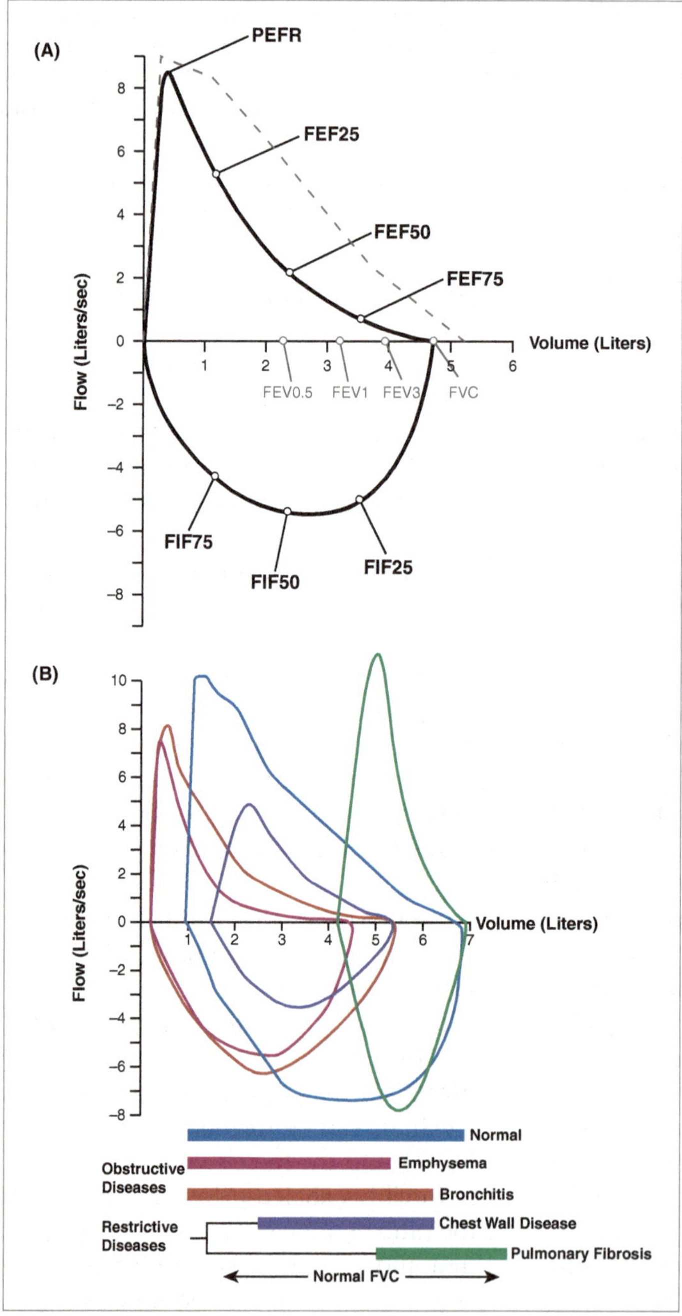


**Figure 7.2** Normal (A) and abnormal (B) flow volume loops with pulmonary function tests.

measures included in these specific spirograms include forced inspiratory flow (FIF) and forced expiratory flow (FEF) to compare expected and abnormal findings. Flow volume loops indicate normal lung function, obstructive disease, or restrictive disease. While pulmonary function tests include measures of peak flow, the additional measures to determine lung volume and capacity that are included in spirometry make it a reliable, effective, powerful tool to diagnose and treat pulmonary disorders.

# RED FLAGS IN HISTORY AND PHYSICAL EXAM (BOX 7.1)

- Shortness of breath
- Difficulty breathing
- Breathlessness
- Left chest, arm, neck, or jaw pain
- Tachypnea
- Retractions
- Skin color changes
- Wheezing
- Confusion
- Hemoptysis
- Drooling and/or any swelling of the lips or throat

**Box 7.1 Red Flags in Subjective History That Indicate Risk for Pulmonary Embolus**

- Sudden onset of pleuritic chest pain
- Breathlessness
- Dizziness or syncope
- Recent long-distance travel
- Prolonged immobility
- History of trauma to lower extremities or pelvis surgery in the last 3 months
- Previous deep vein thrombosis, emboli, malignancy
- Comorbid heart failure or chronic lung disease
- Pregnancy
- Use of hormonal contraception
- History of smoking and/or vaping

# POPULATION HEALTH AND LIFE-SPAN CONSIDERATIONS

## INFANTS AND CHILDREN

- Infants and children have shorter airways, which means that upper airway sounds are frequently transmitted to lower airways making the respiratory assessment more challenging.

- The respiratory rate of infants can vary with temperature, activity, feeding, and even with sleep. When calculating respiratory rate, be sure to count for a full minute to calculate the normal respiratory rate because of these variations.
- Infants are obligate nose breathers and so any congestion can greatly affect their respiratory effort, evident by fussiness or decreased feedings. Nose breathing can also contribute to difficulties in the respiratory assessment due to transmitted airway sounds.
- In infants, it is normal to find them sneezing or hiccupping; however, stridor, grunting, or periodic spasms of coughing may indicate distress.
- Due to a thin chest wall, children's breath sounds may sound louder, harsher, and more bronchial than an adult.

## OLDER ADULTS

- As a person becomes older, the amount of mucus produced throughout the body decreases and this can be evident with dry mucus membranes in the nares, throat, and in the respiratory tract.
- Because of changes in the respiratory system of the older adult, expect to find an increased anteroposterior diameter of the chest wall, and slight hyperresonance of the lungs fields with percussion.
- There is also a decreased amount of chest expansion and more reliance on the diaphragm for breathing. This can be due to muscle weakness, calcification of the rib articulations, general physical disability, or a sedentary lifestyle.
- Older adults with pneumonia are more likely to present with atypical symptoms. Typical symptoms of pneumonia are fever, cough, chest pain, headache, muscle pain, and dyspnea. However, the older adults may present with altered mental status, decreased alertness, or acute confusion, and may complain of poor appetite, fatigue, and/or have had recent falls.

## OTHER CONSIDERATIONS

- The mucosa of dark-skinned individuals can appear gray with central cyanosis. Cyanosis on the skin may be difficult to detect, but it may be appreciated on the membranes around the lips, gums, and nail beds. These areas may have a purple appearance instead of the blue appearance seen in Caucasians. The skin around the eyes might also acquire a bluish or purplish tinge.
- Obesity causes substantial changes to the mechanics of the lungs and chest wall due to the presence of adipose tissue around the rib cage, abdomen, and visceral cavity. This reduces the patient's functional residual capacity and expiratory reserve volume. These mechanical changes cause asthma and asthma-like symptoms such as dyspnea, wheezing, and airway hyperresponsiveness.

## KEY DIFFERENTIALS

- Chronic obstructive pulmonary disease
- Pneumonia
- Pulmonary emboli
- COVID-19
- Bronchitis
- Bronchiolitis
- Pneumothorax
- Lung cancer
- Tuberculosis
- Asthma
- Cystic fibrosis
- Influenza
- Pertussis
- Post-viral cough (sometimes termed post infectious cough)
- Upper respiratory infection
- Postnasal drip
- Congestive heart failure
- Medication side effect
- Nicotine addiction

## REFERENCE

Molnar, C., & Gair, J. (2015). *Concepts of biology* (1st Canadian ed.). Victoria, BC, Canada: BC campus. Retrieved from https://opentextbc.ca/biology.

## KNOWLEDGE CHECK: RESPIRATORY SYSTEM

**1.** Which term BEST describes the low-pitched breath sounds usually auscultated over peripheral lung fields bilaterally in adults?

**A.** Bronchial
**B.** Bronchovesicular
**C.** Tracheal
**D.** Vesicular

**2.** Which objective findings are indicative of acute respiratory distress in an older adult? (Select all that apply.)

**A.** Confusion
**B.** Eupnea
**C.** Retractions
**D.** Sleep apnea
**E.** Tachypnea

**3.** A 40-year-old presents with productive cough after initially having "cold symptoms." The individual denies anosmia, headache, GI symptoms, or dyspnea, and is a non-smoker. Their objective exam reveals no changes in vital signs and a few, scattered, expiratory wheezes to auscultation bilaterally. Which statement is true regarding the diagnosis of bronchitis for this individual?

**A.** Bronchitis is usually bacterial in origin and is likely to cause pneumonia
**B.** Bronchitis is usually viral and is diagnosed from history and physical exam
**C.** The diagnosis requires chest x-ray and sputum cultures for accuracy
**D.** The diagnosis requires pulmonary function tests for accuracy

**4.** Parents have concern for their 3-month-old, who has had 2 days of upper respiratory infection symptoms, a decrease in appetite, tachypnea, low-grade fever, and occasional expiratory wheezing. The MOST LIKELY diagnosis for this infant is:

**A.** Aspiration pneumonia
**B.** Bacterial pneumonia
**C.** Bronchiolitis
**D.** Bronchitis

**5.** Which history findings are risk factors for pulmonary embolus? (Select all that apply.)

**A.** Currently pregnant
**B.** Chronic lung disease
**C.** Underweight
**D.** Use of e-cigarettes
**E.** Wrist fracture in childhood

*(See answers next page.)*

**1. D) Vesicular**

Vesicular breath sounds are soft in intensity, low-pitched, and normally heard over peripheral fields bilaterally. Tracheal breath sounds are loud, high-pitched, and heard over the upper aspect of the trachea and anterior aspect of the neck. Bronchial breath sounds are also louder and higher in pitch, auscultated over the lower aspect of the trachea and the manubrium. Bronchovesicular breath sounds are of intermediate intensity and pitch and are usually heard over the major bronchi in the mid-chest area anteriorly or between the scapulae posteriorly.

**2. A, C, E) Confusion, Retractions, Tachypnea**

Objective findings that indicate acute respiratory distress in older adults include confusion, tachypnea, hypotension, cyanosis or color change, inadequate chest rise, and suprasternal, substernal, or intercostal chest wall retractions. Eupnea is a term for normal respirations. Sleep apnea can predispose older adults to respiratory distress; however, it is not an indication of acute distress.

**3. D) The diagnosis requires pulmonary function tests for accuracy**

Acute bronchitis is a lower respiratory tract infection most often viral in origin; symptoms include productive, persistent cough after initial symptoms of the common cold. The diagnosis of bronchitis is made from history and physical exam. An immune-competent adult under the age of 65 with normal vital signs and without significant changes in their lung exam is not likely to have pneumonia. The individual in this case had no additional symptoms of COVID-19 (e.g., new loss of smell (anosmia), headache, fever, dyspnea, or GI symptoms) and no indication of risk for lung cancers.

**4. C) Bronchiolitis**

Bronchiolitis is an acute viral infection that is common in infants and young children. History includes prodromal viral upper respiratory tract infection (URI) symptoms, followed by increased respiratory effort, wheezing, and cough. Bronchitis, also viral in nature, affects the larger airways and is more common in older children and adults. While pneumonia can result from aspiration and/or bacterium, most commonly pneumonias are viral in nature, and cause cough and high-fever or low body temperatures in infants.

**5. A, B, D) Currently pregnant, chronic lung disease, use of e-cigarettes**

Pulmonary emboli are primarily a complication of thrombosis in the deep venous system of the lower extremities. Causes are multifactorial; patients who are predisposed include those who are pregnant, have comorbid heart or lung disease, and/or are smokers. Obesity, not being underweight, is a risk factor. While surgery, trauma, and immobilization are risk factors, those risks persist for three months and are not lifetime risks. Additional risk factors include use of combined oral contraception, malignancy, and inherited clotting disorders.

6. Hyperresonance to percussion of the chest wall of an adult can indicate:

   **A.** Chronic obstructive pulmonary disease
   **B.** Community-acquired pneumonia
   **C.** Lung tumor suggestive of cancer
   **D.** Pleural effusion

7. Which three assessments are components of a constellation of signs and symptoms that indicate lobar pneumonia? (Select THREE.)

   **A.** Anosmia
   **B.** Bradypnea
   **C.** Crackles to auscultation
   **D.** Egophony (E to A changes)
   **E.** Increased tactile fremitus

8. A 4-year-old presents to the emergency department with acute onset of high fever, difficulty swallowing, hoarseness, and sore throat. The child has respiratory stridor, no cough, and copious oral secretions. The advanced practice nurse should suspect:

   **A.** Aspiration pneumonia
   **B.** Asthma
   **C.** Epiglottitis
   **D.** Viral tonsillitis

9. The bacterium responsible for the highest mortality in adults with community-acquired pneumonia is:

   **A.** *Chlamydia pneumoniae*
   **B.** *Mycoplasma pneumoniae*
   **C.** *Respiratory syncytial virus*
   **D.** *Streptococcus pneumoniae*

10. Which statement BEST defines asthma?

    **A.** Chronic obstruction of airflow causing daily symptoms that worsen over time
    **B.** Chronic airway inflammation worsened by acute bronchospasm in response to triggers
    **C.** Mucociliary dysfunction caused by genetic susceptibility causes increased risk of infection
    **D.** Relatively fixed airway constriction as a result of air trapping, smoking, and infection

*(See answers next page.)*

**6. A) Chronic obstructive pulmonary disease**

Hyperresonance is a very loud sound that is slightly lower in pitch and longer in duration compared to resonance. It can be heard when percussing the chest wall of children or very thin adult patients. It can also be appreciated when the lungs are overinflated with air as a result of asthma, or COPD. When pneumonia, a lung tumor, or pleural effusion are present, the lung fields are more likely to have consolidation; dullness to percussion is noted with abnormalities that cause consolidation within lung fields.

**7. C, D, E) Crackles to auscultation, egophony (E to A changes), increased tactile fremitus**

Lobar pneumonia is consolidation that involves an entire lobe of the lung, resulting from alveolar fluid accumulation, infiltration, and exudate. Physical findings include crackles and rales to auscultation, increased tactile fremitus to palpation, dullness to percussion, and abnormalities in transmitted voice sounds. Positive bronchophony, egophony, and whispered pectoriloquy can indicate consolidation in an area of the lung and are part of a constellation of signs and symptoms that indicate lobar pneumonia, including tachypnea, fever, cough, and dyspnea. Anosmia, loss of smell, is a neurological symptom that is an early indicator of COVID-19 infection. Bradypnea, abnormally slowed respiratory rate, is associated with cardiac abnormalities, medications, toxins, head injuries, and altered consciousness.

**8. C) Epiglottitis**

Inflammation of the epiglottis is a medical emergency that requires recognition of the signs of impending airway obstruction; these include acute onset of fever, dysphonia, dysphasia, drooling, and distress. While acute exacerbations of asthma and aspiration pneumonia can also cause respiratory distress, the presenting symptoms differ and include wheezing, coughing, and chest tightness. Viral tonsillitis can cause significant fever and sore throat but would not be correlated with drooling or stridor.

**9. D) *Streptococcus pneumoniae***

Bacterial pathogens that cause common community-acquired pneumonia include *Streptococcus pneumoniae, Haemophilus influenzae,* and *Moraxella catarrhalis.* While rates of pneumococcal pneumonia have declined as a result of vaccination, Strep pneumonia remains the most common bacterial cause and is responsible for the highest number of deaths in the United States and globally. Bacterial pathogens that cause atypical pneumonia include *Legionella, Mycoplasma pneumoniae,* and *Chlamydia pneumoniae.* Viral causes of pneumonia include influenza A and B viruses, respiratory syncytial virus, adenoviruses, and coronaviruses.

**10. B) Chronic airway inflammation worsened by acute bronchospasm in response to triggers**

Asthma is a disease of chronic airway inflammation; the narrowed airways produce extra mucous and are susceptible to bronchospasm from triggers such as exercise, pollen, dust mites, mold, pet dander, respiratory infections, stress, and environmental temperatures. Unlike COPD, the inflammation is reversible (i.e., not fixed or progressive). For individuals with COPD, obstruction of airflow causes daily symptoms that worsen over time. Individuals with cystic fibrosis can also have symptoms of asthma; the disease process of cystic fibrosis differs, however, in that the mucociliary dysfunction caused by the disorder causes increased risk of bronchiectasis.

# Nervous System

## KEY HISTORY CONSIDERATIONS

- Headaches
- Movement problems, including gait
- Dizziness
- Weakness
- Seizures
- Forgetfulness
- Difficulty concentrating and thinking
- Changes in personality or behavior
- History of trauma or car accidents
- History of concussion or head injury
- History of substance use disorder
- History of cardiovascular disease including stroke, high blood pressure, and blood clots
- Family history of neurological disorders
- Nicotine, alcohol, or recreational drug use

## PHYSICAL EXAMINATION

### GENERAL SURVEY AND INSPECTION

1. Vital signs should be assessed and compared to past measurements to identify any possible disease or pre-disease markers.
2. A height, weight, and body mass calculation should be completed and compared to previous visits, if possible, to identify signs of chronic disease or weight loss.
3. Note the patient's demeanor, affect, and ability to articulate and communicate.
4. Observe the patient's gait, balance, coordination, or tremors.
5. Listen to the patient's response to questions, which provides information regarding the patient's ability to follow directions.
6. Inspection of the face includes attention to shape, features, facial expression, symmetry of the eyebrows, eyes, ears, nose, and mouth, and position of facial features such as nasolabial fold and inspecting for facial muscle atrophy and tremors (for more information, see Chapter 4, "Head, Neck, and Lymphatics").

# MENTAL STATUS EXAM

1. Observe the patient's level of consciousness.
2. Assess the patient's orientation to person, place, and time.
3. Observe the patient's speech and language. Latency, volume, rate, rhythm, intonation, and prosody of speech should be noted.
4. Assess the patient's short-term memory.
5. More detail on the mental status exam is included in Chapter 14, "Mental Health and Substance Use."

## MENTAL STATUS EXAM ABNORMAL FINDINGS

Decreased level of consciousness:

- Levels of consciousness are defined as:
  - **Alert:** Awake with a normal level of consciousness.
  - **Lethargic:** Sleepy, sluggish, and requires stimulation to maintain an awake state.
  - **Stuporous:** Cannot be aroused to a fully awake state. The patient may respond semi-purposefully to stimulation.
  - **Comatose:** No purposeful response to any type of stimulation.

Abnormalities of speech or language include:

- **Aphasia:** A disorder of language that manifests as problems with comprehension, fluency, naming, arithmetic, and/or writing. This is typically caused by a stroke or other brain disorder that involves the language areas of cortex.
- **Verbal apraxia:** A disorder of language where the motor skills that are needed to correctly form the sounds of speech, even when they know which words they want to say, are affected.
- **Dysphonia:** A disorder of voice production caused by abnormal larynx or vocal cord function.
- **Dysarthria:** A disorder of articulation caused by abnormal motor control of the pharynx, palate, tongue, lips, and/or face.

Additional considerations in speech and thought as they relate to abnormalities in mental health are discussed in Chapter 14, "Mental Health and Substance Use."

Abnormalities of short-term memory and cognitive impairment can be assessed using a Mini-Cog.

- The Mini-Cog is a screening test for short-term memory loss associated with cognitive impairment. The clinician should give the patient a list of three simple items, for example: apple, hat, ball. The clinician should ask the patient to repeat them immediately and remember them for 5 minutes. Then the clinician should ask the patient to draw a clock face on a piece of paper with the hands pointing to a certain time. Then ask the patient to recall the three items.
  - Recall of 0 items indicates cognitive impairment.
  - Recall of 1 to 2 items with an abnormal clock face indicates cognitive impairment.
  - Recall of 1 to 2 items with a normal clock face indicates no cognitive impairment.
  - Recall of all 3 items indicates no cognitive impairment.
- Causes of cognitive impairment include such conditions as dementia, traumatic brain injury, stroke, and Parkinson's disease. Cognitive impairment can range in severity from mild to severe depending on the extent and location of injury.

# CRANIAL NERVE (CN) EXAM

## OLFACTORY (I)

The olfactory nerve is tested by asking the patient to identify familiar odors.

1. Make sure the patient's nares are clear and have the patient occlude one naris at a time. Have the patient close their eyes and hold an open vial under their nose. Ask the patient to breathe deeply. Use a different aroma to test the other side. Repeat two to three times with two to three different odors. Patients are expected to perceive an odor on each side and to identify it.

## OPTIC (II)

Testing for optic nerve function includes testing of distant and near vision, ophthalmoscopic examination of optic fundi, with special attention to the optic disc and testing visual fields by confrontation and extinction.

1. Test each eye separately and both eyes together.
2. In those patients with partial vision loss, testing of both eyes can reveal a visual field deficit, testing with one eye will miss this finding. Refer to Chapter 5, "Eyes, Ears, Nose, and Throat," for more on the eye exam.

## OCULOMOTOR, TROCHLEAR, AND ABDUCENS (III, IV, AND VI)

The oculomotor, trochlear, and abducens nerves are tested with movement of the eyes through the six cardinal fields of gaze.

1. Stand in front of the patient and direct them to focus on your finger, which should be in their direct line of vision. Ask them to follow your finger. You will then lead them through the six cardinal fields of gaze. The eye movements should be smooth and transition to each field without difficulty.
2. Exam techniques for visualization of pupil size, shape, response to light, accommodation, and opening of the upper eyelids, are described in Chapter 5, "Eyes, Ears, Nose, and Throat." The pupils should be equal, round, and reactive to light and accommodation. Direct and consensual light reflexes should be observed.

## TRIGEMINAL (V)

The primary function of CN V is to provide sensory and motor innervation to the face.

Motor function:

1. Observe the face for muscle atrophy, deviation of the jaw to one side, and muscle twitching.
2. Ask the patient to clench their teeth tightly as the muscles over the jaw are palpated, evaluating tone. Facial tone should be symmetric, without tremor.

Sensory function:

1. The three trigeminal nerve divisions are evaluated for sharp, dull, and light touch sensations. Have the patient close their eyes, then touch each side of their face at the scalp, cheek and chin alternately using the sharp and smooth edges of a broken tongue blade or paper clip. Ask the patient to report whether each sensation is sharp or dull. Then stroke the face in the same six areas with a cotton wisp asking the patient to report sensation. Discrimination of all stimuli is expected over all facial avoid.

## FACIAL (VII)

The facial nerve has both sensory and motor functions. It controls facial movements, taste, and movement of the lacrimal, submaxillary, and submandibular glands. It is also responsible for the sense of taste on the anterior two-thirds of the tongue.

1. Ask the patient to form specific facial expressions to test for facial symmetry. Ask the patient to raise the eyebrows, squeeze eyes shut, wrinkle the forehead, frown, smile, show their teeth, purse their lips, and puff out their cheeks. Facial movements should be symmetric, coordinated, and smooth.

## VESTIBULOCOCHLEAR (VIII)

This cranial nerve is responsible for hearing and maintaining body balance.

1. Assess hearing with the whisper test. Ask the patient to repeat numbers whispered into one ear while blocking or rubbing your fingers next to the opposite ear.
2. An audiometry examination can also be completed if a more thorough examination is necessary.
3. Vestibular function is tested with the Romberg test, which tests position sense. The clinician has the patient stand with the feet together and eyes open. Ask the patient to close their eyes for 30 to 60 seconds without support. Make sure to guard the patient to ensure they do not fall during the exam. Observe the patient's ability to maintain an upright posture. Minimal swaying is a normal finding.

## GLOSSOPHARYNGEAL (IX), VAGUS (X)

The glossopharyngeal nerve tests the ability of the patient to identify sour and bitter tastes on the posterior third of each side of the tongue, gag reflex and ability to swallow, inspection of the palate and uvula, and speech sounds.

1. Observe the patient swallowing. Swallowing should be smooth and without difficulty.
2. Listen to the patient's speech. The voice should be clear and free from hoarseness.
3. Sensory function of taste may be completed during the CN VII evaluation.
4. Glossopharyngeal nerve function is simultaneously tested during the evaluation of the vagus nerve for nasopharyngeal sensation (gag reflex) and the motor function of swallowing.
5. The gag reflex is initiated by touching the patient's posterior pharyngeal wall with a tongue depressor while observing for upward movement of the palate and contraction of the pharyngeal muscles. The uvula should remain midline. Drooping or absence of an arch on either side of the palate is abnormal.
6. Motor function is evaluated with inspection of the soft palate for symmetry. Have the patient say "ah" and observe the movement of the soft palate. If there is damage to the vagus or glossopharyngeal nerve, the palate does not rise, and the uvula will deviate from midline. To complete testing, have the patient sip and swallow water. The patient should be able to swallow easily.
7. Listen to the patient's speech for hoarseness, nasal quality, or difficulty with guttural sounds.

## SPINAL ACCESSORY (XI)

Evaluation of the spinal accessory nerve includes evaluation of the size, shape, and strength of the trapezius and sternocleidomastoid (SCM) muscles.

1. To test the trapezius muscle, stand behind the patient and observe for atrophy or flickering movement of the skin (a symptom of disease of the nervous system).
2. Place a hand on each shoulder and ask the patient to shrug upward and observe the strength and contraction of the muscles.
3. To test the SCM muscle, ask the patient to turn their head to each side against the clinician's hand, observing the contraction of the opposite SCM and the force of movement against the hand.

## HYPOGLOSSAL (XII)

The hypoglossal nerve innervates all but one of the muscles of the tongue.

1. Inspect the patient's tongue while at rest on the floor of the mouth and while protruded from the mouth observing for size and shape. Have the patient move their tongue in and out of the mouth, side to side, and curled upward and downward without difficulty.
2. Muscle strength of the tongue is tested by asking the patient to push the tongue against the cheek as the clinician applies resistance with an index finger or hand (Figure 8.1).
3. Assess lingual speech sounds (l, t, d, n) by listening to the patient's speech.

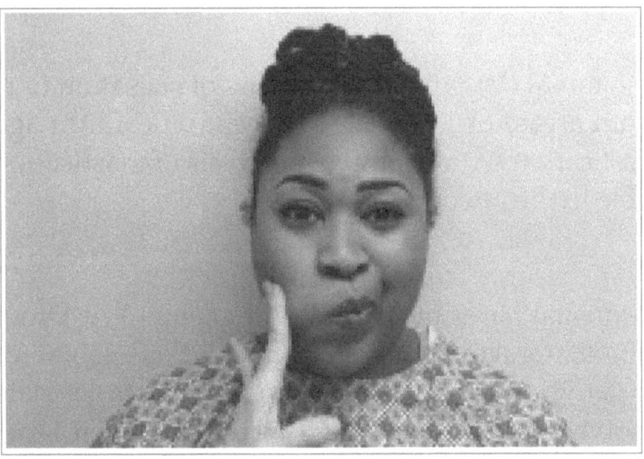

**Figure 8.1** Testing muscle strength of the tongue.

## CRANIAL NERVE ABNORMAL FINDINGS

### *Olfactory (I)*

- CN I is considered abnormal if the patient is unable to discriminate odors or reports a complete loss of smell. This can be due to nasal congestion from conditions like allergic rhinitis or upper respiratory infections. COVID-19 is a common cause of anosmia. Neurologic causes due to damage or deterioration of the olfactory center of the brain include brain tumors, diabetes, Huntington's disease, multiple sclerosis, Alzheimer's disease, or Parkinson's disease. Head and nose injuries, some chemicals and medications, and cocaine addiction can also cause damage to CN I.

### *Optic (II)*

- Damage to the optic nerve can present with partial or complete vision loss to one or both eyes and/or loss of pupillary constriction. The severity and type of vision loss depend on where the damage occurs. Common causes of injury to the optic nerve are glaucoma due to increasing pressure in the eye, optic neuritis due to infection or autoimmune disorders, atrophy due to poor blood flow to the eye, disease, trauma, or exposure to toxic substances.

### *Oculomotor, Trochlear, and Abducens (III, IV, and VI)*

- Uncoordinated or having the inability to move the eye(s) in a specific direction are abnormal findings. Extraocular eye movements that appear jerky or appear involuntary such as nystagmus are also abnormal. CN III is also responsible for reaction to light and accommodation. Ptosis, double vision, difficulty moving the eye, mydriasis, or if the eyes turn down and out indicates a problem with CN III. The inability to look down while the eye is adducted, sometimes causing double vision, indicates damage to CN IV. Lastly, the inability of the eyes to move laterally or medial eye deviation would indicate pathology of CN VI.
- The two most common causes of palsies to CN III, IV, and VI are lack of blood flow or nerve compression. Lack of blood flow is typically due to various disease states such as hypertension or diabetes. Nerve compression is typically due to more serious causes such as an aneurysm, tumor, or brain herniation due to head trauma. Children can be born with a third and fourth nerve palsy, although they can still be induced due to infection, stroke, tumor, or head trauma.

### *Trigeminal (V)*

- Damage to the trigeminal (V) can present as loss of sensation to the face (in the forehead, cheek, or chin areas) or loss of the corneal reflex. Damage can also result in problems with mastication with complete paralysis of mastication muscles or deviation of the mandible to the affected side.

### *Facial Nerve (VII)*

- Observe for tics, unusual facial movements, or asymmetry. Drooping of one side of the mouth, loss of unilateral eye closure, a flattened nasolabial fold, and/or sagging of the lower eyelid are signs of muscle weakness or neurological dysfunction of CN VII. Patients cannot move the upper and lower part of their face on one side with a facial nerve palsy. Only the lower portion of the face is affected if there is a central nerve lesion of CN VII.
- Loss of taste to the anterior two-thirds of the tongue would also indicate CN VII dysfunction.
- Causes of CN VII dysfunction include Bell's palsy, stroke, tumor, basal skull fracture, Ramsay Hunt syndrome, necrotizing otitis externa, acoustic neuroma, and COVID-19.

### *Vestibulocochlear (VIII)*

- Progressive, often unilateral, hearing loss or tinnitus is often the presenting sign when CN VIII is affected. As noted in Chapter 5, "Eyes, Ears, Nose, and Throat," hearing loss is either conductive or sensorineural. Causes of sensorineural hearing loss are presbycusis, noise exposure, hereditary, ototoxicity, sudden idiopathic hearing loss, autoimmune hearing loss, Meniere's disease, vestibular schwannoma, or infection.

*Glossopharyngeal (IX), Vagus (X)*

- Dysphagia, hoarseness of the voice, loss of taste to the posterior one-third of the tongue, loss of the gag reflex, glossopharyngeal neuralgia, or deviation of the uvula from midline are all signs of CN IX and/or CN X dysfunction.
- Compression of the nerve, tumors, trauma, aortic aneurysms, and inflammation can be the cause of the dysfunction.

*Spinal Accessory (XI)*

- Impaired neck rotation, drooping shoulders, shoulder pain, "winging" of the shoulder blades, and weakness of the sternocleidomastoid and/or trapezius muscle can signify CN XI dysfunction. Causes of CV XI dysfunction are typically iatrogenic and most commonly from surgery of the lateral cervical region.

*Hypoglossal (XII)*

- There will be asymmetry, atrophy, and fasciculation of the tongue on the affected side with CN XII dysfunction. Causes are typically due to trauma, dissection of the internal carotid artery, and tumors.

# PROPRIOCEPTION AND CEREBELLAR FUNCTION EXAM

## COORDINATION AND FINE MOTOR SKILLS

1. Observe the patient's body position during movement and at rest.
2. Look for involuntary movements (tics or tremors), muscle bulk, muscle strength, muscle tone, and the patient's coordination.

## RAPID RHYTHMIC ALTERNATIVE MOVEMENTS

1. Ask the seated patient to pat their knees with both hands, alternately turning the palms up and down and gradually increasing the speed of movements.
2. Alternatively, ask the patient to touch the thumb to each finger on the same hand from the little finger and back. One hand is tested at a time, gradually increasing the speed of one hand touching the thumb to the little finger. The clinician should model the movements for the patient before having the patient complete them. The patient should be able to accomplish these movements smoothly and rhythmically.
3. The patient's movements should be accurate, rapid, and smooth during both of these tests.

## ACCURACY OF MOVEMENTS

- Test accuracy of the patient's movements with the use of the finger to nose test. Have the patient keep their eyes open. Ask the patient to use an index finger to touch their nose, then touch the clinician's index finger, which should be positioned approximately 18 inches from the patient to allow full arm extension. The clinician moves their finger position several times during the test which is then repeated on the other hand. The patient should be able to touch their nose then the clinician's finger with accuracy and smoothness.
- The heel to shin test is an alternative method to test accuracy of movement. This test can be performed with the patient sitting or supine. The clinician asks the patient to

run the heel of one foot up and down the shin of the opposite leg and repeat the test with the other heel. The patient should be able to move the heel up and down the shin in a straight line without deviating to the side.

## BALANCE

- Complete the Romberg test (see vestibulocochlear cranial nerve (VIII) section).
- Other methods of evaluating balance are as follows:
  1. Have patient stand with feet slightly apart and push the shoulders with enough effort to throw them off balance (be ready to catch patient if needed). The patient should be able to quickly recover balance.
  2. Request the patient to close their eyes, hold their arms at the sides of the body and stand on one foot, repeating the test on the opposite foot. Slight swaying is normal, and the patient should be able to maintain balance on each foot for 5 seconds.
  3. With their eyes open, have the patient hop in place on one foot and then the other (tests proximal and distal muscle strength). The patient should be able to hop on one foot for 5 seconds without loss of balance.

## GAIT

1. Have the patient walk across the room or down the hall and turn and come back, observing posture, balance, swinging of the arms, and intact movement.
2. The patient should then walk heel to toe in a straight line (tandem walking), walk on their toes, then on their heels.
3. Lastly, have the patient do a knee bend.

These tests assess for gait abnormalities which increase fall risk.

- Testing for pronator drift should also be completed. Ask the patient to stand for 20 to 30 seconds with their eyes closed and both arms straight forward with palms up. The patient is then instructed to keep their arms out and their eyes shut. The clinician taps the arms briskly downward. The arms normally return smoothly to the horizontal position, which requires muscular strength, coordination, and good position sense.

## PROPRIOCEPTION AND CEREBELLAR FUNCTION ABNORMAL FINDINGS

- Abnormal body position may be due to mono-or hemiparesis from stroke.
- Involuntary movements can occur with numerous neurological conditions. Tremors, tics, myoclonus, chorea, athetosis, dystonia, and hemiballismus are types of involuntary movements. These can be the result of a benign (e.g., essential tremor) or a pathological condition (e.g., Parkinson's disease). The type of identified involuntary movement will determine differential diagnoses and possible etiologies.
- Dysdiadochokinesia is the inability to perform rapid, alternating movements often due to cerebellar disease. This can be seen in the upper extremities, the lower extremities, and in the muscles that control speech. Stiff, slow, or jerky clonic movements when the patient is attempting to complete the rapid, alternating movements test are abnormal. These patients may also have a noted change in balance and walking, difficulty with speaking, difficulty with stopping or starting movements, or poor coordination in the arms, hands, and legs. Hereditary ataxias, congenital malformation, neurodegenerative disorders, systemic disorders, multiple sclerosis, strokes,

ataxic dysarthria, and traumatic brain disorders, among other conditions, could be the cause of the dysdiadochokinesia.

- Repeatedly missing the clinician's finger during the finger to nose test, being unable to complete or having marked inaccuracy during the heel to shin test, or having loss of balance during the Romberg test can also indicate cerebellar disease.
- If there is loss of balance during the Romberg test (e.g., the patient staggers or loses balance), postpone other tests of cerebellar function which require balance.
- Observe for instability or need to continually touch the floor with the opposite foot or a tendency to fall. Difficulty hopping may be related to weakness, lack of position sense, or cerebellar dysfunction.
- An uncoordinated gait with reeling and instability is ataxic, which is seen in cerebellar disease, loss of position sense, and intoxication. Tandem walking may reveal ataxia, distal leg weakness and is a sensitive test for corticospinal tract damage. See Table 8.1 for an explanation of gait disturbances.
- With loss of position strength, arms will drift sideward or upward, which is a positive test for pronator drift (Figure 8.2). The patient may not notice the displacement.

**Table 8.1 Abnormal Gait Pattern Characteristics**

| Gait Pattern | Characteristics |
|---|---|
| Antalgic | Limited time of weight-bearing on the affected side; limping |
| Ataxic/cerebellar gait | Clumsy, staggering movements with wide-base gait; titubation present at rest |
| Choreiform/hyperkinetic gait | Nondirectional, jerky, involuntary movements in all extremities |
| Dystrophic/waddling gait | Legs wide apart/weight shifted side-to-side in waddling motion related to weak hip adductor muscles |
| Neuropathic/steppage/equine gait | Seen in patients with foot drop (weakness of foot dorsiflexion); patient attempts to lift leg high enough, so the toe does not drag on the floor |
| Parkinsonian | Stooped posture with head and neck forward and flexion at the knees/rigid body/short shuffling steps/difficulty initiating steps and stopping/bradykinesia |

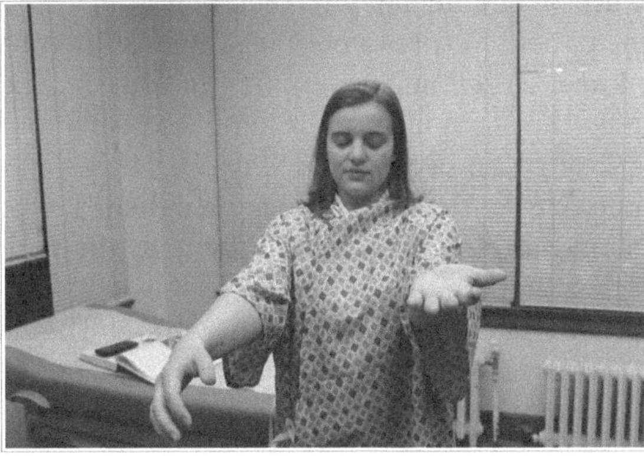

**Figure 8.2** Positive pronator drift test.

## MUSCLE STRENGTH EXAM

Normal muscle strength varies, so the standard of normal should allow for age and sex. The patient's dominant side is usually stronger than the non-dominant side, although differences may be hard to detect.

- Muscle strength is tested by asking the patient to actively resist the clinician's movement. Muscle strength is graded 0 to 5. Refer to Table 8.2 for details of muscle strength grading.

**Table 8.2 Muscle Strength Scale**

| Grade | Level of Function |
|---|---|
| 0 | No movement |
| 1 | Trace movement |
| 2 | Full passive range of motion |
| 3 | Full range of motion against gravity, no resistance |
| 4 | Full range of motion with resistance, though weak |
| 5 | Full range of motion, full strength |

- Muscle strength testing methods include:
  - **Biceps and brachioradialis at the elbow flexion and extension:** The patient pulls and pushes against the clinician's hand.
  - **Extension at the wrist:** The patient makes a fist and resists as the clinician presses down.
  - **Grip strength:** The clinician asks the patient to squeeze two of their fingers as hard as possible and not let them go.
  - **Finger abduction:** Patient's hand is positioned down with fingers spread. The clinician instructs the patient to prevent them from moving fingers as they try to force them together.
  - **Thumb opposition:** The clinician asks the patient to touch the top of the little finger with the thumb against resistance.
  - **Muscle strength of the trunk:** Flexion, extension, rotation, and lateral bending.
  - **Flexion at the hip:** The clinician places their hand on the patient's mid-thigh and asks the patient to raise their leg against their hand.
  - **Adduction at the hips:** The clinician puts their hands on the bed between the patient's knees and asks the patient to bring both legs together.
  - **Abduction at the hips:** The clinician puts their hands on the outside of the patient's knees and asks the patient to spread both legs against their hands.
  - **Extension at the knee:** The clinician supports the knee in flexion and requests the patient to straighten the leg against their hand. Expect a forceful response as the quadriceps is the strongest muscle in the body.
  - **Flexion at the knee:** The clinician positions the patient's leg, so the knee is flexed with the foot resting on the bed. The clinician tells the patient to keep the foot down as they try to straighten the leg.
  - **Foot dorsiflexion and plantar flexion at the ankle:** The clinician requests the patient to pull up and push down against their hand. Heel and toe walk assesses foot dorsiflexion and plantar flexion, respectively.

### MUSCLE STRENGTH ABNORMAL FINDINGS

- Decreased bilateral muscle strength can be a result of de-conditioning, muscle/joint pain, aging, muscle tear/strain, chronic disease, aging, neuromuscular disorders, and autoimmune disorders.
- Abrupt onset, unilateral muscle strength is more worrisome due to the possibility of a stroke.
- Weak grip is seen in cervical radiculopathy, ulnar peripheral nerve disease, carpal tunnel syndrome, arthritis, and epicondylitis.
- Weak finger abduction occurs in ulnar nerve disorders.

## REFLEX EXAM

### SUPERFICIAL REFLEXES

- **Plantar reflex:** Using the end of a reflex hammer, stroke the lateral side of the foot from heel to ball, then across the foot to the medial side with the result of plantar flexion of the toes. This is a normal sign.
- **Abdominal reflex:** With the patient supine, stroke the four abdominal quadrants of the abdomen with the end of a reflex hammer. Stroking downward and away from the umbilicus elicits the lower abdominal reflexes, which respond with a slight movement of the umbilicus toward the area of stimulation. The reflex response should be equal and bilateral.
- The corneal reflex is the response of involuntary blinking when the cornea is touched. CNs V and VII are involved in this response.
- The cremasteric reflex can be elicited by stroking the superior medial side of the thigh. This will cause the contraction of the cremaster muscle, which will elevate the scrotum/testicle on that side.

### DEEP TENDON REFLEXES

Deep tendon reflexes (DTRs) include the biceps, brachioradialis, triceps, patellar, and Achilles reflexes. The patient should be in a seated position. Test each reflex and compare it to the other side of the body. The reflex response should be symmetric, visible, and palpable. DTRs are obtained by positioning a limb with a slightly stretched tendon and quickly tapping the tendon to be tested with a percussion hammer. The expected response is a sudden contraction of the muscle. Each reflex is scored as 0 to 4+ (Table 8.3).

**Table 8.3 Deep Tendon Reflex Grading**

| | |
|---|---|
| Grade 0 | No response |
| Grade 1+ | Sluggish or diminished response |
| Grade 2+ | Active or expected response (normal) |
| Grade 3+ | Brisk/slightly hyperactive |
| Grade 4+ | Brisk/hyperactive |

- **Biceps reflex:** With the patient's arm bent at a 45-degree angle at the elbow, palpate the biceps tendon and place your thumb over the tendon and your fingers under the elbow. Then strike your thumb with the reflex hammer to elicit contraction of the biceps muscle causing flexion of the elbow. The main spinal nerve roots involved are C5 and C6.

- **Brachioradialis reflex:** With the patient's arm bent at a 45-degree angle at the elbow, rest the patient's arm on yours. The patient's hand should be slightly pronated. The clinician directly strikes the brachioradial tendon 1 to 2 inches above the wrist with the reflex hammer. A normal response is forearm pronation and elbow flexion. The main spinal nerve root involved is C6.
- **Triceps reflex:** With the patient's arm flexed at a 90-degree angle, support the patient's arm just above the antecubital fossa and palpate the antecubital fossa. Then directly strike the triceps tendon with a reflex hammer just above the elbow. A normal response is extension of the elbow. The main spinal nerve root involved is C7.
- **Patellar reflex:** With the patient's knee flexed to a 90-degree angle, support the patient's upper leg with your hand to allow the patient's lower leg to hang. Strike the patellar tendon just below the patella. A normal response is extension of the lower leg. The main spinal nerve root involved is L4.
- **Achilles reflex:** With the patient sitting and the knee flexed to a 90-degree angle, keeping the ankle in a neutral position, hold the patient's foot in your hand. Strike the Achilles tendon at the level of the ankle malleoli. A normal response is plantar flexion of the foot. The main spinal nerve root involved is S1.

If deep tendon reflexes are symmetrically diminished or absent, use a technique of isometric contraction of other muscles, which might increase reflex activity. For example, when eliciting the patellar or Achilles reflexes, ask the patient to join their hands together and pull away from each other. This distraction by the patient will often allow their other muscles to relax, allowing a greater response from the DTR.

## REFLEX EXAM ABNORMAL FINDINGS

### *Superficial Reflexes*

- The plantar reflex is abnormal if there is plantar extension of the toes.
- Absence of the corneal reflex can signify damage to CNs V and/or VII. Patients who wear contact lenses may have a blunted response due to desensitization over time.
- If the abdominal reflex is absent, an upper motor neuron lesion should be considered on the side of the absence.
- Testicular torsion, upper/lower motor neuron lesions, L1/L2 spinal cord injury, and ilioinguinal nerve injury can cause absence of the cremasteric reflex.

### *Deep Tendon Reflexes*

- DTRs have high specificity but low sensitivity when ruling out neurological conditions. They can be influenced by a variety of factors, including age, metabolic factors such as thyroid dysfunction or electrolyte abnormalities, medications, illicit drugs, and anxiety level of the patient.
- DTRs may be diminished/hyperactive by abnormalities in muscles, sensory neurons, lower motor neurons, and the neuromuscular junction; acute upper motor neuron lesions; and mechanical factors such as joint disease. As a rule, disease/injury of the lower motor neuron (e.g., nerve roots or peripheral nerves) will cause a diminished or absent reflex. Disease/injury of the upper motor neuron (e.g., spinal cord, brainstem, or brain) will cause a hyperactive reflex with possible clonus. Diminished or hyperactive reflexes are often a normal finding. They are typically only significant when there are other neurological symptoms/signs present, the reflex amplitude is

asymmetric, or the reflex amplitude is different compared with reflexes seen at a higher spinal level.

- Hyperactive reflexes are often normal; however, associated clonus should never be interpreted as a normal finding.

## SENSORY FUNCTION EXAM

Evaluation of the sensory system requires testing of several kinds of sensation such as pain and temperature (spinothalamic tracts); position and vibration (posterior columns); light touch (spinothalamic tracts and posterior columns); and discriminative sensations which depend on pain, temperature, position, vibration, and light touch (the cortex).

1. Evaluate sensation by asking the patient to identify stimuli on the hands, distal arms, abdomen, feet, and legs. Each sensation procedure is tested with the patient's eyes closed. Contralateral areas of the body are tested, and the patient is asked to compare sensations side to side. Normal findings include:
   a. Minimal differences side to side
   b. Correct description of sensations (hot, cold, sharp, dull)
   c. Recognition of the side of the body tested
   d. Location of sensation and recognition if proximal or distal to the site previously tested

When testing, the clinician focuses on the areas that have numbness, pain, motor, or reflex abnormalities.

- Compare symmetric areas on two sides of the body including arms, legs, and trunk. With pain, temperature, and touch sensation, compare distal to proximal areas of the extremities.
- Test fingers and toes first for vibration and sensation. If these tests are normal, the clinician can assume the more proximal areas are normal.
- Evaluation of light touch and superficial pain can be evaluated together.
- Monofilament testing is another important sensory testing tool commonly used in the evaluation of diabetic and peripheral neuropathy. Testing with a 5.07 monofilament should be done on several sites of the foot for all patients with diabetic and peripheral neuropathy. The monofilament should be felt without bending the monofilament.
- **Monofilament testing:** With the patient's eyes closed, the clinician places the monofilament on several sites of the plantar surface of each foot and one side of the dorsal surface of the foot in a random pattern. The clinician applies pressure for 1.5 seconds to each site without repeating a test site. The correct amount of pressure is applied when the filament bends.

### PRIMARY SENSORY FUNCTIONS

- **Light touch:** Lightly touch the skin with a cotton wisp and ask the patient to respond when and where the sensation is felt.
- **Proprioception joint position sense:** Assess the great toe of each foot and a finger on each hand. Hold the joint to be tested by the lateral aspect, in the neutral position and

move the toe up and down. Hold the toe on its sides and not on the top and bottom to avoid providing pressure cues that invalidate the test. Ask the patient to identify the joint position.

- **Vibration:** Use a low-pitched tuning fork (128 Hz which has slower reduction of vibration). Place the stem of a vibrating tuning fork against a bony prominence at the toe or finger joint and ask the patient to identify when and where the buzzing sensation is felt.
- **Superficial pain:** Alternate the sharp and smooth edges of a broken tongue blade, Wartenberg wheel, or paper clip on the skin. The patient is asked to identify each sensation as sharp or dull and where the sensation is felt.
- **Temperature:** Testing skin temperature is omitted if pain sensation is normal. If there are sensory deficits, use test tubes filled with hot and cold water. Ask the patient to identify if the sensation is hot or cold and where the sensation is felt.

## PRIMARY SENSORY FUNCTION ABNORMAL FINDINGS

- Loss of one modality in a conduction system is often associated with the loss of the other modalities conducted by the same tract in the affected area.
- Impaired sensation or inability to feel light touch, superficial pain, vibration, temperature, or proprioception can occur due to a variety of neurological conditions including but not limited to brain tumor, peripheral neuropathy, stroke, spinal cord injury, nerve palsies, and traumatic brain injury.
- Monofilament testing is positive if the patient cannot feel the monofilament in entirety or in a specific location on the foot. This is often seen in peripheral neuropathy secondary to diabetes.

## SPECIAL TESTS

### *Cortical Sensory Function*

Cortical sensory or discriminatory sensory function tests assess the patient's ability to interpret sensation. Patients with lesions in the sensory cortex or posterior spinal cord would be unable to complete these tests. The patient's eyes should be closed during testing.

- **Stereognosis:** Tests the patient's ability to identify a familiar object by touch. Place a key or coin in the patient's hand. The patient's ability to identify the object is a normal response.
- **Two-point discrimination:** Using two ends of a paper clip, alternate touching the patient's skin at various locations with one or two points of the paper clip. The patient's ability to identify one- or two-point touch is a normal response.
- **Extinction phenomenon:** Simultaneously touch two areas on each side of the body (such as the cheek or hand) with the broken end of a tongue blade. The patient should be able to discriminate the number of touches and where they are felt bilaterally.
- **Graphesthesia:** With the blunt end of a reflex hammer or applicator, draw a number or shape on the palm of the patient's hand. Repeat the test using a different figure on the other hand. The patient should be able to identify the shape or number.

Other special tests are used when the clinician suspects meningeal irritation, which can occur with meningitis or subarachnoid hemorrhage.

- **Brudzinski's sign:** The clinician should not use this test if there is injury or fracture of the cervical vertebrae or cervical cord. With the patient lying flat, the clinician puts their hands behind the patient's head and flexes the neck forward, attempting to touch the patient's chin to his/her chest. Normally the patient can easily bend the head and neck forward.
- **Kernig's sign:** With the patient lying flat, flex the patient's leg at the hip and knee, then slowly extend the leg and straighten the knee. Normally, the patient should feel some discomfort behind the knee with extension. A positive test reveals pain with knee extension.

***Special Test Abnormal Findings***

- An inability to identify the object in stereognosis or distinguish the figure in graphesthesia signifies a defect in higher intellectual functioning and is associated with cortical damage.
- When a patient has a lesion in their sensory cortex in the parietal lobe, the patient may only report feeling one finger touch their body, when in fact they were touched twice on opposite sides of their body, simultaneously.
- With extinction, the stimulus not felt is on the side opposite of the damaged cortex.
- A Brudzinski's sign is considered positive when the patient bends the hips and knees in response to neck flexion and is seen in meningeal irritation.
- Kernig's sign is positive when there is pain with extension of the knee and signifies meningeal irritation.

## RED FLAGS IN HISTORY AND PHYSICAL EXAM

- Unilateral weakness
- History of cancer or immunosuppression
- History of trauma, fall, or loss of consciousness
- History of previous stroke or transient ischemic attack (TIA)
- Family history of a progressive neurological disorder
- Reported progressive neurological dysfunction
- Face drooping
- Arm weakness
- Sudden numbness or weakness of the face, arm, or leg, especially unilateral
- Sudden confusion, trouble speaking, or understanding speech
- Sudden trouble seeing in one or both eyes, abrupt vision loss, or double vision
- Sudden trouble walking, dizziness, or loss of balance/coordination
- Sudden severe headache
- Abrupt onset of motor and sensory deficits
- Seizure
- Paralysis
- Syncope
- Memory loss
- Status epilepticus
- Loss of already attained cognitive or developmental abilities
- Meningitis triad (fever, headache, neck stiffness)

# POPULATION HEALTH AND LIFE-SPAN CONSIDERATIONS

## INFANTS AND CHILDREN

Major brain growth occurs in the first year of life with myelinization of the brain and nervous system. Infection, biochemical imbalance, or trauma may disrupt development and growth, producing devastating results with eventual brain dysfunction. Neurologic impulses are provided by the brainstem and spinal cord at birth. Infants have a set of reflexes, called the "primitive reflexes," which are seen during infancy and typically disappear at various times during the first year of life. As the infant's brain develops, the involuntary reflexes are replaced by voluntary movements. These primitive reflexes diminish as the brain develops, and advanced cortical functions and voluntary control become prominent. These reflexes are detailed below.

- **Asymmetrical tonic neck reflex (fencer position):** The clinician rotates the infant's head to one side and this produces an involuntary extension of his/her limbs on the same side and a flexion of the limbs on the opposite side. This reflex typically fades around 4 months of age.
- **Moro (startle) reflex:** Supporting the infant's head, body, and legs, the clinician suddenly lowers the body causing the arms to abduct and extend, followed by relaxed flexion, the legs should flex. This should be symmetrical. This reflex typically disappears by 6 months of age.
- **Stepping reflex:** The clinician holds the infant under the arms, allowing one of the infant's feet to touch the surface of the examination table. The clinician observes for flexion of the hip and knee. The foot should touch the table while the other foot steps forward. This reflex typically disappears by 2 months of age.
- **Palmar reflex grasp:** The clinician places a finger in the infant's hand, pressing against the palmar surface of the hand. The infant flexes all fingers to grasp the clinician's finger. This reflex typically disappears by 3 months of age.
- **Plantar reflex grasp:** The clinician touches the sole of the infant's foot at the base of the toes causing the toes to curl. This is also termed the Babinski reflex. This reflex typically disappears by 8 months of age.
- **Rooting reflex:** When the clinician strokes the infant's cheek, the infant turns their head in that direction, usually looking for food. This reflex disappears around 3–4 months of age.
- As a child's central nervous system matures, the primitive reflexes should become extinguished. Retained primitive reflexes are often an indication of birth injury, head trauma, or cerebral pathologies such as cerebral palsy.
- Asymmetry of the Moro reflex can indicate a hemiplegia, brachial plexus palsy, or a clavicular or humeral fracture on the affected side.

## OLDER ADULTS

- Cerebral neurons decrease with aging both in the brain and spinal cord.
- Slowing of thought, memory, and thinking is a normal part of aging, although this varies from one individual to the next.
- Older adults experience decreased sensory functions of smell, taste, and vision.
- Presbycusis is more common with aging.
- The rate of nerve impulse conduction decreases, causing the older adult to experience slower responses to stimuli, unsteady gait, sleep disturbances, decreased level of cognition, diminished appetite, and decreased range of motion.
- Sarcopenia is the age-associated loss of muscle mass and function, which results in decreased muscle strength and power.
- Posture may change and become mildly forward flexed.
- Gait speed may be slowed due to shortened length and decreased arm swing.
- DTRs may be diminished.
- Fine motor movement and coordination may decrease.

# KEY DIFFERENTIALS

- Alzheimer's disease
- Amyotrophic lateral sclerosis (ALS)
- Bell's palsy
- Brain tumor
- Cerebral palsy
- Cerebrovascular event
- Concussion
- Dementia
- Epilepsy
- Guillain-Barré syndrome
- Headache (migraine, cluster, tension)
- Huntington's disease
- Hydrocephalus
- Meningitis
- Multiple sclerosis
- Muscular dystrophy
- Myasthenia gravis
- Parkinson's disease
- Spina bifida
- Spinal cord injury
- Traumatic brain injury
- Trigeminal neuralgia

## KNOWLEDGE CHECK: NERVOUS SYSTEM

1. Which cranial nerves control extraocular movement of the eyes? (Select all that apply.)

   A. II optic
   B. III oculomotor
   C. IV trochlear
   D. V trigeminal
   E. VI abducens

2. Which two cranial nerves are best assessed by asking an individual to open their mouth, protrude their tongue, and say "ah" while observing the soft palate, uvula, and posterior pharynx? (Select TWO.)

   A. VII facial
   B. VIII vestibulocochlear
   C. IX glossopharyngeal
   D. X vagus
   E. XII hypoglossal

3. A 75-year-old female presents with new onset of headache, facial numbness, slurred speech, and dizziness. Her smile is asymmetrical, and she can close both eyes tightly. What is the MOST LIKELY etiology?

   A. Bell's palsy
   B. Benign paroxysmal positional vertigo
   C. Migraine headache
   D. Stroke

4. A 40-year-old woman is having recurrent episodes of disabling vertigo, lasting 30 minutes, and accompanied by roaring tinnitus, aural pressure, and low-frequency hearing loss. Physical exam reveals no nystagmus with the Dix-Hallpike test, and the Romberg test reveals significant instability. What is the MOST LIKELY diagnosis?

   A. Age-related vestibular dysfunction
   B. Benign paroxysmal positional vertigo
   C. Meniere's disease
   D. Vertebrobasilar atherothrombotic disease

5. When reviewing the medical record of a patient diagnosed with Alzheimer's disease, the clinician notes that patient is aphasic. Which behavior supports this finding?

   A. Difficulty with motor function
   B. Unable to be oriented to person, place, and time
   C. Unable to speak or comprehend speech
   D. Wandering and confusion during the evening hours

*(See answers next page.)*

**1. B, C, and E) III oculomotor, IV trochlear, VI abducens**

Assessment of cranial nerves III, IV, and VI includes the pupillary light reflex, pupillary accommodation, and ocular movements, as these motor nerves innervate the muscles of the eyes. CN II transmits visual information from photoreceptors in the retina to the brain. CN V has sensory and motor divisions responsible for jaw movement, facial expression, and facial sensations.

**2. C and D) IX glossopharyngeal, X vagus**

Cranial nerves IX and X are responsible for the sensory and motor functions of the soft palate, pharynx, larynx, and esophagus. Coordinated swallowing, breathing, and speaking rely on functions of these cranial nerves. CN VII provides motor innervation of facial muscles required for facial expression and sensory innervation of the tongue. CN VIII functions primarily to maintain body balance and hearing. CN XII innervates muscles of the tongue and is assessed by examining the tongue and its movements.

**3. D) Stroke**

Symptoms of stroke include loss of balance, headache, dizziness, blurred vision, facial drooping, arm weakness, and slurred speech. Unlike stroke, Bell's palsy would affect the entire side of the face, and the individual would have difficulty with closing the eye on the affected side. New onset of migraine-type symptoms and vertigo in an older adult should be considered a red flag for stroke.

**4. C) Meniere's disease**

Signs and symptoms of Meniere's disease include hearing loss, tinnitus, and minimally two episodes of significant vertigo lasting 20 minutes or longer; a positive Romberg is consistent with Meniere's. The negative Dix-Hallpike makes the diagnosis of benign paroxysmal positional vertigo (BPPV) unlikely. Vestibular disorders and dysfunction that may cause disabling vertigo are unrelated to age. Vertigo is the hallmark symptom of ischemia in the basilar artery; symptoms would also include diplopia, gaze paralysis, and paralysis or weakness of all extremities.

**5. C) Unable to speak or comprehend speech**

All of the signs and symptoms listed are consistent with the diagnosis of Alzheimer's dementia. The assessment of aphasia specifically refers to the impairment of language, affecting the production or comprehension of speech.

6. A 30-year-old female presents with fatigue, blurred vision, numbness and weakness in extremities, and urinary incontinence. Which three physical exam components should be prioritized based on her presentation and differential diagnoses? (Select THREE.)

   **A.** Coordination testing
   **B.** Cranial nerves II to XII
   **C.** Gait assessment
   **D.** Tinel test
   **E.** Vibratory sensation

7. Which findings suggest acute bacterial meningitis in otherwise healthy adults?

   **A.** Fever, nuchal rigidity, and altered mental status
   **B.** Rash on hands and feet in addition to oral vesicular lesions
   **C.** Recurrent petit mal or focal seizures
   **D.** Vomiting, lymphadenopathy, and parotitis

8. Which statement is true about the Moro reflex in newborns?

   **A.** Allows the infant's head to turn slightly results in a fencing pose response
   **B.** Any fanning of toes in response to startle indicates abnormality in the newborn
   **C.** Reflex is elicited when the sole of foot touches hard surface and stepping motions result
   **D.** Sudden stimulus causes a reflex that includes extension of upper limbs followed by flexion

9. What is the expected response when testing the triceps reflex?

   **A.** Extension of the elbow
   **B.** Flexion and supination of the forearm
   **C.** Flexion of the hand
   **D.** Pronation of the hand

10. The daughter of a 70-year-old male asks the advanced practice nurse if her father may be showing early signs of Parkinson's disease, as he is increasingly having hand tremors. What additional symptoms would support the daughter's intuition?

    **A.** Absence seizures recently diagnosed as epilepsy
    **B.** Acute confusion and significant memory decline
    **C.** Confusion and disorientation in the evening hours
    **D.** Slowness of movements that impair activities of daily living

*(See answers next page.)*

**6. A, B, C) Coordination testing, cranial nerves II to XII, gait assessment**

The individual is presenting with symptoms consistent with multiple sclerosis (MS), and is within the age range and gender most at risk. The neurologic assessments to prioritize include the cranial nerve exam, and cerebellar testing, which include coordination testing (finger-to-nose or finger-to-finger testing) and the assessment of gait. Vibratory sensation testing would be more appropriate if diabetes were being considered as a cause of the numbness in extremities. The Tinel test is appropriate for individuals with possible carpal tunnel syndrome.

**7. A) Fever, nuchal rigidity, and altered mental status**

Fever, headache, altered mental status, and neck stiffness are considered the "classic" symptoms that occur with acute bacterial meningitis in otherwise healthy adults who are not at extremes of age. Newborns and infants are more likely to present with seizures. Parotitis (salivary gland enlargement) in addition to symptoms of headache, fever, and vomiting is suggestive of viral meningitis caused by the mumps virus. Vesicular lesions found in the mouth and/or on the hands and feet are suggestive of hand, foot, and mouth disease caused by the Coxsackie virus.

**8. D) Sudden stimulus causes a reflex that includes extension of upper limbs followed by flexion**

The Moro reflex, which occurs when an infant is startled, results in a symmetrical extension of the infant's extremities while forming a C shape with the thumb and forefinger, followed by a return to a flexed position with extremities against the body. Other newborn reflexes include the tonic neck reflex that results in the fencing pose, the Babinski reflex, which causes fanning out of toes in response, and the stepping reflex, which is observed when the infant is held upright, and one foot touches lightly to a flat surface.

**9. A) Extension of the elbow**

There are three deep tendon reflexes of the upper extremities, triceps, biceps, and brachioradialis. In response to striking the triceps tendon, the muscle contracts causing the elbow to extend. The normal biceps reflex results in elbow flexion. Striking the brachioradialis tendon results in flexion and supination of the forearm.

**10. D) Slowness of movements that impair activities of daily living**

Tremors, rigidity, and slowness of movements are motor symptoms associated with PD; these symptoms eventually impair activities of daily living and predispose individuals to loss of balance and falls. Confusion and disorientation in the evening hours (sun downing) is more common in dementia. While many chronic neurocognitive disorders can lead to dementia, including PD, the decline is slow and progressive; acute confusion or delirium usually indicates a more urgent or emergent condition. Dementia symptoms in individuals with PD usually present in later stages, after significant motor decline. The most common cause of epilepsy in older adults is stroke-related seizure, not PD.

# Musculoskeletal System

## KEY HISTORY CONSIDERATIONS

- Muscle pain
- Joint pain
- Spinal pain (cervical, thoracic, lumbar)
- Edema
- Joint laxity, stiffness, or instability
- Limited or decreased range of motion
- Limited or decreased strength/weakness
- Recent changes in mobility or function
- Impact of mobility issues on their quality of life
- Previous or current history of injury or illness
- Exercise and sports history
- History of falls or blunt force impact
- Gait abnormalities

The approach to examining the musculoskeletal system is the same for all joints and/or limbs that are being examined. The techniques listed below apply to any affected area or joint of the body. More location-specific exams will follow.

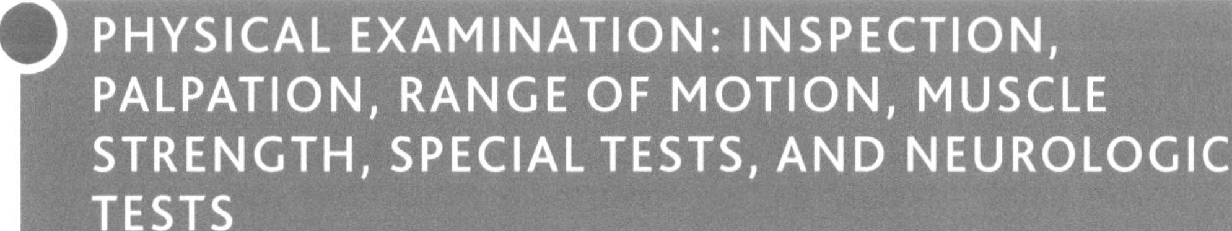

## PHYSICAL EXAMINATION: INSPECTION, PALPATION, RANGE OF MOTION, MUSCLE STRENGTH, SPECIAL TESTS, AND NEUROLOGIC TESTS

### INSPECTION

1. The patient's posture should be erect. The spine should be straight with the normal "S" curvature. Shoulders and hips should be symmetric. Hips, knees, and ankles should be in a straight line.
2. Joints should be observed from the anterior, posterior, medial, and lateral aspects. The contralateral side should be compared for side-to-side differences. Muscles, joints, and bony prominences should be symmetric.
3. Observe alignment of the joint, muscle, and bone at rest and in motion. The patient should not articulate pain during the exam or range of motion tests.
4. Inspect skin in affected and surrounding areas.

5. The patient's gait should be symmetric, smooth, and rhythmic with a natural appearing swing and a coordinated, alternating propulsive (or retropulsive) motion of the lower extremities.

## PALPATION

1. Palpate the affected and surrounding areas for tenderness, calor, or edema. Include the joints, soft tissue, tendons, ligaments, muscles, body prominences, and bursae (if applicable). Solid knowledge of the bony landmarks and underlying anatomy along with precise palpation is invaluable. Bony prominences, muscles, and surrounding tissues should be firm, non-tender, and free from temperature anomalies.
2. Have the patient complete active range of motion of the affected joint. Range of motion is the full movement potential of a joint. Range of motion (ROM) should be completed with every musculoskeletal visit. Most joints will have a contralateral joint in which to compare motion and angles. Normal ROM values are noted in each section below. ROM should be free of pain and without crepitus or contracture. Joints should appear stable.
3. Complete strength testing. Muscle strength is graded on a scale of 0 to 5. A score of 0 indicates no movement, and a score of 5 indicates full muscle strength. See Table 9.1 for muscle strength grading. It is important to test strength bilaterally. Normal strength is defined as full resistance to opposition and is graded as a 5/5. Strength should be equally bilateral.

**Table 9.1 Muscle Strength Scale**

| Grade | Level of Function |
|---|---|
| 0 | No movement |
| 1 | Trace movement |
| 2 | Full passive range of motion |
| 3 | Full range of motion against gravity, no resistance |
| 4 | Full range of motion with resistance, though weak |
| 5 | Full range of motion, full strength |

4. Complete any special tests for the specific joint or area of the body that is of concern. There are countless special tests described in the literature. Few have been vigorously vetted for their efficacy. As a result, there will rarely be one test used to identify pathology. It is more useful to use a cluster of tests to assist in identifying issues. As with other exam skills, use of proper technique is essential to derive useful information from the special tests. Be sure to focus not only on proper patient positioning but on proper hand position and clinician position to ensure reliable and valid tests.
5. The musculoskeletal and neurological systems are closely aligned. Ensuring the neurological system is intact is essential to a comprehensive musculoskeletal exam. See Chapter 8, "Nervous System," for more information about neurological tests.

### INSPECTION AND PALPATION: ABNORMAL FINDINGS

- Gross deformity, edema, bleeding, bruising, asymmetry, misalignment, hypertrophy, or atrophy are abnormal findings, and an underlying cause should be identified based on the history and additional objective information. Gross deformity, edema, bleeding, bruising, asymmetry, and misalignment often occur together and typically are due to injury. Edema suggests synovial inflammation or joint effusion. Older age, undernutrition, and certain medical conditions, such as spinal muscular atrophy, paralysis, peripheral nerve lesions, or muscular dystrophy, can cause muscle atrophy. Skin should also be observed for scars as these can provide clues to past surgeries or injuries.

- Listen for joint crepitus. This is a popping or grinding on palpation when a joint is moved. This may come from abnormal cartilage, tendons, or bone grinding on bone.
- Temperature or color changes in a joint, appendage, or limb is abnormal. Warmth over a joint or extremity can indicate inflammation or infection such as deep vein thrombosis, cellulitis, gout, or septic arthritis. Coolness of a limb, especially if unilateral, can indicate peripheral arterial disease or compartment syndrome. Skin color changes can indicate peripheral vascular disorders or vasomotor disorders like Raynaud's phenomenon.
- Tenderness over a particular bony landmark, ligament, or tendon can help to determine potential differential diagnoses. Once an area of tenderness is localized, the rest of the exam can be used to narrow down differential diagnoses. Localized tenderness suggests inflammation, injury, or infection.
- Any strength testing that is graded less than a 5/5 is abnormal, especially if it is unilateral. Weakness can be indicative of several diagnoses, including neurologic injury, a tendon/ligament injury, muscle strain or overuse syndrome, or even arthritis if the strength is limited due to pain. If weakness is noted, it is important to investigate further, asking if the weakness is due to pain, injury, or true weakness.
- If active ROM is abnormal or the patient cannot complete it, help the patient complete passive ROM. Decreased range of motion suggests one or more of the following:
  - Intraarticular joint problems causing pain with both active and passive ROM
  - Tendon or muscle problems causing weakness or pain with active ROM
  - Prolonged overuse syndrome of any cause
- Gait abnormalities can be multifactorial, due to injury, or seen with various chronic disease states. It is important to determine if the gait abnormality is a result of a musculoskeletal problem, a neurological problem, or a combination of both. An antalgic gait is a compensatory gait used to avoid pain. It is frequently seen in musculoskeletal disorders affecting the lower extremities, including the hip, knee, ankle, or foot. The gait alteration is typically accompanied by shortened steps, and the patient usually has a cane, walker, or crutches. The gait pattern should normalize when the pain resolves. It will not resolve if the pain is due to underlying chronic disease such as arthritis.

## CERVICAL SPINE

### INSPECTION

1. Observe the patient's posture and head position. Note any deformities, asymmetries, increased or decreased cervical lordosis, or excessive thoracic kyphosis. These abnormalities can be inherited or caused by conditions such as achondroplasia, obesity, torticollis, osteoporosis, spondylolisthesis, and kyphosis.

## PALPATION

1. Palpate each spinal process. Tenderness over the midline of the cervical spine when palpating the spinal processes can be indicative of a vertebral fracture.
2. Palpate the soft tissue including the paraspinal musculature, the sternocleidomastoid muscle, and the trapezius muscle. Pain with palpation of these muscles can indicate cervical muscle strain.

## RANGE OF MOTION

- Do not test cervical range of motion if unstable spine injury is suspected.
- Cervical range of motion should include flexion, extension, lateral rotation to the left and right, and lateral bending to the left and right. The majority of flexion/extension occurs between the occiput and C1, with the majority of rotation occurring between C1 and C2.
- Cervical spine ROM normal values:
  - **Flexion:** 45 degrees
  - **Extension:** 55 degrees
  - **Lateral rotation:** 70 degrees
  - **Lateral bending:** 40 degrees

## SPECIAL TESTS OF THE CERVICAL SPINE

- A proper cervical spine exam would also include cranial nerve (CN) testing (specifically CN XI) and reflex testing of the biceps (C5), brachioradialis (C6), and triceps (C7). See Chapter 8, "Nervous System," for more information on these exams.
- **Spurling test:** This test looks to identify if a nerve root is being compressed due to intervertebral disc pathology. Passively extend and rotate the patient's neck to the affected side. Slowly start applying axial pressure by pressing down on the top of the patient's head (Figure 9.1). Radicular pain extending down the arm on the same side as the test is considered a positive test. Be sure to rule out cervical instability, vertebral artery injury, and vertebral fracture before performing. It should not be performed in an acute trauma setting.

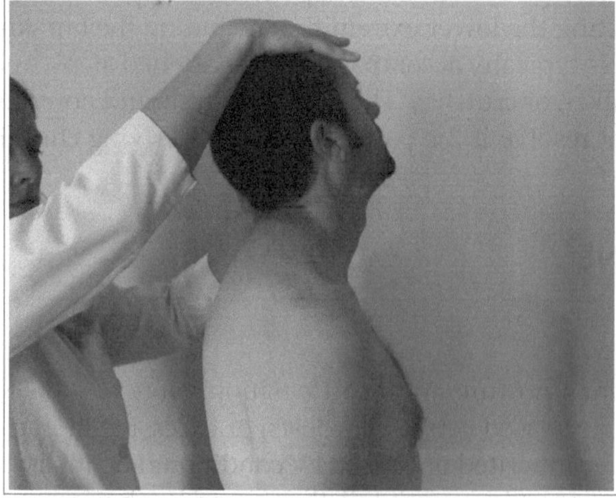

**Figure 9.1** Spurling test.

- **Extension-rotation test:** This test is best used to determine facet joint etiology. Move the patient into cervical extension, then laterally flex and rotate to the same side. Repeat with the contralateral side. The test is considered positive if the maneuver increases pain or causes numbness/tingling on the side of the neck being tested.

## THORACIC/LUMBAR SPINE

### INSPECTION

1. Inspect the spine, looking for increased lumbar lordosis, kyphosis, and side curvature of the spine (scoliosis).
2. Spinal curvature is best examined by having the patient flex forward while observing the spinous processes. The spinal processes should form a straight line. Deviations from midline can indicate scoliosis. Scoliosis is often accompanied by uneven shoulder height, uneven hip height, and a winged scapula.
3. Observe the iliac crests, gluteal folds, posterior superior iliac spines (PSIS), and the anterior superior iliac spines (ASIS) while the patient is standing. Note any differences in height between the left and right sides.
4. While the patient is supine, measure from the ASIS to the medial malleolus to check for true leg length discrepancies. This can then be compared to apparent leg length discrepancies as measured from the umbilicus to the medial malleolus to evaluate for possible pelvic obliquity.

### PALPATION

1. Palpation of the lumbar and thoracic spines should include individual spinous processes, the iliac crests (approximately at L4–L5 interspace), bilateral ASIS, greater trochanters, ischial tuberosities, and bilateral PSIS. The umbilicus often lies near the L3–L4 interspace. Look for any step-off deformities. The transition from one spinous process to the neighboring ones should be smooth, with a slight divot between each.

### RANGE OF MOTION

- Lumbar spine ROM normal values:
  - **Flexion:** 40 to 60 degrees
  - **Extension:** 20 to 35 degrees
  - **Lateral bending:** 15 to 20 degrees
  - **Lateral rotation:** 5 to 20 degrees

### SPECIAL TESTS OF THE LUMBAR SPINE

- **Straight leg raise:** This test looks to identify lumbar radiculopathy. Have the patient lie supine. Lift one leg at a time to 90 degrees or as far as the patient can tolerate. Place your other hand on the knee to ensure full knee extension. The test is considered positive if there is pain between 30 and 70 degrees of hip flexion that radiates below the knee. To further confirm neurologic etiology, slightly lower the leg and dorsiflex the foot; this will often also reproduce the radicular symptoms.

- **Valsalva maneuver**: This test looks to identify if the pain is coming from the spinal canal. With the patient sitting, have them take a deep breath and bear down as if trying to have a bowel movement. Localized or radicular pain is considered a positive test.
- Have the patient stand and observe them from the front. Note the symmetry of the patient's shoulders. The shoulders should be even. Uneven shoulder height can be a clue to scoliosis. Ask the patient to turn around and bend at the waist. The clinician should stand behind the patient and observe the patient from the rear. The spine should be straight without curvature and centered over the sacrum. Angles of less than 10 degrees can often be followed with periodic radiographs. Angles of up to 30 degrees, typically show no lasting effects into adulthood. Angles over 50 degrees will lead to complications later in life. In more severe cases of scoliosis, a unilateral rib hump and winged scapula may be present, as noted above. Routine screening for scoliosis is not recommended.

# SHOULDER

## INSPECTION

1. When inspecting the shoulder, evaluate the patient's arm swing. Does it appear equal or does the motion seem limited on one side? Movements should be smooth and coordinated. Use the contralateral side for comparison, not just during inspection, but when testing range of motion, strength, and special tests.
2. Look for any muscle atrophy (indicative of a nerve palsy or extreme deconditioning), deformity (fracture or dislocation), winging scapula (scoliosis), Popeye deformity (loss of the superior attachment of the biceps tendon), or scars (post surgery or injury).

## PALPATION

1. **Palpate the bony landmarks:** Scapula (including the coracoid process, acromion process, spine of scapula, superior and inferior angles of the scapula, and the medial and lateral borders of the scapula); clavicle (including sternal end, acromial end, entire shaft); and humerus (including the deltoid tuberosity, the greater tuberosity [lateral], the bicipital groove, and the lesser tuberosity [medial]).
2. **Palpate the joints and ligaments:** Sternoclavicular joint, the acromioclavicular (AC) joint, the sternoclavicular ligament, and the acromioclavicular ligament. Palpation of the rotator cuff should include the following:
   a. **Supraspinatus tendon:** Below the anterior lateral acromion
   b. **Infraspinatus tendon:** Below posterolateral acromion
   c. **Teres minor:** Inferior to the infraspinatus
   d. **Subscapularis insertion:** Lateral to coracoid at the anterior shoulder
   e. **Spine of the scapula:** Origin of the infraspinatus
3. **Palpate the areas of soft tissue:** Insertion point of the rotator cuff muscles at greater tuberosity; the axilla borders; the serratus anterior muscles; the pectoralis major muscles; the upper, middle, and lower trapezius; the deltoid (anterior, middle, and posterior bellies); the sternocleidomastoid; the biceps insertion and belly; and the latissimus dorsi muscles.
4. When palpating the musculature, feel for tenderness and tone, and compare the muscles to the contralateral side.
5. Have the patient perform the Apley's scratch test. Ask the patient to abduct and externally rotate their arms, then reach behind their back and touch the contralateral

scapula. Next, have the patient abduct and internally rotate their arm, then ask the patient to reach behind their back as if tucking in their shirt, and reach as far up their back as possible. Compare range of motion bilaterally.

6. To test active horizontal adduction, have the patient abduct their arms to 90 degrees, flex the elbow to 90 degrees, then reach across the front of their body and touch the contralateral AC joint.
7. To test for full abduction range of motion, have the patient externally rotate their arm to allow the humeral head to clear under the acromion.

## RANGE OF MOTION

***Passive Range of Motion Normal Values***

- **Abduction:** 180 degrees (approximately 2/3 of motion comes from glenohumeral joint, 1/3 from thoracoscapular joint)
- **Adduction:** 45 degrees
- **External rotation:** 90 degrees
- **Internal rotation:** 90 degrees
- **Forward flexion:** 180 degrees
- **Extension:** 50 degrees
- **Horizontal adduction:** 45 degrees

Test all shoulder movements and compare bilaterally.

## SPECIAL TESTS OF THE SHOULDER

Shoulder tests should be completed in clusters, in contrast to completing a single test, to improve the reliability of results.

- **Hawkins-Kennedy test:** This test helps to identify shoulder impingement, particularly of the supraspinatus. While holding the patient's elbow at 90 degrees with one hand, and their wrist with the other hand, flex the shoulder to 90 degrees, then internally rotate (Figure 9.2). Pain and apprehension are considered positive tests.

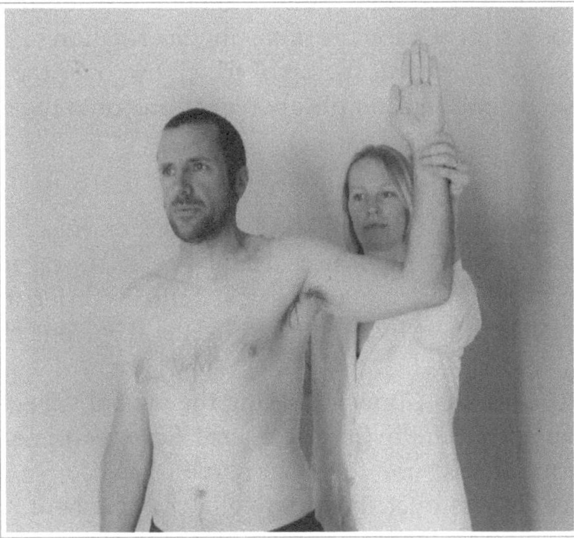

**Figure 9.2** Hawkins–Kennedy test.

- **Neer test:** This test also looks to identify supraspinatus impingement. While stabilizing the patient's scapula, passively forward flex the arm while the arm is in the pronated position. Pain and apprehension are considered positive tests.
- **Empty-can test:** This test helps to identify supraspinatus weakness due to a tear, impingement, or a nerve injury. Have the patient abduct both of their arms to 90 degrees in the scapular plane (approximately 30 degrees of horizontal adduction). Next, have them internally rotate the shoulder, so their thumbs are pointing to the ground. Then, have the patient try to actively resist adduction. A positive test is an inability to hold the arm in the testing position.
- **Painful arc test:** Ask the patient to forward flex the arm in 30 degrees of horizontal adduction. Ask them to slowly move their arms overhead to 180 degrees. Pain in the 60–120 degrees of flexion range is considered positive. Pain will often be worse with internal rotation and somewhat relieved with external rotation. A positive test is indicative of subacromial impingement.
- **External rotation resistance test:** This test is used to identify rotator cuff pathology, particularly of the infraspinatus and teres minor. While standing in front of the patient, have them flex their elbow to 90 degrees, then have them try to externally rotate the shoulder while providing resistance. Pain or weakness is considered a positive result. The test can be repeated with the arm abducted to 90 degrees.
- **Lag test**: This test also looks to identify rotator cuff pathology. With the patient seated, have them flex their elbow to 90 degrees, then abduct to 90 degrees. Move them 5 degrees less of full external rotation then ask them to hold the position. An inability to hold the position when support is removed is considered a positive test.

## ELBOW

### INSPECTION

1. Examine the elbow in both flexion and extension.
2. Identify the carrying angle with the elbow in extension. A normal carrying angle is between 5–15 degrees valgus. An increase in the angle is known as "cubitus valgus." Cubitus varus is a decrease in that angle, also known as "gunstock deformity"; in children, this can be a sign of a fracture affecting the rotation of the distal end of the humerus. Also, look for edema at the tip of the elbow, over the olecranon fossa, as olecranon bursitis is a common complication of falling onto the tip of the elbow.

### PALPATION

1. **Palpate the bony landmarks:** Medial and lateral epicondyles, origins for the wrist flexors and extensor bundles, the medial and lateral supracondylar lines of the humerus, the olecranon, the olecranon fossa, the ulnar border, and the radial head. The radial head is felt about an inch distal to the lateral epicondyle during pronation and supination.
2. Palpate the soft tissue of the elbow, including the medial side of the elbow, feeling for the origin of the flexor bundle (pronator teres, flexor carpi radialis, palmaris longus, and flexor carpi ulnaris), and the ulnar nerve.
3. Palpate for any tenderness over the ulnar collateral ligament. On the lateral side, palpate the extensor bundle (brachioradialis, extensor carpi radialis longus, and the extensor carpi radialis brevis) and feel for any tenderness over the radial collateral

and the annular ligaments. The hand should be moved anteriorly to find the insertion of the biceps tendon and the brachial artery, which lies just medial to the biceps insertion point. The median nerve is found medial to the brachial artery.

## RANGE OF MOTION

### *Passive Range of Motion Normal Values*

- **Flexion:** 135 degrees
- **Extension:** 0 to 5 degrees hyperextension
- **Supination:** 90 degrees
- **Pronation:** 90 degrees

## SPECIAL TESTS OF THE ELBOW

- **Cozen test:** This test looks to identify lateral epicondylitis, also known as "tennis elbow." With the elbow stabilized and the hand pronated and in a fist, have the patient extend their wrist against resistance. Pain over the lateral epicondyle is considered a positive test.
- **Golfer's elbow test:** This test looks to identify medial epicondylitis, or golfer's elbow. Again, with the elbow stabilized, have the patient supinate their hand and close their fist. Next, have the patient flex their wrist against resistance. Pain over the medial epicondyle is considered a positive test.
- **Varus stress test:** This test looks to identify injury to the radial (lateral) collateral ligament of the elbow. With the wrist stabilized, apply a varus force to the medial side of the elbow while it is flexed to 20 or 30 degrees. Pain or excess motion compared to the contralateral side is considered a positive test.
- **Valgus stress test**: This test seeks to identify injury to the ulnar (medial) collateral ligament of the elbow. With the elbow flexed to 20 or 30 degrees and the wrist stabilized, apply a valgus force to the lateral elbow. Pain or excess motion compared to the contralateral side is considered a positive test.
- **Tinel's sign**: This test looks to identify compression of the ulnar nerve. With the elbow relaxed and the wrist supported, tap the ulnar nerve as it courses through the ulnar notch (Figure 9.3). Tingling or pain along the ulnar distribution is considered a positive test.

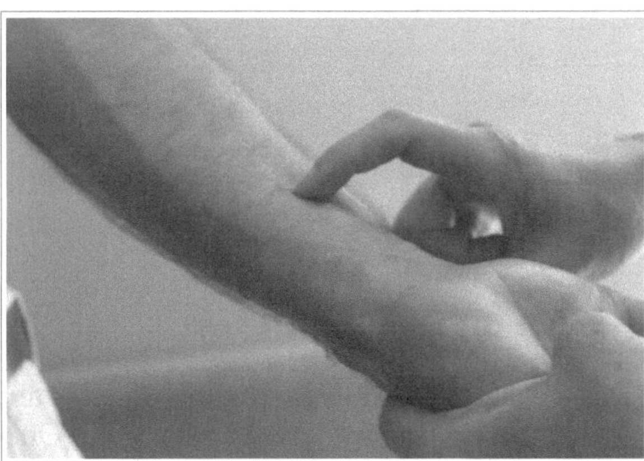

**Figure 9.3** Tinel's sign.

## WRIST/HAND

### INSPECTION

1. Inspect the wrist and hand. Ensure all five fingers are present. Missing digits or parts of digits are not always noticeable at first glance. Observe the creases on the hands. Note the thenar eminence, the thick muscle belly at the base of the thumb, and the hypothenar eminence at the base of the little finger.
2. Inspection of the fingers and nails is also essential for a thorough exam. With the fingers extended, look for rotation or crossing over of the fingers. This could be a sign of a phalange or metacarpal fracture. With a closed fist, the fingers should lay next to each other and again, not cross one another.

### PALPATION

1. Palpate the styloid processes of both the radius and the ulna. Then, move to the anatomical snuffbox, the depression on the radial side of the wrist bordered by the abductor pollicis longus and the extensor pollicis brevis tendons. Tenderness in this area is a sign of a possible scaphoid fracture. Feel for fullness and good muscle tone in the thenar and hypothenar eminences.
2. Palpate the entire length of each metacarpal, again feeling for any tenderness or deformity. Finish the bony palpation at the fingers with each phalange and interphalangeal joint.

### RANGE OF MOTION

#### *Passive Range of Motion Normal Values*

- **Wrist extension:** 70 degrees
- **Wrist flexion**: 80 degrees
- **Radial deviation**: 20 degrees
- **Ulnar deviation**: 30 degrees
- **MCP flexion**: 80 to 90 degrees
- **MCL extension**: 30 to 45 degrees
- **PIP flexion**: 100 degrees
- **PIP extension**: 0 degrees
- **DIP flexion**: 90 degrees
- **DIP extension**: 20 degrees
- **Finger abduction:** 20 degrees
- **Finger adduction**: 0 degrees
- **Thumb MCP flexion:** 50 degrees
- **Thumb MCP extension:** 20 degrees
- **Thumb abduction:** 70 degrees
- **Thumb adduction:** 0 degrees

### SPECIAL TESTS FOR THE WRIST AND HAND

- **Finkelstein test:** This test helps to identify tenosynovitis of the abductor pollicus longus and extensor pollicus brevis tendons, also known as "DeQuervain's syndrome." With the forearm stabilized, have the patient grasp their thumb in their fist, then perform ulnar deviation of the hand. Pain over the tendons is considered a positive test. Be sure to slowly deviate the hand, as this test, when positive, can be exquisitely painful.

- **Phalen's test**: This test looks to identify median nerve pathology, particularly carpal tunnel syndrome. Have the patient sit with the dorsum of their hands touching, in maximal wrist flexion, applying force through the wrists, for 1 minute (Figure 9.4). Numbness or tingling in the median nerve distribution is considered a positive test.

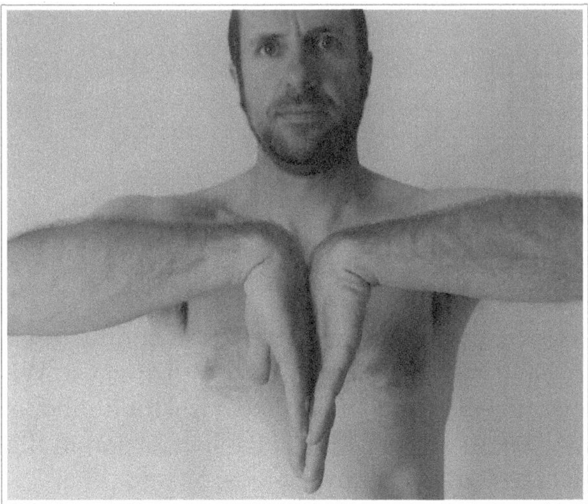

**Figure 9.4** Phalen's test.

- **Varus/Valgus test:** As with the elbow, the collateral ligaments in the fingers can be tested with a varus or valgus force applied while the joint is relaxed and supported. Pain or excess motion compared to the contralateral side is considered a positive test. This test is particularly useful at the MCP joint of the thumb to identify skier's thumb, or a tear of the ulnar collateral ligament at the base of the thumb with increased motion or pain with a valgus force.

# HIP

## INSPECTION

1. Inspect the hips.
2. Inspect the bony landmarks, including the levels of the iliac crests, PSIS, ASIS, gluteal folds, and medial malleoli, to determine the symmetry of the lower limbs, leg length, or possible pelvic obliquity.
3. Note the bony landmarks while the patient is standing and lying supine.
4. A measurement from the ASIS to the medial malleolus is considered a true leg length measurement and should be done bilaterally for comparison. A measurement from the umbilicus to the medial malleolus is considered an apparent leg length measurement and can be compared to the true leg length measurement to help identify possible soft tissue adaptations that can result in apparent leg length differences even when true ones do not exist.

## PALPATION

1. Palpate the hip. True hip joint pathology typically presents as pain and tenderness in the groin. Pain on the lateral hip, over the greater trochanter, is more commonly a trochanteric bursitis or abductor tendonitis, possibly related to a tight IT band or gluteal musculature.

2. Palpate the ischial tuberosities deep in the gluteal folds as this is the origin of the hamstrings and a common area of injury.

## RANGE OF MOTION

***Passive Range of Motion Normal Values***

- **Flexion:** 120 degrees
- **Extension:** 20–30 degrees
- **Abduction**: 40 degrees
- **Adduction:** 20 degrees
- **Internal rotation:** 30 degrees
- **External rotation:** –60 degree

## SPECIAL TESTS FOR THE HIP

- **Thomas test**: This test is used to identify hip flexor contracture and tightness. With the patient supine, have them bring one knee to their chest. When completing this maneuver, it is imperative for the clinician to control for lumbopelvic movement (i.e., pelvic tilt) (Vigotsky, Lehman, et al., 2016). Passive flexion in the contralateral leg is considered a positive test on the contralateral side.
- **FABER test:** This test looks to identify hip flexor, sacroiliac, or hip intra-articular pathology. FABER stands for **F**lexion, **AB**duction, and **E**xternal **R**otation. With the patient supine, have them flex, abduct, and externally rotate the hip until the ankle rests upon the contralateral knee. Then, apply downward pressure, moving the knee closer to the table (Figure 9.5). Pain or decreased range of motion is considered a positive test.

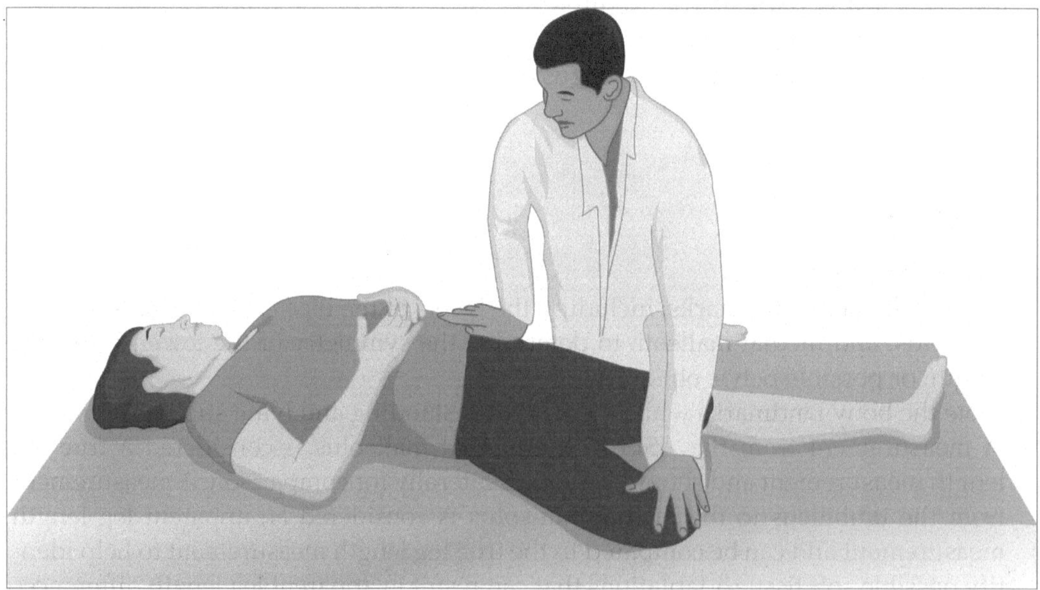

**Figure 9.5** FABER test.

- **Log roll:** This test looks to identify intra-articular pathology, particularly symptomatic arthritis. With the patient supine, hold the ankle or knee and passively internally and externally rotate the leg. Pain in the groin is considered a positive test.

- **Stinchfield test:** This test identifies intra-articular hip pathology. With the patient supine, have them flex the hip to 30 or 45 degrees. Apply a downward pressure on the ankle with the patient resisting. Pain in the groin is considered a positive test.
- **Trendelenburg's test:** This test looks to identify weakness of the abductor musculature. Have the patient stand on one leg for 10 seconds, then switch legs. Weakness of the gluteus medius on the standing side will lead to a dip of the pelvis on the unsupported side. If this is seen, it is considered a positive test.
- The Barlow-Ortolani maneuvers are designed to test for hip dislocations and subluxations in 0- to 1-year-olds. With the infant supine, flex the hips and knees to 90 degrees. The clinician's thumbs should rest on the medial side of the knees, fingers resting on the greater trochanters. Adduct the thighs and put gentle pressure through the femurs, trying to shift them out of the acetabulums. A clunk is considered positive. For the next step, slowly abduct the thighs and use the fingers to put pressure on the trochanters to guide the femoral head back into position. Again, a clunk is considered a positive test and could be a sign of hip subluxation or dislocation. If dysplasia is suspected within the first 6 months of life, an ultrasound evaluation is preferred to x-ray. If any tests are abnormal, refer to a pediatric orthopedic clinician for intervention(s) and/or treatment options.

## KNEE

### INSPECTION

1. Inspect the knee. Look for any deformity, asymmetry, and/or edema.
2. Look for genu valgus (knock knee) and genu varus (bow-legged). A prominent tibial tuberosity can be a sign of Osgood–Schlatter's disease, which is common in adolescence.

### PALPATION

1. Palpate the knee. On the lateral side of the knee, palpate the fibular head, lateral joint line, lateral femoral condyle, IT band and insertion on Gerdy's tubercle, biceps femoris insertion, and the lateral collateral ligament. On the medial side, palpate the medial joint line, MCL origin and insertion, pes anserine, and muscle bellies of the semitendinosus and semimembranosus. Feel anteriorly for the patella and its borders, the tibial tuberosity, and the patellar and quadriceps tendons. On the posterior side, feel in the popliteal fossa for a possible fluid collection, known as a "Baker's cyst." This can be a sign of a meniscus tear. Often, meniscus tears will refer to pain to the popliteal fossa.

### RANGE OF MOTION

*Passive Range of Motion Normal Values*

- **Flexion:** 130 to 140 degrees
- **Extension:** 0 to 5 degrees hyperextension

### SPECIAL TESTS FOR THE KNEE

- **Valgus stress test:** This test helps to identify injury to the medial collateral ligament. With the patient supine and relaxed, hold the ankle of the patient and apply a valgus stress to the lateral knee. Test in full extension and in 20 to 30 degrees of knee flexion. Pain or excessive laxity is considered a positive test.

- **Varus stress test:** This test looks to identify injury to the lateral collateral ligament. With the patient supine and relaxed, hold the ankle of the patient and applying a varus stress to the medial knee. Test in full extension and in 20 to 30 degrees of knee flexion. Pain or excessive laxity is considered a positive test.
- **Anterior drawer test:** This test helps to identify injury to the anterior cruciate ligament. With the patient supine, have them flex their hip to 45 degrees and flex their knee to 90 degrees, resting their foot on the table. Next, the clinician should sit on the patient's foot to stabilize the leg and place their hands behind the proximal tibia, resting their thumbs on the tibial tuberosity. Use the index fingers to ensure relaxation of the hamstring muscles. Apply an anterior force. Increased anterior translation is indicative of an ACL tear.
- **Posterior drawer test**: This test looks to identify injury to the posterior cruciate ligament. With the patient supine, have them flex their hip to 45 degrees and flex the knee to 90 degrees, resting their foot on the table. Next, sit on the patient's foot to stabilize the leg. Hands should be placed behind the proximal tibia, resting the thumbs on the tibial tuberosity. Use the index fingers to ensure relaxation of the hamstring muscles. Apply a posterior force. Increased posterior translation is indicative of a PCL tear.
- **Lachman test**: This test is used to identify a tear to the ACL. With the patient supine and relaxed, place the outside or proximal hand over the distal thigh and inside hand, or distal hand, over the proximal tibia. Allowing the hip to externally rotate can help ensure the patient is relaxed. Next, apply anterior translation force on the tibia with the distal hand while stabilizing the thigh with the proximal hand (Figure 9.6). Excessive anterior tibial translation is indicative of an ACL tear. This test can be challenging if the patient is guarding.

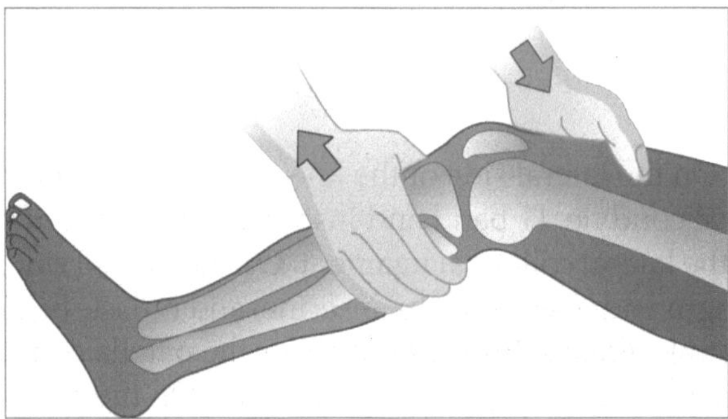

**Figure 9.6** Lachman test.

- **McMurray's test:** This test identifies meniscus pathology. With the patient supine, use one hand to grasp the patient's ankle and the other hand to stabilize the patient's knee. With the knee flexed, externally rotate the tibia and apply a valgus force while extending the knee. Next, move the knee from flexion while internally rotating the tibia and applying a varus force. Pain or clicking over the medial or lateral joint lines is considered a positive test.
- **Apprehension test**: This test looks to identify patellar laxity or subluxations/dislocations. With the patient supine and relaxed, place the knee in full extension. Next, apply a lateral force to the medial border of the patella. Pain or guarding is considered a positive test.

- **Ballottement test**: This test looks for joint effusion in the knee. Joint effusion is mostly caused by trauma to the knee. The patient should lay in the supine position with the legs extended. The clinician should place one hand superior to the patella and use the other hand to apply downward pressure in an anterior to posterior "milking" motion. If there is fluid present, the clinician will feel it against their lower hand. Then gently push down on the patella. If the patella can be depressed, it means that it was "floating" in fluid and signifies a positive test.
- **Bulge sign:** This is another test commonly used to test for knee effusion. Gently press slightly medial to the patella. Then move the hand in an ascending motion and apply pressure firmly on the lateral aspect of the knee. A positive test would be if a "bulge" is seen on the medial aspect of the knee after the lateral pressure was applied. This would indicate that a moderate amount of fluid is present. A medial aspect that does not bulge but tensely reflects lateral pressure is consistent with a large amount of fluid.

## ANKLE/FOOT

### INSPECTION

1. Start with inspecting the patient's footwear. Shoes can provide information on wear patterns and show where a person is putting pressure on their feet throughout their gait cycle. This can provide information about possible foot deformities or gait patterns.
2. Observe the foot and ankle of the patient both in standing and sitting positions. Look for deformities and asymmetries as with any other joint. It is important to note any areas of calluses or corn formations. Calluses can indicate abnormal weightbearing or improperly fitting shoes. The skin should be the thickest around the heel, at the lateral border, and over the metatarsal heads.
3. Look at the arches in the patient's feet. The arches should be more pronounced when the patient is not bearing weight.
4. Observe the metatarsals. There are also several toe deformities, including claw toes, hammertoes, and mallet toes, that should be noted on inspection.

### PALPATION

1. Palpate the medial side of the ankle and foot. Palpate over the medial malleolus, then down the foot to the navicular bone (most prominent bone on the medial side). Palpate the medial head of the talus, which is just proximal to the navicular bone. Move down the foot to the first metatarsal then distally to the first phalange and the interphalangeal joint. On the lateral side, start palpation at the lateral malleolus, then move inferiorly to palpate the peroneus longus and brevis. Just distal to the lateral malleolus is the area of the anterior talofibular ligament. Palpate down the foot and feel for the styloid process of the fifth metatarsal. This is a common area of avulsion or stress fractures. Lastly, palpate the shaft of the metatarsals and phalanges, feeling for the metatarsophalangeal (MTP) and interphalangeal (IP) joints.
2. On the posterior foot, palpate the Achilles tendon and its insertion site, feeling for any crepitus or nodularity. Then, move to the plantar surface and the calcaneus. Continue moving distally and palpate the metatarsal shafts and heads, feeling for any tenderness.

3. Palpating for pedal pulses. The posterior tibial artery can be palpated just posterior to the medial malleolus, and the dorsalis pedis artery can be palpated between the extensor hallicus longus and the extensor digitorum longus tendons. Absent or diminished pedal pulses can indicate peripheral vascular disease, compartment syndrome, or other pathology.

## RANGE OF MOTION

***Passive Range of Motion Normal Values***

- **Dorsiflexion**: 20 degrees
- **Plantarflexion:** 50 degrees
- **Inversion:** 30 degrees
- **Eversion:** 20 degrees
- **Abduction:** 10 degrees
- **Adduction:** 20 degrees
- **1st MTP flexion:** 45 degrees
- **1st MTP extension:** 70 degrees

## SPECIAL TESTS FOR THE ANKLE/FOOT

- **Squeeze test**: This test is used to identify syndesmotic (or high) ankle injuries or fractures. With the patient relaxed, squeeze the proximal tibia and fibula together. Pinpoint pain or pain distally is considered a positive test.
- **Talar tilt:** This test identifies ligamentous ankle injury. With the patient relaxed and the foot in a neutral position, passively move the foot into an adducted position, pain or increased motion is considered positive and a sign of damage to the lateral ankle ligaments. Next, passively move the foot into an abducted position. Pain or increased motion is considered a positive test.
- **Thompson test:** This test is used to evaluate the integrity of the Achilles tendon complex. With the patient prone or seated with the foot unsupported, squeeze the belly of the gastrocnemius. With an intact complex, the foot should use passively plantar flex when the calf is squeezed. No plantar flexion of the foot is considered a positive test.

# RED FLAGS IN HISTORY AND PHYSICAL EXAM

- Cervical spinal injury or trauma
- History of cancer
- Associated neurological deficits
- Saddle anesthesia
- Loss of bowel or bladder control
- Paralysis
- Weakness (especially unilateral with an acute onset or progressive)
- Gross deformity
- Associated unintended weight loss
- Point tenderness
- Extreme pain or pain that reoccurs over time
- Absence of pulses

# POPULATION HEALTH AND LIFE-SPAN CONSIDERATIONS

## INFANTS AND CHILDREN

- The skin on the spine should be inspected at birth for any abnormalities, including hairy patches, café-au-lait spots, or doughy lipomata. These findings could be indicative of underlying neurological pathology such as spina bifida.
- The majority (about 90%) of peak bone mass is acquired by girls by age 18 and in boys by age 20, making childhood the best time to ensure bone health through proper nutrition and exercise.
- Apophyses are weak and vulnerable to both macro- and micro-trauma and a common site of injury for children.
- Epiphyseal plates (growth plates) and the epiphysis (end of the bone) are also very vulnerable to injury. Roughly 1/3 of pediatric injuries are located within or near the growth plate.
- Isolated ligament injury is rare in children younger than 14. Children's ligaments are stronger than the physes and epiphyses, so bone or growth plate fractures or ligamentous bony avulsions are more common.
- The growing adolescent skeleton is even more susceptible to both overuse and acute injury. Increases in height and body mass increase the incidence of sport and exercise-related injury.
- Gower's sign is a sign of muscle weakness in the proximal hip muscles and is commonly associated with muscular dystrophy. Gower's sign is noted when the child moves from sitting on the floor to standing. In a positive test, the child will move from hands and knees to hands and feet, then move hands to knees to help push themselves to a standing position (Figure 9.7).

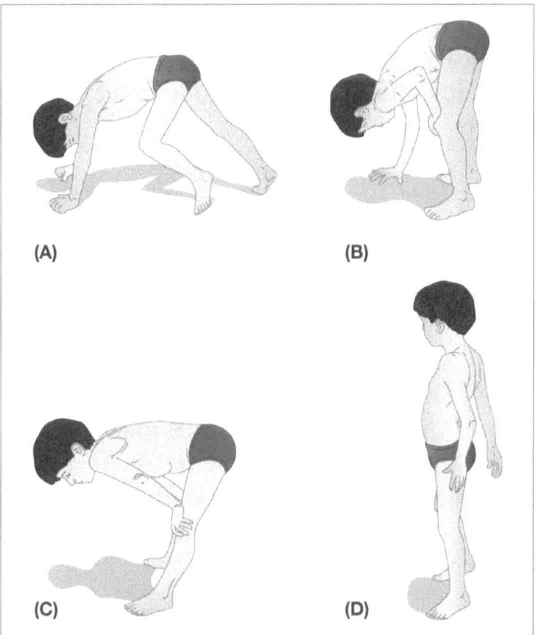


**Figure 9.7** Gower's sign. In a positive test, the child will move from hands and knees (A) to hands and feet (B), then move hands to knees (C) to help push themselves to a standing position (D).

## OLDER ADULTS

- As people age, their muscle mass decreases even with regular exercise. Muscle fibers shrink and may lose tone.
- Older adults lose bone mass and bone density especially women following menopause. Bone fractures and breaks become more common due to osteopenia and osteoporosis.
- Many joints such as hips, knees, and fingers began to lose cartilage.
- Joints become stiffer and less flexible due to degenerative changes in cartilage and loss of joint fluid.
- Changes in gait and posture often occur. Posture may become more stooped, and walking patterns become shorter and shorter.
- Spinal discs become thinner and lose fluid. This contributes to a shortened spine and decreased height.
- A hip fracture can be life-threatening in the elderly.

## OTHER CONSIDERATIONS

- Men have more muscle mass and on average, are physically stronger and faster than women. Men have an average of 26 pounds more skeletal muscle mass than women. However, men's muscles tend to fatigue more easily than women's.
- Women have a wider pelvis and a larger hip width to femoral length. This makes their body mechanisms different from their male counterparts and putting them at greater risk for certain injuries.
- Women are at increased risk for musculoskeletal injuries specifically tearing a knee ligament, spraining an ankle, developing osteoarthritis of the knee, fracturing a hip (due to osteoporosis), and tearing an anterior cruciate ligament.
- African Americans tend to have longer limbs and a higher center of gravity compared to Caucasians. Asians and Caucasians tend to have longer torsos which makes their centers of gravity lower.
- African Americans have higher bone density, followed by Caucasians and Hispanics. Asians have the lowest bone density.

# KEY DIFFERENTIALS

## SPINE (CERVICAL)

- Acute meningitis
- Acute whiplash
- Angina pectoralis
- Carotid insufficiency
- Cervical facet syndrome
- Cervical strain and sprain
- Radiculopathy
- Spine instability
- Spinal stenosis
- Spondylosis
- Torticollis

## SPINE (LOWER)

- Ankylosing spondylitis
- Compression fractures
- Herniated disc
- Infection
- Malignancy
- Muscle strain
- Sciatica
- Spinal stenosis
- Spondylolisthesis
- Scoliosis*

## HAND/WRIST

- Bone fracture
- Carpal tunnel syndrome
- Dupuytren contracture
- DeQuervain's tenosynovitis
- Ligament tears
- Overuse syndrome
- Sprained wrist
- Trigger finger (trigger thumb)

## ELBOW

- Biceps tendinopathy
- Cubital tunnel syndrome
- Lateral epicondylitis (tennis elbow)
- Medial epicondylitis (golfer's elbow)
- Olecranon bursitis
- Osteochondral defect
- Posterior impingement
- Radial head subluxation (nursemaid's elbow)
- Radial tunnel syndrome
- Triceps tendinopathy
- Ulnar collateral ligament injury

## SHOULDER

- AC joint sprain
- Adhesive capsulitis (frozen shoulder)
- Biceps tendonitis
- Bone fracture/break (clavicle, humerus)
- Glenohumeral or AC joint arthritis
- Subacromial bursitis
- Subacromial impingement
- Tear (rotator cuff, labral, proximal biceps)

## HIP

- Developmental dysplasia of the hip*
- Femoroacetabular impingement
- Hip impingement syndrome
- Hip labral tear
- Iliopsoas bursitis
- Legg-Calve-Perthes disease*
- Piriformis syndrome
- Septic arthritis
- Slipped fapital femoral epiphysis*
- Stress fracture
- Trochanteric bursitis

*Seen mostly in the pediatric population.

## KNEE

- Bursitis
- Chondromalacia patella
- Ligament tears (anterior cruciate ligament, posterior cruciate ligament, lateral collateral ligament, medial collateral ligament)
- Medial plica syndrome
- Meniscus tear
- Patellar sublaxation/dislocation
- Patellar tendonitis
- Patellofemoral syndrome
- Popliteal cyst
- Osgood-Schlatter disease
- Osteoarthritis
- Overuse syndromes

## FOOT/ANKLE

- Achilles tendonitis
- Ankle sprain
- Bunion
- Clubfoot*
- Plantar fasciitis
- Stress fracture

## OTHER

- Gout
- Muscular dystrophy*
- Osteoporosis/osteopenia
- Osteoarthritis
- Rheumatoid arthritis

*Seen mostly in the pediatric population.

# REFERENCE

Vigotsky, A. D., Lehman, G. J., Beardsley, C., Chung, B., &Feser, E. H. (2016). The modified Thomas test is not a valid measure of hip extension unless pelvic tilt is controlled. *PeerJ 4*, e2325. doi:10.7717/peerj.2325.

# KNOWLEDGE CHECK: MUSCULOSKELETAL SYSTEM

1. A 50-year-old states that she thinks that she has rheumatoid arthritis "like her mom." Which physical findings would MOST indicate that she may have rheumatoid arthritis?

   **A.** Her back and hips are stiff and have decreased range of motion
   **B.** She is experiencing stiffness and pain in her knees throughout the day
   **C.** She is experiencing painful inflammation in her hands, fingers, knees, and feet
   **D.** The joints in her right hand are enlarged, stiff, and non-tender to palpation

2. A positive straight leg raise usually indicates:

   **A.** Hip or trochanteric bursitis
   **B.** Lumbar nerve root irritation
   **C.** Muscle strain and/or spasm
   **D.** Poor posture or conditioning

3. A 13-year-old complains of knee pain that began during the basketball season. The advanced practice nurse is considering Osgood-Schlatter disease as the likely diagnosis. All of the following assessments are typical of Osgood-Schlatter disease, except:

   **A.** Nighttime knee pain
   **B.** Pain is worse after vigorous activity
   **C.** Pain with palpation of the tibial tuberosity
   **D.** Swelling just below the patella

4. Tinel's test to assess for entrapment of the median nerve in the carpal tunnel is performed by having the individual seated and:

   **A.** Asking them to approximate their wrists and apply pressure for 1 minute
   **B.** Asking them to place their hands in a praying position for 1 minute
   **C.** Lightly tapping or percussing the palmar surface of the wrist
   **D.** Requesting them to raise both hands above their shoulders

5. The physical exam of an infant 24 hours after C-section delivery for breech presentation reveals asymmetry of gluteal, inguinal, and thigh skin folds. Which assessments are a priority for this infant?

   **A.** Barlow-Ortolani maneuvers
   **B.** Curvature of cervical and thoracic spine
   **C.** Flexibility and mobility of both ankles
   **D.** Talar tilt and Thompson tests

*(See answers next page.)* 

**1. C) She is experiencing painful inflammation in her hands, fingers, knees, and feet**

Rheumatoid arthritis (RA) is a chronic inflammatory disorder that affects numerous joints, causing painful swelling, redness, warmth, and deformity. Individuals with osteoarthritis (OA) will also experience stiffness and joint deformities, but they are unlikely to experience overall symptoms. RA is common in hands and fingers and is bilateral; OA is less symmetrical and often affects the spine and hips.

**2. B) Lumbar nerve root irritation**

The straight leg raise (SLR) is a maneuver done when an individual has low back pain to assess for lumbosacral nerve root irritation or impingement. Muscle strain, muscle spasms, and poor muscle tone are common causes of low back pain that do not correlate with radiculopathies and would not result in pain with the SLR. Hip or trochanteric bursitis causes inflammation that is also not reproduced with the SLR. Disc herniation, prolapse or protrusion, malignant intraspinal lesions, osteomyelitis, and sciatica can lead to radiculopathy; pain associated with these disorders is reproduced with the SLR.

**3. A) Nighttime knee pain**

Osgood-Schlatter disease is a common cause of knee pain in adolescents, caused by the extra stress that physical activity causes during growth spurts. Symptoms include anterior knee pain, with swelling and tenderness to palpation of the tibial tuberosity just below the patella where the patellar tendon attaches to the tibia. Nighttime knee pain is more common with conditions like arthritis; rest helps resolve the symptoms of Osgood-Schlatter disease.

**4. D) Requesting them to raise both hands above their shoulders**

Carpal tunnel syndrome is a condition causing pain, numbness, and tingling in the hand because of median nerve compression. Tinel's test involves percussing or tapping the wrist at the area where the median nerve is compressed to reproduce the symptoms. There are other tests that can also reproduce symptoms, including Phalen's test (holding flexion of the wrists), the Reverse Phalen's test (maintaining extension), and raising the hands in the air, above the level of the shoulders.

**5. A) Barlow-Ortolani maneuvers**

Asymmetry of the gluteal, inguinal, and thigh skin folds are signs of developmental dysplasia of the hip (DDH). Risk factors for DDH include breech position in utero, and female gender. Barlow-Ortolani maneuvers are designed to test for hip dislocations and subluxations in infants from birth through one year of age; if smooth movement is interrupted by a "clunk" with either maneuver, referral to a pediatric orthopedic clinician is indicated for DDH evaluation and treatment. Assessing spinal curvature is a priority for evaluation of scoliosis. Assessing ankle position and mobility is a priority for an infant with suspected talipes equinovarus or congenital clubfoot. The Talar tilt and Thompson tests are special tests to evaluate for ankle strains or fractures.

6. A 13-year-old male has a 3-month history of pain in left knee, thigh, and groin, which has significantly worsened despite limited participation in physical activities. He has no known injury, is overweight, and has been limping. His history is most consistent with the diagnosis of:

   **A.** Adolescent growth spurt
   **B.** Duchene muscular dystrophy
   **C.** Osgood–Schlatter disease
   **D.** Slipped capital femoral epiphysis

7. An individual reports "twisting my ankle" while jogging on an uneven surface. Which finding indicates need for an ankle x-ray, based on Ottawa ankle rules?

   **A.** Lateral ankle discoloration and swelling
   **B.** Moderate pain with weight bearing for 24 hours after the injury
   **C.** Pain in the mid-foot and bony tenderness at the navicular bone
   **D.** Pain with internal rotation of the foot and ankle

8. A 34-year-old truck driver reports a sharp pain in the lower back that worsens with ambulation. The symptoms began after a strenuous 3-day drive. The patient has difficulty walking on the heels and shows weakness in the extensors of the big toes. The MOST LIKELY diagnosis is:

   **A.** Compression fracture
   **B.** L5 or S1 root irritation
   **C.** Upper lumbar disc herniation
   **D.** Spondylosis

9. The advanced practice nurse notes a positive anterior drawer sign when evaluating the knee of a female college athlete, which suggests an unstable knee joint related to:

   **A.** Ligament damage
   **B.** Meniscus tear
   **C.** Patellar dislocation or subluxation
   **D.** Weak quadriceps muscle

10. Which three special tests of the shoulder together indicate supraspinatus nerve impingement, injury, or weakness? (Select THREE.)

   **A.** Empty can test
   **B.** Cozen test
   **C.** Finkelstein test
   **D.** Hawkins-Kennedy test
   **E.** Neer test

(*See answers next page.*)

**6. D) Slipped capital femoral epiphysis**

Slipped capital femoral epiphysis (SCFE) occurs most often in patients aged 8 to 14 years, who typically present with hip, thigh, or knee pain, and a limp. Risk factors for SCFE include male gender and being overweight or obese. Cues to the diagnosis include worsening symptoms despite rest. Pain and limping indicate a disease process not consistent with normal growth and development. Signs and symptoms associated with Duchene muscular dystrophy, progressive muscle weakness and degeneration, are more likely to present earlier in childhood. A teen with Osgood–Schlatter disease is more likely to have knee pain that worsens with activity and resolves with rest.

**7. C) Pain in the mid-foot and bony tenderness at the navicular bone**

Indications for ankle radiographs, according to Ottawa ankle rules, include (1) pain in the malleolar zone and bony tenderness on the posterior edge of the lateral or medial malleolus, (2) pain in the mid-foot zone and bony tenderness at the base of the fifth metatarsal or at the navicular bone. In addition, inability to bear weight both immediately and in the emergency department are indicators. Notice that discoloration, swelling, and pain with weight bearing or movement are findings associated with ankle injuries, and are non specific for fracture.

**8. B) L5 or S1 root irritation**

Compression or inflammation of the L5 and/or S1 spinal nerve root may cause radiculopathy symptoms or sciatica, characterized by pain, generally felt as a sharp, shooting, and/or searing feeling in the buttock, thigh, leg, foot, and/or toes that worsens with ambulation. Numbness and weakness in the foot and/or toes are associated with nerve root irritation. The age and occupation of the individual indicate that compression fracture (often caused by osteoporotic changes and in older adults) is less likely. Disc herniation is more likely in the lower rather than upper back area and is also more likely in older adults. Spondylosis is degenerative and worsens with age.

**9. A) Ligament damage**

The anterior drawer test is a special test of the knee that helps to identify injury to the anterior cruciate ligament. To identify meniscus pathology, a McMurray's test would be indicated. To test patellar subluxation or dislocation, an apprehension test would be indicated. Weak quadriceps muscle predisposes adolescent athletes to Osgood-Schlatter disease; palpation of the tibial tubercle to assess knee pain would be indicated.

**10. A, D, E) Empty can test, Hawkins–Kennedy test, Neer test**

Shoulder tests should be completed in clusters to improve reliability of results. The Empty can, Hawkins–Kennedy, and Neer tests help to identify supraspinatus impingement. The Cozen test is used to identify lateral epicondylitis. The Finkelstein test helps to identify tenosynovitis of the abductor pollicis longus and extensor pollicis brevis tendons, also known as "De Quervain's syndrome."

# 10

# Gastrointestinal and Renal Systems

## KEY HISTORY CONSIDERATIONS

- Location and severity of abdominal pain
- Pattern of bowel movements
- Ability to tolerate oral intake
- Pain, discomfort, or change in urination
- History and pattern of growth and development
- History of unintentional weight loss
- History of systemic symptoms
- Current pregnancy or chance of pregnancy
- Currently sexually active
- Typical dietary intake
- Smoking history/tobacco use

## PHYSICAL EXAMINATION: INSPECTION, AUSCULTATION, PERCUSSION, PALPATION, AND SPECIAL TESTS

### INSPECTION

1. Observe the patient's overall appearance, posture, and position.
2. Observe the patient for increased discomfort with movement. Observe the patient with coughing, walking, or sudden movement of the bed.
3. Inspect the abdomen from the side as well as while looking down at the abdomen for symmetry and contour.
4. Inspect the skin on the chest, abdomen, back, and genitourinary areas.

#### INSPECTION: ABNORMAL FINDINGS

- Patient appears toxic, in significant pain, or has abnormal vital signs.
- Increased pain with sudden movement is a clue to peritonitis. Patients with peritonitis typically prefer to lay still.
- **Skin changes:** If the abdomen, back, or genital region have any ecchymosis, rashes, venous patterns, or discolorations, further examination is necessary.
    - Ecchymosis on the abdomen can be highly suggestive of internal abdominal conditions and provide clues as to the underlying etiology.

        - Grey Turner's sign (flank ecchymosis) and Cullen's sign (umbilical ecchymosis) are rare findings that have been thought to be important clues to abdominal hemorrhage, acute pancreatitis, or ectopic pregnancy.
        - When there is bruising on the trunk or genital region, abuse should also be considered. The patient's age, risk factors, and history, in addition to the appearance and pattern of bruising, should be considered when determining if this is a possibility.
    - Dilated abdominal wall veins are a clue to portal hypertension.
    - Scars can provide information about past abdominal conditions and surgeries.
    - Jaundice is another important visual finding that should be noted as well as abdominal venous patterns. These visual findings may suggest liver involvement of various etiologies.

Rashes on the abdomen and/or genitals can be many different conditions. See Chapter 3, "Integumentary System," for further information about skin rashes.

- **Masses, nodules, and hernias:** Asking the patient to raise their head off the exam table allows the abdominal muscles to contract and allows the clinician to assess for previously undetected masses, bulges, or nodules. A pulsatile mass around the umbilicus is typically an abdominal aortic aneurysm.
- A protuberant abdomen may be caused by obesity, tumors, pregnancy, or distention by gas or fluid.

## AUSCULTATION

1. Auscultation for bowel sounds does not provide additional assessment information and is not evidence-based.
2. Auscultate for bruits over the aorta, iliac, renal, and femoral arteries if the patient has any of the following risk factors: early-onset hypertension (before age 30), the presence of an arterial bruit and hypertension, accelerated hypertension, medication-resistant hypertension, renal failure, flash pulmonary edema, or renal failure after initiation of an Angiotensin-converting enzyme (ACE) inhibitor (ACE inhibitor) or an Angiotensin II receptor blocker (ARB). Patients without hypertension should not have auscultation for asymptomatic bruits because bruits frequently are a normal finding.

### AUSCULTATION: ABNORMAL FINDINGS

- Abdominal bruits are heard in up to 20% of healthy people and are more common in those under 40. Continuous bruits (across systole and diastole) or a bruit heard away from the midline are more concerning and deserve a more focused assessment.
    - Bruits over the renal arteries may be a sign of renal artery stenosis.
    - Bruits over the femoral arteries may be a sign of peripheral vascular disease.
- Friction rubs may also be heard over the liver and spleen due to inflammation of the peritoneal surface of these organs from a mass or tumor.

## PERCUSSION

1. Percuss lightly in all four quadrants of the abdomen (Figure 10.1). Generalized tympany can be found over most of the abdomen due to gas. Dullness occurs over fluid, organs, masses, or a distended bladder. Percussion should not elicit pain.

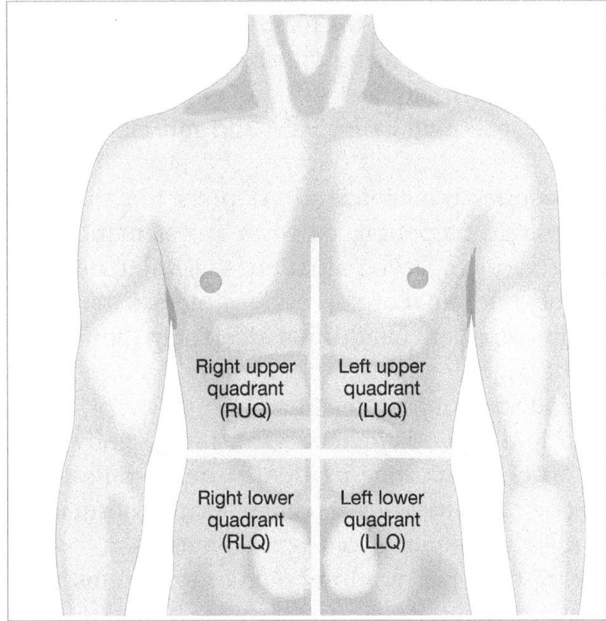


**Figure 10.1** Four quadrants of the abdomen to describe the location and symptoms of pain.

2. If the chief concern and patient history are suggestive of conditions affecting the kidneys, percuss the right and left costovertebral angle. Direct fist percussion can be used. This is when the clinician directly strikes the costovertebral angle using the ulnar surface of the fist. Conversely, indirect fist percussion may be used by placing the palm of the right hand on the back and striking this hand with the ulnar surface of the fist of the left hand.

### PERCUSSION: ABNORMAL FINDINGS

- Gentle percussion that causes pain and tenderness suggests some underlying pathology. Patient history and location of pain should help identify possible diagnoses.
- Tenderness or pain with percussion of the kidney(s), referred to as costovertebral angle tenderness (CVA tenderness), can indicate kidney inflammation due to conditions like pyelonephritis or can be musculoskeletal in nature such as a lower back strain. The patient history would be important to discern which body system was affected.

## PALPATION

1. Palpate all four quadrants for tenderness or masses. Start with light palpation of the abdomen, moving in a systematic way through all four quadrants. The clinician should place the palmar surface of their hand lightly on the abdomen with fingers outstretched and close together. Press down on the abdominal wall no more than one centimeter with light palpation. The clinician should keep the hands low and parallel to the abdomen; keeping the hands high and pointing downward increases the likelihood of the patient tensing the abdomen. Use a light and circular motion. The abdomen should normally feel soft and smooth. Palpate the painful areas last as examining these areas will cause pain and muscle tension that skew palpation findings.
2. Deep palpation requires the clinician to depress the abdomen five to eight centimeters. Similar to light palpation, move in a systematic way throughout all four quadrants of the abdomen. Deep palpation is useful in helping to determine potential enlargement of abdominal organs and/or masses that may not be large enough to detect with light palpation. In addition, deep palpation may reveal tenderness not evident with light palpation. When performing deep palpation, note any masses, organomegaly, tenderness, and pulsations.
3. Palpate the aorta to detect aortic aneurysm. Press gently inward in the epigastric region slightly left of the midline to identify aortic pulsations. Place one hand on each side of the aorta and measure its diameter. The normal aorta is <3 cm.
4. Palpate for inguinal lymph nodes or inguinal masses.
5. If the patient has right upper quadrant pain or symptoms suggestive of either liver or gallbladder enlargement, it is appropriate to palpate for the liver border and gall bladder. The liver edge normally lies under the rib cage at the right midclavicular line. To palpate for the liver, the clinician should place their right hand on the patient's right lower quadrant (Figure 10.2). As the patient inhales, the edge of the liver will descend – the clinician should feel for it hitting their fingers. Repeat, moving the right hand up an inch at a time, until the liver edge is felt or the costal margin is reached. If the liver's edge is felt, observe the consistency, regularity, and tenderness as it moves under the fingers. With deep inspiration, some normal livers are palpable but typically they are not felt. The liver edge, if felt, is usually rubbery and soft in texture. A gallbladder can be felt behind the smooth liver border in the right upper quadrant of the abdomen. If the gall bladder is palpable, it is an abnormal finding.
6. If the clinician has concern for spleen enlargement, palpating for the spleen is important. This is done in the same way that liver palpation is completed. Palpate for the spleen from the left side or by reaching across the patient. Beginning in the left lower quadrant, ask the patient to inhale as you move your fingers up the abdomen. Feel for the spleen hitting your fingertips. If it is not felt, move your hand up an inch at a time, and repeat until you reach the costal margin. A normal spleen should not be palpated.

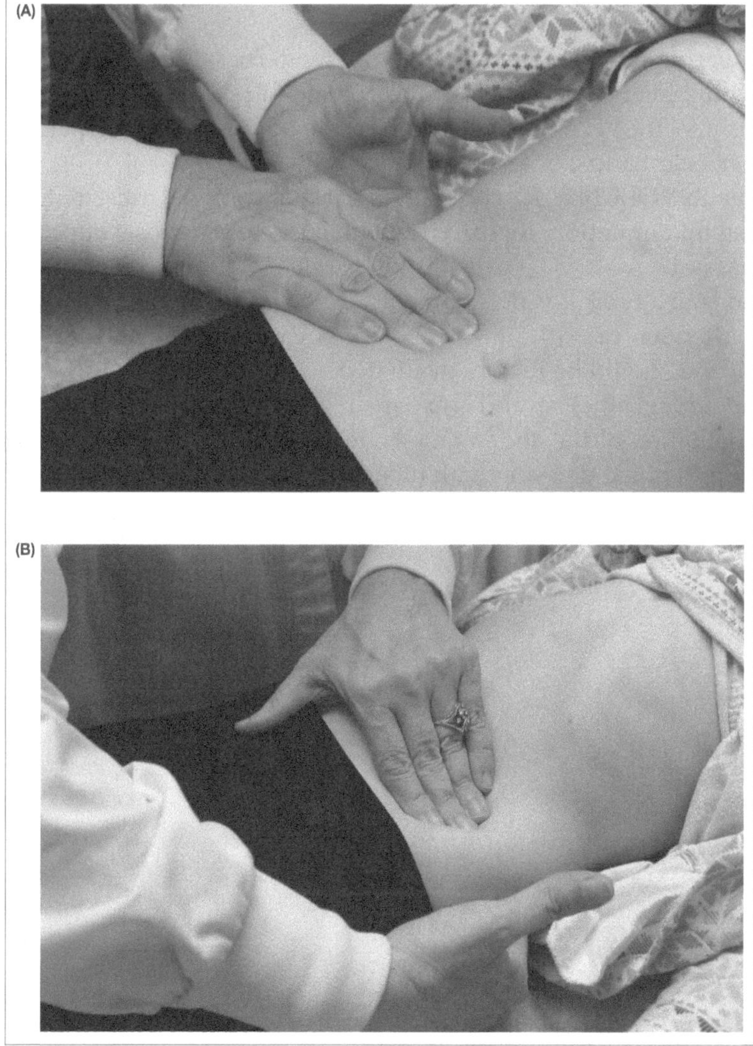


**Figure 10.2** Palpation of the (A) right kidney and (B) left kidney.

7. Palpation of the kidneys should be considered if the patient is having symptoms suggestive of urinary or renal etiology. To palpate the right kidney, stand at the right side of the patient, and place one hand on the patient's right flank, and the other hand at the right costal margin. Press the two hands together and ask the patient to take a deep breath. The kidney edge may be felt between the fingers or not palpated at all; both findings are normal. To palpate the left kidney, reach across the patient and behind the left flank with the left hand. Press the right hand into the abdomen while asking the patient to inhale. Press firmly between the two hands; there should be no change with inhalation.

## PALPATION: ABNORMAL FINDINGS

- Exam findings of guarding, rigidity, rebound tenderness, percussion tenderness, and pain with coughing nearly double the likelihood of peritonitis.
- Guarding is a VOLUNTARY contraction of the abdominal musculature due to tenderness, fear, cold hands, or anxiety.
- Rigidity is an INVOLUNTARY contraction of the abdominal musculature in response to peritoneal inflammation. Rigidity alone makes the diagnosis of peritonitis almost four times as likely.
- Lymph nodes are typically non-palpable. Any lymph nodes that are hard, fixed, matted, non-tender, or >10 mm in size are suggestive for infection or underlying malignancy and should be further evaluated.
- An aortic aneurysm is > 3 cm and is expansible, meaning it will push the hands apart.
- Pain with palpation of the abdomen can be a variety of conditions. Location of the pain can help to guide decision-making and evaluation. See Figure 10.3 for possible diagnoses based on the location of the abdominal pain or discomfort.

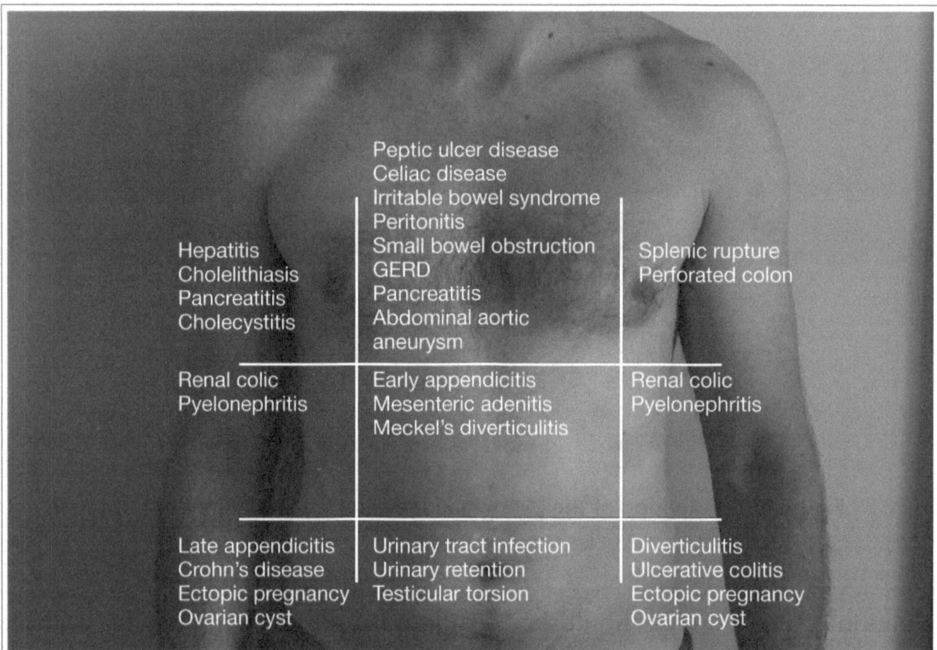


**Figure 10.3** Differential diagnoses according to localization of abdominal pain.

- **Hepatomegaly:** An enlarged liver can occur in a variety of conditions including but not limited to cancer, congestive heart failure, cirrhosis, alcohol misuse, hepatic steatosis, and polycystic liver disease. A firm, cirrhotic liver is more likely to be palpable than a normal liver. If the liver edge is palpated, feel carefully for clues of cirrhosis. The cirrhotic liver is firmer than normal and may have palpable irregularity or nodules.
- If a gallbladder is palpable during an abdominal exam, this is an abnormal finding. A palpable and tender gallbladder suggests acute cholecystitis and has a positive likelihood of detecting obstruction of the bile ducts. Compared with the smooth liver, an enlarged gallbladder feels like a firm mass. If palpable, an inflamed gallbladder is exquisitely tender making palpation difficult due to abdominal muscle guarding.

- **Splenomegaly:** If the spleen is palpated, it is enlarged. Common causes of splenomegaly are portal hypertension, hematologic malignancies, and infectious diseases.

## SPECIAL TESTS FOR THE ABDOMEN

### SCRATCH TEST

The scratch test may be used to detect liver size. To perform this technique, place a stethoscope just beneath the xiphoid process while using the finger to scratch the abdominal surface (Figure 10.4). Note the differences in sound transmission over solid and hollow organs; when the liver is reached, the sound of the finger scratching the abdominal surface becomes louder. The scratch test has shown high reproducibility and moderate agreement between the scratch test findings and ultrasound; although, obesity can jeopardize these results.

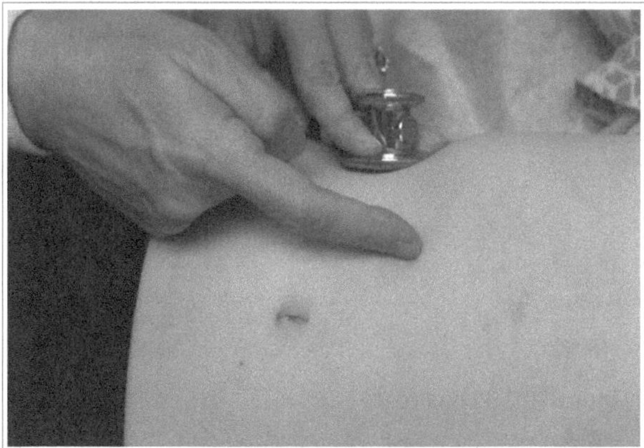

**Figure 10.4** Scratch test.

### McBURNEY'S POINT

Anatomically, McBurney's point is the location of the appendix in most adults: 1/3 of the distance from the right anterior superior iliac spine to the umbilicus. Tenderness at this point is a more specific finding of appendicitis than general RLQ tenderness.

### MURPHY'S SIGN

Murphy's sign is a finding of acute cholecystitis. The clinician palpates under the right costal margin in the midclavicular line and observes as the patient inhales. Murphy's sign is present if the patient has cessation of their breath and increased tenderness as the inflamed gallbladder hits the clinician's finger. It is a more specific finding of cholecystitis than having right upper quadrant tenderness.

### REBOUND TENDERNESS OR BLUMBERG'S SIGN

Palpate the abdomen by applying slow and steady pressure to the suspected area followed by abrupt removal of the pressure. The test is considered positive if pain is worsened upon release of the hands (verses application of the pressure) when the underlying structure(s) shift back into place. A positive sign indicates peritoneal irritation. The odds of appendicitis triple in children who exhibit rebound tenderness and reduce the likelihood of its occurrence if rebound tenderness is absent.

## ROSVING'S SIGN

Deeply palpate the left iliac fossa. If pain is felt in the right iliac fossa, this is considered a positive Rovsing's sign. Historically, a positive Rovsing's sign has been associated with an acute appendicitis.

## PSOAS TEST

With the patient in the supine position, place one hand just above the patient's right knee. Ask the patient to raise the leg while applying downward pressure on the leg (Figure 10.5). Pain can indicate irritation of the psoas muscle due to inflammation of the appendix. Some sources indicate a positive test can indicate a retrocecal (behind the cecum) appendicitis presentation due to retroperitoneal inflammation.

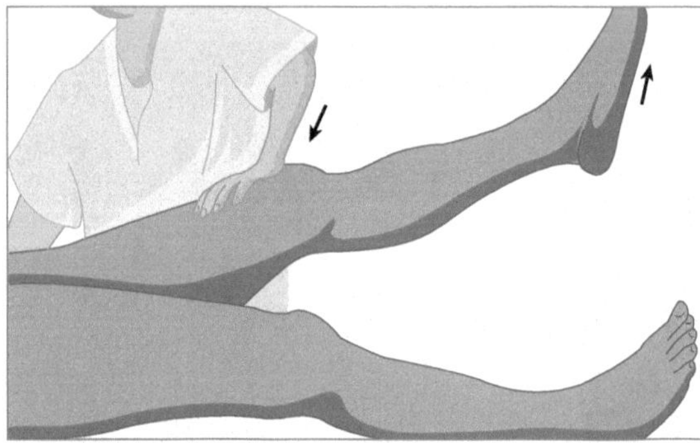

**Figure 10.5** Psoas test.

## HEEL DROP TEST (ALSO CALLED THE MARKLE TEST OR HEEL JAR TEST)

Have the patient stand on their toes, then ask them to abruptly release back onto their heels, creating a jarring sensation to the body. If there is pain in the right lower quadrant, this is a positive test and contributes further information toward a possible diagnosis of appendicitis.

## DIGITAL RECTAL EXAMINATION (DRE)

Digital rectal exams (DREs) are sometimes warranted when a patient has specific gastrointestinal or urinary concerns. Otherwise, DRE is not performed as a routine part of abdominal exams. To complete this exam, the individual should be unclothed from the waist down and in a gown and/or covered with a drape. Ideal positioning for the exam is either with the individual standing with a forward bend at the waist, or side lying with knees to chest. Separate the buttocks and inspect for fissures, hemorrhoids, bleeding, skin tags, and rashes. Lubricate the index or middle finger of a gloved hand. The clinician should inform the patient a finger will be inserted into the rectum. Ask the patient to take a deep breath, relax and breathe out while gently inserting the examining finger into the anal canal. If the patient is a male, palpate the prostate anteriorly, noting its size, symmetry, and texture. A normal prostate is walnut-sized, symmetrical, and smooth with a cartilaginous texture (similar to the tip of the nose). The prostate has a midline groove (sulcus) that should be palpable. Rotate the finger 360° to palpate the span of the rectal wall for masses or irregularities. Stool may be palpated in the rectal vault. Note the consistency (hard or soft). Assess anal tone by asking the patient to tighten their anal sphincter on the finger. Once the patient relaxes, withdraw the finger, and inspect for blood, stool, or mucus.

### FLUID WAVE

If you suspect ascites, test for a fluid wave. Have the patient hold the edge of one hand firmly in the midline. This decreases movement of soft tissue, which can give a false-positive result. Percuss one side of the abdomen with the fingers of one hand while holding the other hand against the opposite side. A positive result is a tap against the hand caused by a wave of ascitic fluid set in motion by percussion. This is a specific finding that supports the presence of ascites.

## RED FLAGS IN HISTORY AND PHYSICAL EXAM

- Bilious emesis
- Deceleration of linear growth
- Delayed onset of puberty
- Dysphagia
- Family history of inflammatory bowel disease, Lynch syndrome, celiac disease, peptic ulcer disease, Barrett's esophagus, or hepatobiliary disease
- Feculent vomiting
- Hematuria
- Hematemesis
- Hepatosplenomegaly
- Nighttime pain or diarrhea
- Oral ulcers
- Perianal skin tags/fissures
- Persistent RUQ or RLQ pain
- Persistent vomiting or diarrhea
- Recurrent unexplained fever
- Rectal bleeding or melena
- Severe flank pain
- Severe groin pain
- Unexplained anemia
- Unintentional weight loss

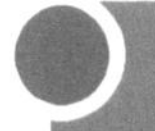

## POPULATION HEALTH AND LIFE-SPAN CONSIDERATIONS

### INFANTS AND CHILDREN

- Newborn jaundice is a common condition. It is a concern if it develops in the first 24 hours after birth, is present for greater than 1 week, or is severe.

- Infants and toddlers often have a protuberant abdomen due to immature development of the abdominal muscles.
- Children can get dehydrated quickly. They often will not have changes in their vital signs until they are moderately to severely dehydrated. Number of oral feedings and the number of wet diapers are important history questions to ask a parent when their child is ill.
- When conducting a newborn abdominal exam, hold the hips and knees in a flexed position to relax the abdominal muscles.
- Inguinal lymph nodes are often palpable in young children.
- If a child is ticklish, have them place their hands on top of your hands during the exam.
- Toxin ingestion needs to be considered in children and adolescents who present with abdominal pain and vomiting.
- Foreign body ingestion should also be a consideration in young children. The symptoms will depend on the characteristics of the foreign body (its size, whether it is sharp or toxic, etc.) and where the foreign body is in the gastrointestinal tract. Most complications from pediatric foreign body ingestion are due to esophageal impaction, with 70% occurring at the upper esophageal sphincter or thoracic inlet. Symptoms commonly seen when the foreign body is located in the esophagus include food refusal, drooling, gagging, sore throat, emesis, hematemesis, dysphagia, stridor, cough, chest pain, or if the child is able to speak, a reported foreign body sensation. If the foreign body is in the stomach or lower intestine, symptoms include abdominal pain, abdominal distension, vomiting, or hematochezia. Unexplained fever can occur when the foreign body is in either the upper or lower GI tract.
- Kidneys are easier to palpate in neonates and children. The right kidney is more often palpated than the left kidney.
- Urinary tract infections (UTI) present differently in children and symptoms vary by age.
- Children under the age of 5 rarely have urinary tract infections. This can be an indication of a structural abnormality of the urinary tract, sexual abuse, or holding their urine for an extended amount of time.

## OLDER ADULTS

- The presentation of an older patient with abdominal pain may be very different from that seen in a younger patient.
- Older patients tend to present later in the course of their illness and have more nonspecific symptoms that do not follow classic patterns. Vital signs can also be misleading due to things like physiological aging differences, chronic conditions, and polypharmacy.
- Abdominal pain, nausea, and/or vomiting may be only signs of a myocardial infraction, so this should always be a differential diagnosis for these conditions.
- Older adults are more likely to have poor outcomes, so they require more aggressive workups when presenting with abdominal pain or gastrointestinal symptoms.

- Up to 30% of older adults have urinary incontinence. This can be due to stress incontinence, urge incontinence, overflow incontinence, functional incontinence, or mixed incontinence. Careful history taking can help determine the type of incontinence that is present.
- Benign prostatic hyperplasia (BPH) is a common condition in older adult men that can cause bladder, urinary tract, or kidney infections due to the blocking of the flow of urine out of the bladder.
- Bladder cancer often presents with painless, intermittent, gross hematuria.

### ADDITIONAL CONSIDERATIONS

- Stretch marks and linea nigra, a blackish-brown vertical line along the midline, are common findings on the abdomen during pregnancy and post-partum.
- With increasing abdominal pressure and stretching, often due to pregnancy, diastasis recti, a condition where the rectus abdominis muscles separate, can occur.
- Patients with solitary kidneys will have kidney enlargement.
- Renal failure often presents with fluid retention causing swelling in the legs, feet, and ankles, shortness of breath, fatigue, and confusion.
- Urinary tract infections are much more common in girls and women due to shorter urethras and close proximity to the anal opening.
- Uncircumcised boys and men more at risk for developing a UTI than those who are circumcised.

## KEY DIFFERENTIALS

### ABDOMEN AND GASTROINTESTINAL TRACT

- Abdominal aortic aneurysm
- Abdominal migraine
- Acute myocardial infarction
- Appendicitis
- Celiac disease
- Cholecystitis
- Cholelithiasis
- Colon cancer
- Crohn's disease
- Diverticulitis/diverticulosis
- Ectopic pregnancy
- Gastroenteritis
- Gastroesophageal reflux disease (GERD)
- Gastroparesis
- Hepatitis
- Irritable bowel syndrome
- Mesenteric adenitis
- Ovarian cyst
- Pancreatitis
- Peptic ulcer disease
- Perforated colon
- Peritonitis
- Pneumonia
- Pregnancy
- Small bowel obstruction
- Splenic rupture
- Testicular torsion
- Ulcerative colitis

## UROLOGICAL SYSTEM

- Autoimmune-disease related kidney disease
- Glomerulonephritis
- Incontinence
- Nephrotic syndrome
- Pyelonephritis
- Polycystic kidney disease
- Renal carcinoma
- Renal colic
- Renal failure (acute and chronic)
- Urinary tract infection
- Urinary retention

# KNOWLEDGE CHECK: GASTROINTESTINAL AND RENAL SYSTEMS

1. An individual has been diagnosed with peritonitis. Which assessment is expected based on this diagnosis?

   **A.** Cannot lie still on the exam table
   **B.** Experiencing polyuria and polyphagia
   **C.** Pain is exacerbated by sudden movements
   **D.** Pain is relieved with use of a heating pad and massage

2. If positive, which assessment or sign helps to confirm the diagnosis of appendicitis?

   **A.** Gray Turner's sign
   **B.** Kehr's sign
   **C.** Kernig's sign
   **D.** Psoas sign

3. Which patient population is LEAST at risk for complications associated with urinary tract infections?

   **A.** Infants
   **B.** Young adult women
   **C.** Pregnant women
   **D.** Older adults

4. An advanced practice nurse assesses the abdomen of an individual with a history of diabetes and hypertension. Arrange the listed abdominal assessment steps in the correct order.

   **A.** Auscultation
   **B.** Inspection
   **C.** Palpation
   **D.** Percussion

5. Which abdominal assessment finding is MOST concerning?

   **A.** Dullness to percussion over the upper abdominal quadrants of an infant
   **B.** Hollow, drum-like sound when percussing the abdomen of a hungry child
   **C.** Linea nigra and diastasis recti of the abdomen noted during postpartum exam
   **D.** Non-tender costovertebral angle to fist percussion in a female patient

*(See answers next page.)*

**1. C) Pain is exacerbated by sudden movements**

Inflammation of the peritoneum (peritonitis) causes abdominal rigidity, pain, fever, nausea, and vomiting. The individual with peritonitis prefers to lie still, as their severe pain is exacerbated with motion or sudden movements. Massage and application of heat would also exacerbate this condition. Assessments would include decreased urinary output and poor appetite, not increased urinary output (polyuria) and increased appetite (polyphagia). Causes of peritonitis include appendicitis, pancreatitis, perforated colon, diverticulitis, cirrhosis, and pelvic inflammatory disease.

**2. D) Psoas sign**

Objective signs that are correlated with appendicitis include right lower quadrant pain, rebound tenderness, guarding, and the psoas sign (pain on extension of the right thigh). Other confirmatory signs of peritonitis include the obturator sign (pain on internal rotation of the right thigh) and Rovsing's sign (pain in the right lower quadrant with palpation of the left lower quadrant). Gray Turner's sign, ecchymosis of the flanks, is an uncommon manifestation of intra-abdominal hemorrhage. Kehr's sign, the occurrence of pain in the tip of the shoulder is considered a classic sign of splenic rupture. Kernig's sign is elicitation of pain with passive extension of the knee, indicating possible meningitis.

**3. B) Young adult women**

Young adult women are the least at risk for complications associated with urinary tract infections (UTIs). Infants, pregnant women, and older adults are more likely to have atypical symptoms and are more at risk for pyelonephritis.

**4. B, A, D, C) Inspection, auscultation, percussion, palpation.**

The order for assessment of the abdomen is: inspection, auscultation, percussion, and then palpation. Inspection is the first step and should include assessment for skin changes. The patient's history of comorbidities necessitates the inclusion of auscultation for bruits over renal and femoral arteries. Percussion occurs prior to palpation to identify any underlying pathology. Light and deep palpation are final steps to assess for masses, organ enlargement, or tenderness.

**5. A) Dullness to percussion over the upper abdominal quadrants of an infant**

Tympany (hollow, drum-like sound) to percussion of the abdomen is the expected finding for individuals in any age group. Dullness to percussion of the abdomen can indicate a mass or solid tumor; although dullness may indicate constipation, especially in the lower left abdominal quadrant, the finding of dullness to percussion across upper quadrants is concerning and requires further assessment. Linea nigra, a blackish-brown vertical line along the midline, is a common finding during pregnancy and post-partum; with increasing abdominal stretching during pregnancy, diastasis recti, a condition where the rectus abdominis muscles separate, is also common. Costovertebral angle tenderness to either direct or indirect percussion would not be an expected finding for any gender or in any age group.

6. Which symptom is MOST often experienced when an individual has persistent gastroesophageal reflux?

   A. Bloating
   B. Diarrhea
   C. Sore throat
   D. Vomiting

7. An individual presents with localized, severe abdominal pain, and has inspiratory arrest with deep palpation of the right upper quadrant under the costal margin during inspiration. Their assessment is highly suggestive of:

   A. Appendicitis
   B. Cholecystitis
   C. Pneumonia
   D. Pyelonephritis

8. The most common clinical presentation of Crohn's disease includes:

   A. Difficulty swallowing and pharyngitis
   B. Painless gastrointestinal bleeding and hematemesis
   C. Painless gastrointestinal ulcers and melena
   D. Weight loss, abdominal pain, and diarrhea

9. An adolescent is suspected to have mononucleosis. Which physical exam finding warrants the most caution regarding rest and return to usual activities?

   A. Fever
   B. Lymphadenopathy
   C. Splenomegaly
   D. Tonsillar enlargement

10. A 30-year-old female presents with urgency to urinate. Which additional assessments are MOST indicative of urinary tract infection for this individual? (Select all that apply.)

    A. Abdominal bloating
    B. Dysuria
    C. Dyspareunia
    D. Hematuria
    E. Urinary frequency

*(See answers next page.)*

**6. C) Sore throat**

The reflux of stomach acid causes irritation of the lining of the esophagus and throat. Common symptoms include retrosternal burning, chest pain, sore throat, difficulty swallowing, hoarseness, and persistent cough. Symptoms may include nausea but are not likely to include bloating, diarrhea, or vomiting.

**7. B) Cholecystitis**

Murphy's sign is a specific finding associated with cholecystitis. This sign is elicited by palpating the abdomen under the right costal margin and observing as the patient inhales. Inspiratory arrest (the cessation of breath) and increased tenderness occur when the inflamed gallbladder moves downward during the maneuver. Murphy's sign would be negative in pyelonephritis, appendicitis, and pneumonia. In addition, appendicitis is more likely to cause right lower quadrant pain,, pyelonephritis is more likely to lead to costovertebral angle tenderness, and any abdominal pain associated with pneumonia is likely to be generalized or non-specific.

**8. D) Weight loss, abdominal pain, and diarrhea**

Crohn's disease is an autoimmune, inflammatory bowel disease associated with intermittent exacerbations of mucosal inflammation and ulceration that can affect all layers of the bowel wall. Severity can range from mild to severe. Key history and physical findings include abdominal pain, severe diarrhea, fatigue and malaise, fever, weight loss, and arthralgia. As the disease process most commonly affects entire GI tract, pharyngitis and dysphagia are not common presentations.

**9. C) Splenomegaly**

Infectious mononucleosis is common in adolescents and children. Typical findings include fever, pharyngitis, malaise, lymphadenopathy, and tonsillitis. While splenomegaly can occur, and does occur in about 50% to 60% of cases, the finding warrants caution regarding return to activities to avoid the risk of splenic rupture, which is a vascular emergency.

**10. B, D, E) Dysuria, hematuria, urinary frequency**

Common symptoms associated with urinary tract infections (UTIs) include urinary urgency, frequency, and pain or discomfort with urination (dysuria). Blood in the urine (hematuria) and/or cloudy urine are associated. Dyspareunia (pain with sexual intercourse), and abdominal bloating are not common symptoms, and are more likely to be associated with vulvar, vaginal, and/or ovarian disease processes that include ovarian cancer, endometriosis, and pelvic inflammatory disease. GI disorders associated with bloating and dyspareunia include constipation and irritable bowel disease.

# Breasts and Axillae

## KEY HISTORY CONSIDERATIONS

- Breast tenderness or pain
- Breast lump
- Spontaneous breast discharge
- Changes in appearance of breast, nipple, or skin on breast
- Dimpling of the breast
- Reported itching of the breast
- Rash on breast
- Presence of axillary or supraclavicular lymphadenopathy
- Current or previous malignant or nonmalignant conditions
- Breastfeeding history (current and past)
- Presence of breast implants, including length of time, type, and complications
- Use of hormone replacement therapy
- Last mammogram
- Menstrual and menopause history
- Family history of breast, ovarian, or colon cancer
- Family history of BReast CAncer (BRCA) mutation
- Nicotine use
- Alcohol intake

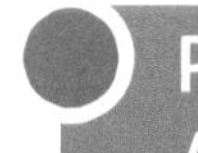

## PHYSICAL EXAMINATION: INSPECTION AND PALPATION

Despite the controversy regarding the population health benefit of clinical breast exam (CBE) for the screening of breast cancer, CBE may identify a small proportion of breast malignancies not detected with mammography, may be requested by an individual as a component of their exam, and can be used to document the presence of palpable masses and cysts in young women who are not typical candidates for mammography.

### INSPECTION

1. With the patient sitting and disrobed to the waist, note breast size, shape, and contour. Size, shape, and contour will vary from person to person.
2. Inspect the breasts and nipples for symmetry.
3. Nipple color varies from pink to black based on the skin color of the patient. Montgomery tubercles are a normal finding on the areola.

4. Have the patient raise their arms overhead, place their hands at the hips, and sit with their hands pressed together; observe for a shift in nipple position, as well as significant asymmetry or any unusual dimpling or bulging of breast tissue.
5. With the patient laying, observe the breasts in this position. This will move the breast tissue into a different position which may cause a lump or another abnormality to be visualized that was not noticeable when in the sitting position.
6. Also in the laying position, ask the patient to raise their hands above their head, inspect the axillary areas. The skin texture should be smooth and free from any lumps or bumps.
7. Venous patterns can be visible and are especially pronounced in pregnancy and during breastfeeding.

### INSPECTION ABNORMAL FINDINGS

- Any changes to the skin of the breasts, including a scaly rash, peau d'orange appearance (orange, red, or purplish appearance of the skin), erythema, or edema are abnormal and could be a sign(s) of breast cancer.
- Alterations in the contour of the breasts should be compared side-to-side. Dimpling, especially when unilateral, in the skin can be a presentation of breast cancer, especially if the malignant lump is growing closer to the overlying skin.
- Nipple inversion can be a normal finding if the patient has always had the inversion. Nipple inversion is worrisome if it is unilateral and/or a new finding.
- Breast dimpling can be a sign of inflammatory breast cancer or fat necrosis.

## PALPATION

1. Have the patient move their shoulders slightly forward and palpate above the clavicle for supraclavicular lymphadenopathy.
2. Palpate axillary lymph nodes while the person is still in a seated position; each arm should be supported while nodes are palpated. Palpation should be completed with the pads of the fingers, using a fluid, circular motion. Care should be taken to ensure the entire surface area of the lymphatic region is palpated, both lightly and deeply.
3. Palpate each breast in the supine position with one hand above the head. The entire breast is examined from the second to sixth ribs and from the left sternal border to the midaxillary line. To assure a thorough assessment, imagine the breast divided into four quadrants with vertical and horizontal lines intersecting at the nipple. The upper outer quadrant encompasses the axillary tail of breast tissue that extends into the axilla. This is the most common location for breast cancer, so special attention should be paid to this area. Palpate in all four quadrants of both breasts by compressing breast tissue between the pads of the three middle fingers and the chest wall.
4. Proper breast palpation technique encompasses the use of the finger pads in a continuous rolling, gliding circular motion in the vertical strip, circular, or wedge pattern. The pressure of the fingers should be varied from light to medium to deep palpation. The areola and the nipple are included inherently in the palpation of the breast. However, nipple expression to assess for the presence of nipple discharge is not recommended unless the patient describes spontaneous discharge that requires evaluation.

### PALPATION ABNORMAL FINDINGS

- Any tenderness, depressions, masses, or deformities discovered during palpation of the breasts is abnormal.
- Thickening of the skin in the axillary area or over the breast can be found in some malignancies and should be considered abnormal.
- A lump that has an irregular shape or that is fixed, hard, and has a pebbly surface is more worrisome for a carcinoma. The lump is often painless but, in some cases, it can be painful. If the lump feels rubbery, moves easily, and/or comes and goes with menstrual cycles, it is more likely to be benign.
- Enlarged lymph nodes that are palpated in the axilla or supraclavicular region are abnormal and need further evaluation. This is especially true for the supraclavicular region. If a lymph node is palpated in this region, malignancy should be suspected until ruled out.
- Accessory or additional mammary tissue remote from the primary breast tissue can occur along "milk lines" anywhere from the axilla to the groin. This is a benign finding. It may present as a soft subcutaneous lump near or in the axillae, as a supernumerary or "third" nipple, or as a mistaken freckle or mole. These areas of the accessory breast tissue can be tender and enlarge in response to the hormonal fluctuations of the normal menstrual cycle and can become full and active with pregnancy and lactation.

## RED FLAGS IN HISTORY AND PHYSICAL EXAM

- Family history of BRCA mutation
- Hard, fixed breast lump
- Spontaneous nipple discharge, especially after menopause

## POPULATION HEALTH AND LIFE-SPAN CONSIDERATIONS

### CHILDREN AND ADOLESCENTS

Puberty typically starts between the ages of 8–13. Breast "buds" are usually the first sign of puberty. The Tanner stages (or the Sexually Maturity Rating Scale [SMR]) are used to objectively classify and track the development of secondary sex characteristics during puberty.

The Tanner stages for the breasts are:

**Stage 1:** Small nipples with no breast tissue.

**Stage 2:** Breast and nipples have just started to grow. The areola has become larger. Breast tissue bud feels firm behind the nipple.

**Stage 3:** Breast and nipples have grown additionally. The areola has become darker. The breast tissue bud is larger.

**Stage 4:** Nipples and areolas are elevated and form an edge toward the breast. The breast has also grown a little larger.

**Stage 5:** Fully developed breast. Nipples are protruding, and the edge between areola and breast has disappeared.

## OLDER ADULTS

- Breast tissue tends to hang more loosely due to atrophy of grandular tissue and the replacement of it by fat.
- Nipples often become smaller, flatter, and lose some of their erectile ability.
- Breast cancer is a disease of aging with age of 62 being the median age of diagnosis.
- More favorable breast cancer subtypes are more prevalent in the older adult population, but aggressive subtypes can still develop.

## OTHER CONSIDERATIONS

- White women are more likely to develop breast cancer than African American, Hispanic, and Asian women.
- African American women are more likely to develop more aggressive, more advanced-stage breast cancer, and are more likely to die due to breast cancer than other races.
- African American women develop inflammatory and triple-negative breast cancers more often than White women.
- Asian and Pacific Islander women have the lowest incidence and death rates of breast cancer.
- Transgender women using hormone treatment may have an increased risk of breast cancer compared to the general male population.
- There are unknown risks associated with residual breast tissue in transgender men who have undergone bilateral mastectomy as well as the possible technical limitations of mammography.
- Pregnant and lactating women have unique considerations. Refer to Chapter 17, "Pregnant Populations," for more information on breast differences in these populations.

# KEY DIFFERENTIALS

- Accessory breast tissue
- Breast cancer
- Candida albicans (thrush) infection
- Duct ectasia
- Ductal or lobular hyperplasia
- Fat necrosis
- Fibroadenomas
- Fibrocystic breast disease
- Galactorrhea
- Gynecomastia
- Inflammatory breast cancer
- Intraductal papilloma
- Invasive ductal carcinomas
- Invasive lobular carcinomas
- Lipoma
- Lobular carcinoma in situ
- Mastalgia
- Mastitis
- Paget's disease of the breast

# KNOWLEDGE CHECK: BREASTS AND AXILLAE

1. A young adult woman presents with breast pain that is bilateral, generalized, and cyclic. Noting no palpable breast masses, the advanced practice nurse can correctly share that the mastalgia:

   **A.** Is likely caused by exercise or trauma
   **B.** Needs to be evaluated by imaging
   **C.** Is related to normal hormonal fluctuations
   **D.** Results from ovarian dysfunction

2. Mastitis is common in women who are:

   **A.** Breastfeeding
   **B.** Obese
   **C.** Perimenopausal
   **D.** Using hormonal contraception

3. The U.S. Preventive Services Task Force (USPSTF) (2016) screening recommendations for women at average risk of breast cancer include:

   **A.** Annual mammography for women age 40 to 74 years
   **B.** Annual mammography for women age 50 years and over
   **C.** Biennial mammography for women age 40 to 74 years
   **D.** Biennial mammography for women age 50 to 74 years

4. According to the American College of Radiology (ACR), which diagnostic imaging test is recommended to initially evaluate a palpable breast mass in women younger than 30 years of age?

   **A.** Magnetic resonance imaging
   **B.** Mammogram
   **C.** Ultrasound
   **D.** No imaging is recommended

5. Which assessment is associated with increased risk for breast cancer in women?

   **A.** Early menopause
   **B.** Late menarche
   **C.** Nulliparity
   **D.** Breastfeeding

*(See answers next page.)*

**1. C) Related to normal hormonal fluctuations**

Mastalgia is extremely common and is experienced by the majority of women during their reproductive years. Cyclic mastalgia, described as heaviness and/or generalized tenderness, is related to normal hormonal fluctuations; in younger women nodularity can be associated. Non-cyclic pain may originate from the chest wall, can be caused by exercise or trauma, and would be more likely experienced as unilateral pain. There is no data to support any strong link between breast pain and malignancy; imaging is not indicated for mastalgia.

**2. A) Breastfeeding**

Infection in breast tissue occurs in up to 10% of women who are lactating and less than 2% of those who are not. Increased risk factors for mastitis include smoking, prolonged breast engorgement, nipple piercings, and post-menopausal status; however, caution is indicated for any individual who is not pregnant and not breastfeeding who presents with mastitis-type symptoms, as inflammatory breast cancers should be ruled out.

**3. D) Biennial mammography for women age 50 to 74 years**

Breast cancer is the second-leading cause of cancer death among women in the United States. The USPSTF guidelines changed in 2016, noting the risks of overdiagnosis and treatment with more frequent mammography in the general population, especially in younger women of average risk. Current recommendations are for biennial screening mammography for women aged 50 to 74 years; the decision to start screening mammography in women prior to age 50 years should be an individual one.

**4. D) No imaging is recommended**

According to the ACR, breast ultrasound should be the primary imaging tool for women with palpable lumps who are pregnant, lactating, or younger than 30 years. For women aged 30 to 39 years, either ultrasound or diagnostic mammography may be used for initial evaluation. MRI is rarely indicated to evaluate a clinically detected finding. For women 40 years old and older, mammography, followed in most cases by ultrasound, is recommended. Imaging performed before biopsy is helpful in characterizing the nature of the mass.

**5. C) Nulliparity**

Factors associated with increased risk for breast cancer include *early* menarche, *late* menopause, never having breastfed, first pregnancy after age 30, never having been pregnant (nulliparity), and obesity; these factors likely increase the exposure to endogenous estrogen over the course of a lifetime.

6. Which finding requires the MOST urgent referral and is likely to require biopsy for diagnosis? (Select all that apply.)

   A. Cyclic breast tenderness in a young adult female
   B. Gynecomastia in an obese pre-adolescent male
   C. Itching, redness, and flaking of the areola in a non-lactating female
   D. Mastitis in a non-pregnant, non-lactating, post-menopausal female
   E. Persistent inverted nipples in a pregnant female

7. Which statement is true about a 1 week old newborn with breast swelling and milk-like discharge?

   A. This is a normal finding only if the newborn is female
   B. This is related to maternal estrogen and is a normal finding
   C. This abnormality can indicate pituitary tumor
   D. This abnormality is related to maternal substance use

8. For which patient should BRCA gene testing be recommended? (Select all that apply.)

   A. A patient with a personal history of breast cancer before age 45
   B. A patient with a personal history of melanoma
   C. A patient with a family history of breast cancer in two or more relatives
   D. A patient with a family history of ovarian and prostate cancer
   E. A patient with a family history of breast cancer after age 65

9. Screening for breast cancer is which level of prevention?

   A. Primary
   B. Primordial
   C. Secondary
   D. Tertiary

10. Which two physical characteristics are MOST LIKELY associated with malignant breast lumps or masses? (Select TWO.)

    A. Bilaterally palpable, mobile
    B. Immobile and fixed to adjacent structures
    C. Palpable and painful just prior to menses
    D. Smooth, rubbery consistency
    E. Unilateral with skin dimpling

*(See answers next page.)*

**6. C, D) Itching, redness, and flaking of the areola in a non-lactating female, mastitis in a non-pregnant, non-lactating, post-menopausal female**

Itching, burning, redness, or flaking of the areola are symptoms of Paget's disease of the breast; biopsy and referral are recommended for prompt diagnosis and treatment. Signs of mastitis in a non-pregnant or non-lactating female should be assumed to be breast cancer until proven otherwise; the post-menopausal age increases the risk of malignancy. All other assessments listed are normal, benign findings, including mastodynia (cyclic tenderness), gynecomastia in pre-adolescent and adolescent males, and persistent (non-acute) nipple inversion.

**7. B) This is related to maternal estrogen and is a normal finding**

Maternal estrogen commonly causes breast swelling and discharge in newborns of either gender. After infancy, galactorrhea (milky nipple discharge) requires further evaluation to assess for elevated prolactin levels, and underlying abnormalities. Causes of galactorrhea in adulthood include medications, pituitary tumor, thyroid disorders, stress, substance use, pregnancy, and chronic renal failure.

**8. A, C, D) Personal history of breast cancer before age 45, family history of breast cancer in two or more relatives, family history of ovarian and prostate cancer**

Recommend BRCA gene testing for individuals who are at increased risk for having an inherited gene mutation, including those with personal history of breast cancer diagnosed before age 45, two or more types of cancer, or ovarian cancer; personal or family history of male breast cancer; two or more relatives diagnosed with breast cancer at any age (or one diagnosed before age 50); one or more relatives with ovarian cancer; two or more relatives with prostate cancer or pancreatic cancer; or one or more relatives with a history of cancer that would meet any of these criteria.

**9. C) Secondary**

Secondary prevention emphasizes early disease detection and targets healthy-appearing individuals with subclinical forms of the disease; pap testing for cervical cancer and mammograms to screen for breast cancer are examples of secondary prevention. Primary prevention consists of measures aimed at susceptible populations to prevent the disease from occurring; immunizations are an example of primary prevention. Tertiary prevention targets those who have diseases to reduce severity and improve outcomes; cardiac rehabilitation is a prime example. Primordial prevention is risk factor reduction targeted towards an entire population through a focus on social and environmental conditions; an example is improving access to safe sidewalks in urban neighborhoods to promote physical activity and reduce the risk of obesity, heart disease, and diabetes.

**10. B, E) Immobile and fixed to adjacent structures, unilateral with skin dimpling**

Malignant breast masses are more likely to be hard, asymmetric, unilateral, and immobile; associated skin dimpling, edema, and nipple retraction are also correlated with breast cancers. Benign breast lumps are more likely to be smooth, soft, or rubbery consistency, and are typically mobile, bilateral, and without associated skin changes. Cyclic breast pain with breast "lumpiness" are common findings in women of reproductive age.

12

# Female Reproductive System

## KEY HISTORY CONSIDERATIONS

- Vaginal discharge
- Abdominal/pelvic pain
- Dysuria
- Dyspareunia
- Infertility
- Vaginal itching
- Vaginal dryness
- Vaginal lesions
- Menstrual history including cycle frequency, duration, flow, and irregularities
- Menopausal history (if applicable)
- Obstetric history
- Dysmenorrhea
- Human papillomavirus (HPV) vaccination status
- Last pap smear and any history of irregular pap smears
- Family history of reproductive cancers including breast, ovarian, cervical, vulvar, vaginal, colon, endometrial, and uterine
- Family history of diethylstilbestrol (DES) use
- Smoking history
- Sexual history (including unprotected vaginal, oral, or anal sex)
- Use of contraceptives and barrier methods for sexually transmitted infection (STI) protection
- Sexual orientation and gender identity

## PHYSICAL EXAMINATION: INSPECTION AND PALPATION

### INSPECTION

#### EXTERNAL GENITALIA EXAM

1. The pelvic exam begins with a thorough exam of the external genitalia. Beginning with the mons pubis, evaluation should include the pattern and quality of hair distribution on both the mons and the labia majora. Inspect for signs of infection. Proceed to inspection of the skin of the mons, labia majora, and perineum.

2. Evaluate the labia and clitoris for development or atrophy. Inspect the introitus, noting its shape—closed or gaping—in the lithotomy position.
3. The openings of the bartholin and skene glands should be inspected for edema, erythema, and purulent discharges. The perineal body should then be assessed. This area begins with the posterior aspect of the labia and extends to the anus. Similar to the inspection of the skin of the mons pubis and labia majora, the inspection of the perineal body should include the items previously described.
4. Finally, the perianal area should be examined.

## INTERNAL GENITALIA EXAM

1. Performing a speculum examination allows for direct visualization of the cervix and the surrounding vaginal walls. A speculum examination for the sole purpose of screening for STIs is not necessary, as other methods for sample collection are available. The appropriately sized speculum should be chosen prior to starting the examination.
2. By convention, the speculum examination is performed first, followed by the bimanual examination. The speculum should be warmed using either warm water or a warming device. Current recommendations suggest that a small amount (dime-sized) of lubricant be applied to the introitus and bills of the speculum for ease of insertion.
3. Begin by separating the labia with the thumb and first finger of the nondominant hand for visualization of the introitus.
4. Palpate the skene and bartholin glands. These should be non-tender, and no discharge should be elicited with palpation.
5. Insert the speculum and rotate the handle of the speculum downward, so the bills are in the inferior/superior position and open the speculum for visualization of the cervix. Open the speculum only as wide as needed for visualization. It is not necessary to open it completely (Figure 12.1).

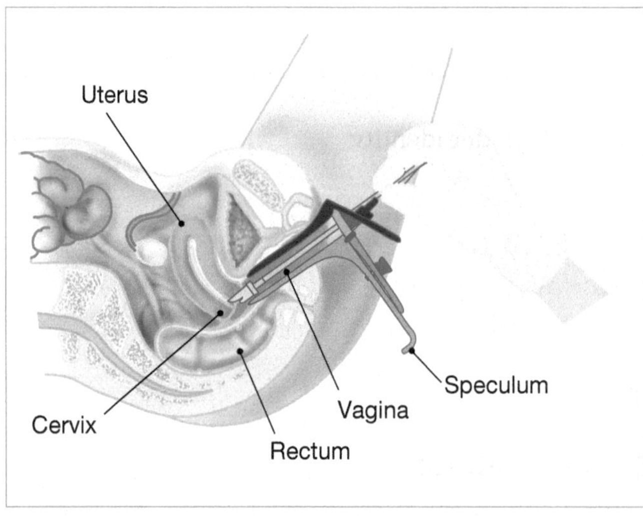


**Figure 12.1** Speculum examination of cervix and vagina

6. The vaginal tissue should be inspected during both insertion and removal of the speculum. If using a plastic speculum, the bills are clear, which can aid in visualization. Use of a metal speculum will require tilting the position of the bills, so visualization

of the entirety of the vaginal vault can be performed. The vagina should be inspected for color, tissue appearance, moisture, or the presence of discharge.

7. The speculum should be positioned to allow for visualization of the entire surface of the cervix.
8. A visual inspection of the cervix should be performed and include the size and shape of the os, color, bleeding, or discharge, the evaluation of the squamocolumnar junction (i.e., transformation zone), and assessment for any lesions or growths.
9. Collection of any necessary specimens can be completed at this time. Carefully completing the collection of endocervical and cervical cells by meticulously following the technique recommended is required if an adequate specimen is to be evaluated for cellular changes. These techniques vary depending on the collection tools used. The transformation zone is the most common area on the cervix for abnormal cells to develop, so collection of cells from this region is imperative when collecting cervical cytology.

## INSPECTION OF ABNORMAL FINDINGS

- The skin inspection of the entire genital region, including the perineum and anus, should evaluate for discoloration or hypopigmentation, erythema, and areas of excoriation. Note any visible ulcerations, pustules, vesicles, growths, lesions, nevi, warts, varicosities, scars, hemorrhoids, or evidence of injury or trauma.
- Skin lesions can indicate an STI. Herpes simplex virus (HSV), genital warts, primary syphilis, scabies, and chancroid can all present with lesions on the genitals and rectum.
- White patches on the skin of the inner vulva, but not involving the vaginal mucosa, can be concerning for vulval lichen sclerosus. It can be localized or spread to surrounding skin.
- Painless white streaks in a lacy or fern-like pattern on the labia majora, labia minora, and/or vaginal introitus are seen with vulval lichen planus. Erosive lichen planus is a more severe form of this condition that causes painful and persistent erosions and ulcers which leads to scarring, adhesions, resorption of the labia minora, and introital stenosis. This can sometimes occur concurrently with lichen sclerosus.
- Any evidence of trauma found on the external or internal genitalia examination should prompt further investigation.
- Visible live lice and/or nits in the pubic hair indicate pubic lice (pediculosis pubis).
- Any moles or lesions on the vaginal wall should be noted and referred to a specialist. Vulvar and vaginal cancer can present with skin changes such as sores, lumps, or ulcers that do not go away. Melanoma of the mucous membranes is often discovered at a late stage.
- Unusual odors can be indicative of an STI, bacterial vaginosis, or vulvocandidiasis.
- Cervicitis is an inflammation of the cervix, most often due to a STI, specifically chlamydia or gonorrhea. The cervix is erythematous and friable on exam. If there are punctate hemorrhages present, characterizing the commonly used term "strawberry cervix," then trichomonas is the likely causative agent.
- Vaginal discharge can be a normal finding, an infectious process, or due to another cause.
  - A sticky, mucous-like, white, odorless discharge occurs around ovulation and is normal.
  - Discharge increases during pregnancy.
  - A white, thick, curd-like discharge is seen with vulvocandidiasis.
  - A thin, white/gray/yellow, malodorous discharge is common with trichomoniasis.

- A yellow, white, or green discharge can be seen in both chlamydia and gonorrhea.
- A thin, white, or gray vaginal discharge with a fishy odor can accompany bacterial vaginosis.
- A retained tampon, genitourinary syndrome on menopause, vaginal atrophy, and/or vaginal fistulas can also cause discharge.
- Rarely, discharge is due to cervical and vaginal cancers.

- Ectropion, nabothian cysts, myomas, and small cervical polyps are commonly encountered on the cervix and are benign findings.
  - Ectropion occurs due to the eversion of the endocervix. This eversion exposes columnar epithelium, causing a reddish appearance around the cervical os. It may cause vaginal discharge and postcoital bleeding. Although benign, malignancy should also be excluded by cervical cytology when ectropion is present.
  - Nabothian cysts are epithelial cysts that may be translucent or opaque, whitish to yellow in appearance. There can be a single cyst or multiple and typically range in size from 3 to 4 cm in diameter. They are typically asymptomatic.
  - A cervical myoma is a single, small firm mass of smooth muscle from the lower uterine segment that can sometimes protrude through the cervical os. They are usually small and asymptomatic but can enlarge and cause symptoms including dysuria, dyspareunia, and/or urethral obstruction.
  - Cervical polyps are reddish-pink growths that typically originate in the endocervical canal and are usually asymptomatic; however, they may cause postcoital bleeding or bleeding between menses.
- Red, blue, or black lesions, termed "powder burns," can be a sign of cervical endometriosis. These lesions do not blanch on compression. Patient may be asymptomatic or report discharge, dysmenorrhea, pelvic pain, or dyspareunia.
- The appearance of cervical cancer will vary based on the stage of the cancer. In early stages, physical findings can appear normal or have the red, inflamed appearance of cervical ectropion. In later stages, the cervix may appear hard, ulcerated, or eroded in appearance.

## PALPATION

### BIMANUAL PELVIC EXAM

1. Based on the United States Preventive Services Task Force (USPSTF) recommendation, there is insufficient evidence to assess the balance of benefits and harms of screening with pelvic examination to detect a range of gynecologic conditions in asymptomatic, nonpregnant women; therefore, conducting pelvic examinations should not be routine practice. The decision to conduct a pelvic exam should be individualized, with the benefits and harms carefully considered in each patient situation.
2. The bimanual pelvic examination is performed to assess the uterus and adnexa. The index and middle finger of the dominant hand are lubricated with a water-soluble lubricant and inserted into the vagina until the cervix is palpable, moving fingers to the posterior fornix, located below the cervix. The nondominant hand is placed on the lower abdomen, above the pubic symphysis. Using the flat surface of the fingers, a sweeping downward motion toward the internal fingers is used to isolate the uterus. The internal fingers direct the uterus up to the fingers, gently compressing the uterus (Figure 12.2). This procedure allows for palpation of the uterine size and position in the pelvis. The size, shape, and symmetry of the uterus should be documented, as well as the position

and consistency of the uterus. In normal circumstances, palpation of the uterus is not painful, and any discomfort should be noted and may warrant further evaluation.

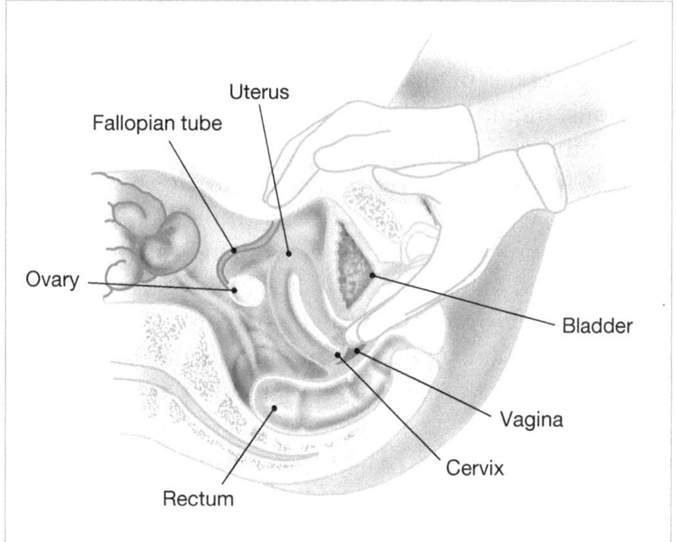


**Figure 12.2** Bimanual examination

3. Palpation of the adnexa serves to assess the ovaries and fallopian tubes. To assess the right adnexa, the clinician shifts the internal fingers to the patient's right side, moving the fingers to the right vaginal fornix. The flat surface of the fingers of the nondominant hand are placed just medial to the right anterior superior iliac spine and directed downward to meet the internal fingers. The goal is to capture the adnexa between the internal and external fingers for palpation. The ovary is approximately 3 × 2 cm and is often compared to the size of a walnut. This maneuver is repeated on the left side for assessment of the left adnexa. The ovaries are not always palpable. The size and mobility of the adnexa, as well as consistency, should be noted if they are palpated. There is a lack of evidence to support using manual palpation to screen for ovarian cancer so it should not be used for this purpose.
4. Cervical motion tenderness (CMT) is performed by placing the index and middle finger on either side of the cervix and gently pulling the cervix first to one side, then the other. This should not cause pain or discomfort.

## RECTOVAGINAL EXAMINATION

1. The rectovaginal examination (RVE) can be used for additional evaluation, if needed, and is typically performed after bimanual examination is completed. It is used to further assess the uterus, uterosacral ligaments, and the rectovaginal septum. Clean gloves should be donned prior to completing the RVE. The first finger of the dominant hand is placed into the vagina, and the middle finger of the same hand is placed into the rectum. Gentle upward pressure of the middle finger allows for the assessment of the rectovaginal septum. The uterosacral ligaments can be palpated by locating them along the posterior wall of the cervix, lateral to the sacrum. A retroverted uterus can also be examined using this method.
2. Examination should evaluate for any abnormalities, including tenderness, nodules, or apparent thickening or thinning.

### PALPATION ABNORMAL FINDINGS

- Enlargement and/or tenderness of the inguinal lymph nodes are a concern for either infection or malignancy of the genitalia.
- Tenderness on bimanual examination, including cervical motion tenderness (CMT), is a cardinal sign of pelvic inflammatory disease (PID). CMT is found in several pathologic conditions, including PID, appendicitis, and ectopic pregnancy. Positive CMT is noted when the patient experiences pain with traction on the adnexa. Interrater reliability for CMT is low, but there is still evidence that suggests its clinical significance in assisting with diagnosis of pelvic inflammatory disorder.
- Palpation of the ovaries in postmenopausal women is always an abnormal finding; if this should be identified on examination, it is highly suggestive of ovarian cancer.
- An enlarged uterus or pelvic mass that can be palpated during an abdominal or pelvic exam can signify pregnancy, uterine fibroids, or malignancies. Adnexal masses can be due to malignancy (ovarian or fallopian tube), ectopic pregnancy, hydrosalpinges, endometriomas, or can be a benign tumor.
- A rectocele can be felt on the DRE. The weakened wall of tissue that separates the vagina from the rectum causes the vaginal wall to bulge.

## SPECIAL TESTS

### AMINE ODOR TEST (KNOWN AS THE WHIFF TEST)

- This test is performed along with other tests to assist in the diagnosis of bacterial vaginosis. A small amount of discharge is removed from the vagina with a cotton swab. Several drops of 10% potassium hydroxide are added to the cotton swab. A strong fishy odor indicates a positive test.

### CERVICAL CYTOLOGY

- For patients 21 to 65 years of age, cervical cancer screening is recommended every 3 years with cervical cytology alone, every 5 years with high-risk HPV testing alone, or every 5 years with co-testing (cervical cytology and high-risk HPV testing).

### CULTURES

- Nucleic acid amplification tests are used to screen for trichomoniasis, gonorrhea, and/or chlamydia. These DNA tests can be performed from specimens collected from a variety of sites, including urine, provider-collected endocervical samples, and clinician or patient-collected vaginal specimens.

### MICROSCOPY

- Microscopy can be used to identify a number of genitourinary conditions. Buds and hyphae indicate the presence of yeast. Clue cells are seen with bacterial vaginosis. Trichomonads can also be visualized under the microscope.

### URINALYSIS

- Urinalysis can be used to rule in or rule out a urinary tract infection and provide additional information related to other potential disease processes. The combination of hematuria, pyuria, and nitrates is diagnostic for a urinary tract infection.

### VAGINAL PH TEST

- Using litmus paper to assess the vaginal pH can also assist in making the correct diagnosis. A small strip can be placed directly on the vaginal wall or a small amount of vaginal discharge can be placed on the litmus strip using a cotton swab. Normal vaginal pH is between 3.8 and 4.5 in premenopausal individuals. The pH in bacterial vaginosis is between 5.0 and 6.0, trichomonas is between 5.0 and 7.0, vulvocandidiasis is less than 4.5. In the absence of bacterial pathogens, a vaginal pH of 6.0 to 7.5 is strongly suggestive of menopause.

## RED FLAGS IN HISTORY AND PHYSICAL EXAM

- Abdominal distention or bloating
- Early satiety with loss of appetite
- Exposure to DES
- Unexplained pelvic or abdominal pain
- Increased urinary urgency or frequency
- Postcoital bleeding
- Postmenopausal bleeding
- Unexplained weight loss or fatigue
- Unexplained change in bowel habits
- Unilateral lower abdominal pain with vaginal bleeding, dizziness, weakness, and positive pregnancy test
- Over 50 years of age with new symptoms of irritable bowel syndrome

## POPULATION HEALTH AND LIFE-SPAN CONSIDERATIONS

### INFANTS, CHILDREN, AND ADOLESCENTS

- Routine genitourinary (GU) exams should be performed during all infant and child wellness examinations. The newborn examination, in particular, should include inspection for congenital malformations, atypical or ambiguous genitalia, and placement and patency of the anus. The pediatric anogenital examination should be performed with a caregiver present.
- Use of a speculum is never indicated in the prepubertal female ano-genital exam unless unexplained vaginal bleeding is present; in that situation, the examination is performed under general anesthesia.
- For adolescents, a chaperone can be a caregiver or another healthcare clinician, but this should be the adolescent's choice. Assess the Tanner state of sexual maturity for female adolescents:

- **Stage 1**: Small nipples with no breast tissue; no pubic hair
- **Stage 2**: Breast and nipples have just started to grow. The areola has become larger. Breast tissue bud feels firm behind the nipple. Initial growth of long pubic hairs. These are straight, without curls, and light in color.
- **Stage 3**: Breast and nipples have grown additionally. The areola has become darker. The breast tissue bud is larger. The pubic hair is more widespread. The hair is darker, and curls may have appeared.
- **Stage 4**: Nipples and areolas are elevated and form an edge toward the breast. The breast has also grown a little larger. More dense hair growth with curls and dark hair. Still not entirely as an adult woman.
- **Stage 5**: Fully developed breast. Nipples are protruding, and the edge between areola and breast has disappeared. Adult hair growth. Dense, curly hair extending toward the inner thighs.

- The following exam findings are highly suggestive of sexual abuse even in the absence of a disclosure of sexual abuse by the child:
  - Acute injuries to genital/anal tissues;
  - Acute lacerations or bruising of labia, perianal tissues, or perineum;
  - Acute laceration of the posterior fourchette or vestibule (not involving the hymen);
  - Bruising, petechiae, or abrasions on the hymen;
  - Acute laceration (tear) of the hymen (partial or complete);
  - Vaginal laceration;
  - Perianal laceration with exposure of tissue below the dermis;
  - Healing (nonacute/chronic) injuries to genital/anal tissues;
  - Perianal scar;
  - Scar of posterior fourchette;
  - Healed hymenal transection between 4 and 8 o'clock, which extends through to the base of the hymen with no hymenal tissue remaining at the location; and/or
  - A missing segment of hymen between 4 and 8 o'clock
  - Traumatic findings can also result from accidental ano-genital injury. However, any history given by the child and/or caregiver should be closely examined for timeliness and plausibility.

## OLDER ADULTS

- The decrease in estrogen levels during the menopause transition results in thinning of the vaginal tissue. This thinning causes decreased elasticity of the tissue, a paler appearance, and more fragile tissue, which can result in vaginal dryness and petechiae. These changes can range from asymptomatic to moderate-to-severe dyspareunia, vaginal discomfort, and irritation. As a result of these changes, speculum examination may be uncomfortable for the postmenopausal patient.

## PREGNANCY

- Refer to Chapter 17, "Pregnant Populations," for more information.

## OTHER CONSIDERATIONS

- Being overweight/obese may be a predictor for early occurrence of menarche.
- Non-Hispanic Black females mature earlier than other races, although sexual development completes at approximately the same age.
- Vaginoplasty is a surgical construction of a vaginal canal and usually involves a penile inversion procedure. The anatomy of the neovagina is a blind cuff and may have a more downward sloping presentation. In the first 3 to 6 months after vaginoplasty, it is imperative to receive clearance from surgeon prior to internal exam and anoscope should be used rather than speculum. Transwomen will need to adhere to a dilation schedule long term to maintain vaginal depth.
  - The prostate will be small and withdrawn in patients on feminizing hormone therapy. For patients who have undergone vaginoplasty, it may be reasonable to assess the prostate digitally through the neovagina as access from the rectum may be obscured by the vaginal wall.
  - The prostate is not removed during vaginoplasty, and infectious prostatitis must be considered for at-risk women.
- Female genital cutting, also referred to as female circumcision or genital mutilation, is a cultural practice, predominantly in Asia and Africa, defined as "all procedures involving partial or total removal of the external female genitalia or other injury to the female genital organs for non-medical reasons." The World Health Organization has defined four classifications of female genital cutting:
  - **Type 1:** Partial or total removal of the clitoral glans and/or the prepuce/clitoral hood.
  - **Type 2:** Partial or total removal of the clitoral glans and the labia minora, with or without removal of the labia majora.
  - **Type 3:** Also known as infibulation, the narrowing of the vaginal opening through the creation of a covering seal formed by cutting and repositioning the labia minora, or labia majora, sometimes through stitching, with or without removal of the clitoral prepuce/clitoral hood and glans.
  - **Type 4:** Includes all other harmful procedures to the female genitalia for non-medical purposes (e.g., pricking, piercing, incising, scraping, and cauterizing the genital area).
- Female genital cutting has no health benefits and causes short- and long-term complications. Immediate complications include severe pain, fever, swelling, bleeding, and urinary problems. Long-term complications include chronic infection, menstrual disorders, dyspareunia, sexual dysfunction, and an increased risk of childbirth complications for mother and baby. These individuals have unique care considerations.

## KEY DIFFERENTIALS

- Bacterial vaginosis
- Bartholin gland cyst
- Cervical cancer
- Cystocele
- Ectopic pregnancy
- Endometriosis
- Genitourinary syndrome of menopause
- Infertility
- Intertrigo
- Lichen planus
- Lichen sclerosus
- Menopause
- Menstrual irregularities
- Ovarian cancer
- Pelvic inflammatory disease (PID)
- Polycystic ovarian syndrome (PCOS)
- Pregnancy
- Premenstrual dysphoric disorder
- Premenstrual syndrome
- Rectocele
- Ruptured ovarian cyst
- Sexually transmitted infections (STIs)
- Stress urinary incontinence
- Uterine fibroids
- Uterine prolapse
- Vulvar cancers and vulvar intraepithelial neoplasia (VIN)
- Vulvovaginal candidiasis

## KNOWLEDGE CHECK: FEMALE REPRODUCTIVE SYSTEM

1. Which BEST describes the signs and symptoms of vaginal candidiasis?

   **A.** Abdominal pain and copious yellow-green vaginal discharge
   **B.** External pruritus, dysuria, and thick white vaginal discharge
   **C.** Foul fishy odor, vaginal irritation, and thin vaginal discharge
   **D.** None of the above, as the condition is commonly asymptomatic

2. During menopause, what happens to levels of luteinizing hormone (LH) and follicle-stimulating hormone (FSH)?

   **A.** Become non-detectable
   **B.** Decrease dramatically
   **C.** Remain the same
   **D.** Increase dramatically

3. The presence of clue cells on a vaginal wet mount exam evaluated with microscopy indicates:

   **A.** Bacterial vaginosis
   **B.** Candida albicans
   **C.** Trichomoniasis
   **D.** Normal vaginal flora

4. Assessment consistent with bacterial vaginosis (BV) includes:

   **A.** Frothy, gray-green cervical discharge with a pH below 4.0
   **B.** Thick, white discharge adherent to inflamed vaginal mucosa
   **C.** Thin, malodorous vaginal discharge with pH above 4.5
   **D.** Vagina itching, dysuria, and severe abdominal pain

5. A 60-year-old woman who is 10 years past menopause presents for her annual women's health exam. Which finding requires urgent or immediate evaluation?

   **A.** Atrophic vaginitis
   **B.** Grade 2 cystocele without straining
   **C.** Palpable left adnexa consistent with ovary 3 x 3 cm size
   **D.** Prolapse of posterior vaginal wall with straining

6. Which risk factor is associated with cervical cancer?

   **A.** Dysmenorrhea
   **B.** Long-acting reversible contraception
   **C.** Polycystic ovarian syndrome
   **D.** Sexual history of multiple partners

*(See answers next page.)* 

**1. B) External pruritus, dysuria, and thick white vaginal discharge**

Women with vaginal candidiasis (yeast infection) have symptoms of thick, white, adherent discharge, vulvar and vaginal itching, dysuria, and often dyspareunia. Pelvic pain with discharge that is copious is more highly correlated with sexually transmitted infections. Women with symptomatic bacterial vaginosis (BV) infections typically report vaginal itching or irritation, white or gray thin vaginal discharge, and presence of a strong fishy odor that is particularly noticeable after intercourse or their menstrual cycle. Vaginal candidiasis may be asymptomatic in women who have recurrent infections, but the condition is commonly symptomatic.

**2. D) Increase dramatically**

Menopause results from loss of ovarian sensitivity to gonadotropin stimulation, which is directly related to follicular attrition. During menopause, as aging follicles become more resistant to gonadotropin stimulation, circulating FSH and LH levels increase dramatically.

**3. A) Bacterial vaginosis**

A vaginal wet mount exam, also called a "wet prep," is a test to identify the cause of vaginal discharge. Microscopy can reveal normal epithelial cells, white blood cells, red blood cells, motile trichomonads, yeast hyphae and spores, and clue cells. Clue cells are epithelial cells that have a stippled appearance and fuzzy margins as a result of adherent bacteria, primarily *Gardnerella vaginalis*; the presence of clue cells indicates bacterial vaginosis.

**4. C) Thin, malodorous vaginal discharge with pH above 4.5**

Women with symptomatic BV infections typically report vaginal itching or irritation, white or gray thin vaginal discharge, presence of a strong fishy odor that is particularly noticeable after intercourse or their menstrual cycle; pH is alkaline. Cervical discharge that is frothy or copious is more highly correlated with sexually transmitted infections, although the pH with trichomoniasis, for example, would be alkaline. Women with vaginal candidiasis (yeast infection) have symptoms of thick, white, adherent discharge, vulvar and vaginal itching, dysuria, and often dyspareunia

**5. C) Palpable left adnexa consistent with ovary 3 x 3 cm in size**

Adnexal fullness or enlargement in a postmenopausal woman would be an abnormal finding consistent with an ovarian mass, requiring a high index of suspicion for malignancy. The presence of a cystocele and/or rectocele may warrant evaluation but are not urgent or emergent findings. Atrophic vaginitis after menopause is common.

**6. D) Sexual history of multiple partners**

Multiple sex partners, having one partner who is high risk, and sexual activity at a young age are all risk factors associated with cervical cancer, most often the result of HPV infection. Additional risk factors include smoking, and do not include menstrual disorders, or use of long-acting, reversible contraception. Untreated polycystic ovarian syndrome can increase the risk of endometrial cancer.

7. A young adult female presents for evaluation of amenorrhea. She is a college athlete, is sexually active, mostly uses condoms for contraception, and has no history of sexually transmitted infections. What is the MOST LIKELY cause of her amenorrhea?

   **A.** Disordered eating
   **B.** Female athlete triad
   **C.** Low percentage of body fat
   **D.** Pregnancy

8. What causes the pain and cramping associated with primary dysmenorrhea?

   **A.** Ovulatory dysfunction
   **B.** Prostaglandin release and synthesis
   **C.** Shedding of abnormal uterine lining
   **D.** Stress and low levels of serotonin

9. Which reason for seeking care is MOST urgent for the woman who recently started taking combined estrogen-progestin oral contraceptive pills?

   **A.** Breast tenderness
   **B.** Nausea
   **C.** Severe headaches
   **D.** Spotting between periods

10. A 40-year-old woman G2P2 presents with a history of heavy and prolonged menstrual bleeding and mild anemia. Her exam reveals an enlarged uterus, and her pregnancy test is negative. Her MOST LIKELY diagnosis is:

    **A.** Bleeding disorder
    **B.** Endometriosis
    **C.** Polycystic ovarian syndrome
    **D.** Uterine fibroids

(*See answers next page.*)

**7. D) Pregnancy**

Women of reproductive age who are sexually active and are not using contraceptive methods consistently are at risk for unintended pregnancy. While the female athlete triad—menstrual dysfunction, low intake, and loss of bone density—is not uncommon in young women participating in sports; this is not as likely as pregnancy for the college-aged female without routine use of contraception. Disordered eating and low percentage of body fat are correlated with the female athlete triad and can be linked to amenorrhea.

**8. B) Prostaglandin release and synthesis**

Primary dysmenorrhea is pain that results during the menstrual cycle from the increased synthesis of prostaglandins in endometrial tissue and the release in menstrual fluid. Non-steroidal anti-inflammatory medications are capable of relieving primary dysmenorrhea because they inhibit prostaglandin synthetase enzymes. Stress, ovulatory dysfunction, and abnormalities in uterine lining are more likely to cause irregular cycles, heavy bleeding, or amenorrhea; these can be causes of secondary dysmenorrhea.

**9. C) Severe headaches**

Use of oral contraceptive pills increases the risk of ischemic stroke and thromboembolism. Use the acronym ACHES (abdominal pain, chest pain, headaches, eye problems, severe calf or thigh pain) to review symptoms to report urgently for anyone beginning use of combined estrogen-progestin oral contraceptive pills. Other side effects of breast tenderness, nausea, mood changes, and abnormal menstrual bleeding commonly resolve during the first three months of use.

**10. D) Uterine fibroids**

Uterine fibroids are benign masses that develop within the uterine wall, are more common in women 30 to 40 years old, and lead to heavy menstrual bleeding and anemia. While endometriosis, bleeding disorders, and polycystic ovarian syndrome can lead to irregular and painful cycles, none are likely to cause uterine enlargement.

# Male Reproductive System

## KEY HISTORY CONSIDERATIONS

- Urethral discharge
- Dysuria
- Nocturia
- Blood in semen
- Painful ejaculation
- Urinary urgency, hesitancy, or weak urinary stream
- Recurrent urinary tract infections
- Testicular lump or lump in the inguinal area
- Infertility
- Perineal or rectal pain
- Anal itching
- Sexual dysfunction (including erectile dysfunction and premature ejaculation)
- Injury to the groin
- Human papillomavirus (HPV) vaccination
- History of undescended testicle
- History of sexually transmitted infections including human immunodeficiency virus (HIV)
- History of diabetes or cardiovascular disease
- History of sexual abuse or interpersonal violence
- History of colonoscopy
- Family history of prostate, urogenital, rectal, or colon cancers
- Exposure to chemical carcinogens
- Nicotine use
- Alcohol intake
- Sexual history (including unprotected vaginal, oral, or anal sex)
- Sexual orientation and gender identity

## PHYSICAL EXAMINATION: INSPECTION AND PALPATION

### INSPECTION

1. Inspect the hair and skin of the groin, pubis, penis, scrotum, and perineum for rashes, lesions, discoloration, or swelling.
2. Note whether the penis is circumcised or uncircumcised.

3. Note the Tanner stage if appropriate. See the "Infants, Children, and Adolescents" section for more details on the Tanner stages.
4. When adults present with genitourinary (GU) concerns and are uncircumcised, retract the prepuce (foreskin) of the penis, then inspect the glans and urethral meatus. The opening of the urethra should be at the tip of the penis.
5. The testes should appear as two discrete oval-shaped organs. Typically, the left testes is slightly lower than the right. The testes may retract up towards the body if the room is cooler.
6. If a rectal examination is necessary, inspect the perineum, anal folds, and anal opening.

### INSPECTION ABNORMAL FINDINGS

- Any ecchymosis, edema, erythema, scars, or lesions on the penis, scrotum, perineum, or anus are abnormal. Lesions can be due to a noninfectious, infectious, or malignant etiology. Noninfectious causes include such conditions as pearly papules, psoriasis, lichen sclerosus, lichen nitidus, lichen planus, tinea cruris, or angiokeratomas. Infectious causes can include a variety of sexually transmitted infections, including HPV, syphilis, herpes simplex virus, chancroid, balanitis, or scabies. Carcinoma in situ and squamous cell carcinoma can also be found in these areas and should be considered.
- Smegma is a white discharge that can develop under the foreskin of uncircumcised men due to the buildup of oil cells and dead skin cells. This is not infectious although it can have the appearance of pus.
- Penile discharge is suggestive of a urethritis, which is typically seen with sexually transmitted infections such as gonorrhea or chlamydia.
- Penile adhesions can occur in circumcised boys if the remaining foreskin is not retracted on a regular basis and the penile shaft skin adheres to the glans of the penis. Adhesions that are untreated can become skin bridges.
- If the urethral opening is on the anterior side of the penis, this is an epispadias. If it is on the posterior side of the penis, it is hypospadias.
- Pubic hair should be inspected for nits, which would indicate pubic lice.
- If there is a protuberant area in the inguinal area, it is likely an inguinal hernia.
- Skin tags, fissures, and hemorrhoids are common findings in the anal area.
- If there is evidence of anogenital injury without a consistent history, especially in children, sexual abuse should be ruled out. Acute injury, perianal scarring, lesions, lacerations, ecchymosis, and healing injury to the genitals or perianal tissue are physical findings that require immediate follow-up.

## PALPATION

1. Palpate the shaft of the penis for nodules, plaques, or other soft tissue masses. The index or middle finger of the clinician's hand should be placed posteriorly while the thumb of the same hand is placed anteriorly.
2. Retract the foreskin if the individual is uncircumcised and gently compress the glans penis between the thumb and first finger to inspect for patency, inflammation, or urethral discharge.

3. The testes should be gently palpated for nodules, hard masses, or abnormal shape. Use the thumbs and index fingers of both hands to gently palpate the entire testicle, while the remaining fingers stabilize the testicle. A normal testis should feel smooth, ovoid, and non-tender. Size and volume can be estimated using an orchidometer.
4. Palpate the epididymis along the posterior aspect of the testis and up along the spermatic cord.
5. Palpate for inguinal lymph nodes.
6. The examination for an inguinal hernia should be performed with the patient in a standing position and the clinician in a seated position facing the patient. With a gloved index or middle finger, gather loose skin from the scrotum and invaginate the scrotal sac with the finger upward along the inguinal canal until the external ring is reached. Ask the patient to cough or bear down similar to when they are having a bowel movement. This maneuver increases the intra-abdominal pressure which will make a hernia more apparent. While the patient bears down, observe and feel the inguinal area for bulging over the femoral canal that can indicate a femoral hernia (Figure 13.1).

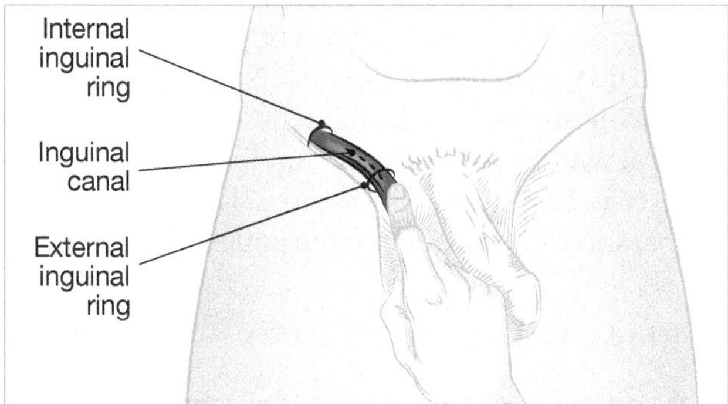


**Figure 13.1** Technique for assessing inguinal hernias.

7. Although not a routine exam, the digital rectal examination (DRE) can be performed to evaluate the lower rectum and prostate. A DRE is typically performed for presenting concerns of unexplained blood in the stool, an abnormal mass in the anus or rectum, a significant change in bowel or bladder habits, change in urinary stream, and/or urethral discharge or bleeding. Otherwise, DRE is not performed as a routine element of male wellness examinations. For the digital rectal examination, the individual should be unclothed from the waist down and in a gown and/or covered with a drape. Ideal positioning for the examination is either with the male standing with a forward bend at the waist or side-lying with knees to chest. Separate the buttocks and first inspect the anal opening. Lubricate the index or middle finger of a gloved hand. Inform the patient that a finger will be inserted into the rectum. Ask the patient to take a deep breath and relax and breathe out while gently inserting the examining finger into the anal canal. Palpate the prostate anteriorly, noting size, symmetry, and texture (Figure 13.2). A normal prostate is walnut-sized, symmetrical, and smooth with a cartilaginous texture (similar to the tip of the nose). The prostate has a midline groove (sulcus) that should be palpable. DRE gives a poor indication of prostatic size.

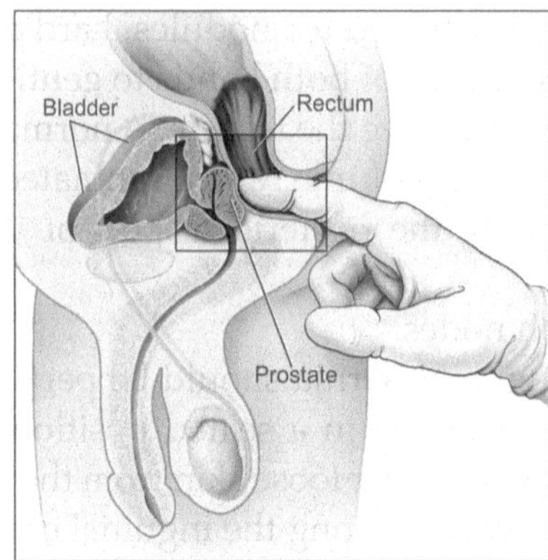


**Figure 13.2** Digital rectal examination, including examination of the prostate.
*Source:* U.S. Department of Health and Human Services, National Institutes of Health, and the National Cancer Institute.

8. Stroking the skin of the anal area, usually with the end of a paper clip, should cause a contraction of the anal musculature ("the anal wink").
9. Rotate the finger 360 degrees to palpate the span of the rectal wall for masses or irregularities. Stool may be palpated in the rectal vault. Note the consistency (hard or soft). Assess anal tone by asking the patient to tighten their anal sphincter on the finger. Once the patient relaxes, withdraw the finger, and inspect for blood, stool, or mucus. A fecal occult blood test can be performed if desired. Re-drape the patient, provide tissues or cleansing cloths, and allow privacy so the patient can clean up and get dressed.

## PALPATION ABNORMAL FINDINGS

- Note any swelling or soft tissue masses within the scrotal sac, epididymis, or spermatic cord. Tenderness or edema in the scrotum can indicate infection such as an orchitis.
- Signs of testicular cancer include a sometimes painful, unilateral, firm lump in the testes, a significantly smaller testicle with a reported history of sudden shrinking, or scrotal edema.
- Fibrosis can occur along the shaft of the penis, which can cause palpable plaques and penile curvature.
- A testicle raised above the normal position accompanied by severe groin or abdominal pain, nausea, vomiting, fever, and a history of injury to the groin is concerning for testicular torsion, which is a surgical emergency.
- A varicocele is abnormally dilated veins in the scrotum. This is often described as feeling like a "bag of worms" on palpation.
- A fluid-filled, well-circumscribed painless growth located above or behind a testicle and on the epididymis is often a spermatocele. Spematoceles are benign cysts that are often pea-sized but can grow to be quite large.
- Enlargement and/or tenderness of the inguinal lymph nodes are a concern for either infection or malignancy of the genitalia.
- If an inguinal hernia is present, a bulging sensation can be visualized, palpated, or felt at the tip of the finger when the patient coughs or bears down during the examination. When the patient is standing, if the upper portion of the mass is not discrete,

it is likely an inguinal hernia. Hernias are typically non-tender and retractable. A hernia that will not retract is termed an incarcerated hernia and is a surgical emergency.
- Tenderness with palpation of the prostate can indicate a prostatitis or orchitis.
- Nodules, masses, induration, asymmetry, or an area on the prostate that is harder than the surrounding areas is abnormal and can be a sign of prostate cancer.
- Nodules or masses on the rectal wall can range from internal hemorrhoids, polyps, or carcinomas. Carcinomas are usually fixed and hard. Occasionally, foreign bodies can also be palpated during the exam and should be gently removed.
- Blood, pus, or black stool signifies an infectious or malignant process. Frank red blood can indicate a fissure, laceration, polyp, hemorrhoid, carcinoma, or a chronic inflammatory bowel disease. Pus in the stool can indicate infection. A small amount of mucus in the stool is normal. Larger amounts can be due to either infectious or noninfectious processes. Infectious causes are primarily bacteria in origin and noninfectious causes are such conditions as inflammatory bowel disease.
- Hard stool can be palpated and is a sign of constipation or fecal impaction.
- Absence of the anal wink can be due to muscle weakness, nerve damage, and spinal cord injury.

## SPECIAL TESTS

### CREMASTERIC REFLEX

- Attempt to elicit the cremasteric reflex when evaluating for certain testicular concerns that cause scrotal pain. The reflex is triggered by stroking the inner thigh with the index and middle finger. An intact reflex will cause the ipsilateral cremaster muscle to contract, thereby raising the testis. In some conditions, like testicular torsion, the cremasteric reflex will be negative because the cremaster muscles surrounding the spermatic cord are twisted and unable to contract. The absence of the cremasteric reflex for individuals presenting with scrotal pain is a useful sign, indicating the need for emergent evaluation.

### TRANSILLUMINATION

- Transillumination is a technique for evaluating the scrotal sac for certain concerns such as scrotal swelling. Perform the procedure by dimming the lights of the exam room and shining a bright light (e.g., penlight, otoscope, or flashlight) through the wall of the scrotum. Fluid will illuminate; soft tissue masses will not.

# RED FLAGS IN HISTORY AND PHYSICAL EXAM

- Sudden onset of testicular pain and swelling
- Transverse testicular lie
- Nausea, vomiting
- Acute abdominal pain (which may be the presenting symptom of testicular torsion in children and adolescents)
- Hematuria
- Palpable bladder

- Fever and flank pain or tenderness
- Erection that will not resolve
- Penile discharge and/or lesions
- Painless testicular lump
- Exquisite tenderness of a testicle
- Exquisite tenderness of the prostate
- Nodularity of the prostate
- Loss of anal reflex
- Loss of cremasteric reflex
- Loss of bowel or bladder control

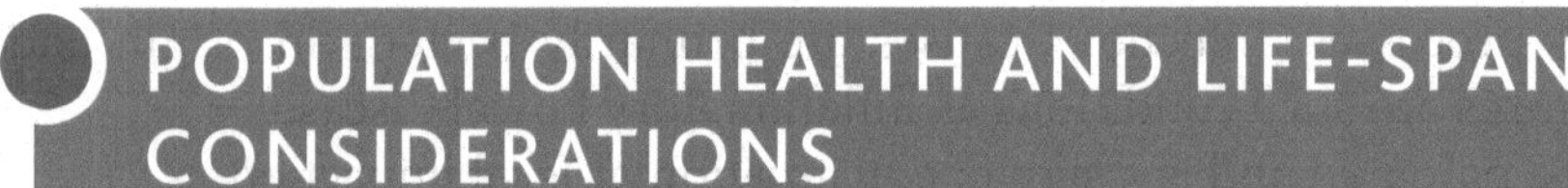

# POPULATION HEALTH AND LIFE-SPAN CONSIDERATIONS

## INFANTS, CHILDREN, AND ADOLESCENTS

- The anogenital examination of the infant or child should be performed with a caregiver present. If the caregiver is unable to be present, a chaperone or another healthcare clinician should be present. Some states have mandatory chaperone laws, so it is important for clinicians to be aware of their respective state laws. For adolescents, a chaperone can be a caregiver or another healthcare clinician, but this should be the adolescent's choice.
- Routine GU exams should be performed during all infant and child wellness examinations. Note that the foreskin of uncircumcised newborns and young infants may be tightly adhered to the glans penis and should never be forcefully retracted. The newborn examination, in particular, should include inspection for congenital malformations, ambiguous genitalia, and placement and patency of the anus.
- The clinician should palpate the scrotal sac for soft tissue masses and to ensure that both testes have descended and can be brought down into the lower third of the scrotal sac. If the testis cannot be palpated in the scrotum, the clinician should palpate the inguinal canal and upper scrotal sac for the testis. Some testes are "retractile," meaning they can move between the inguinal canal and scrotum. A retractile testis can be located and brought down into the lower third of the scrotum. Retractile testes should resolve by puberty.
- For adolescents, the genital examination can produce anxiety. Adolescents can be unsure whether their developing bodies are "normal," and they have a greater need for modesty and privacy during sensitive examinations. Assessment of the adolescent genitalia is similar to the adult, except the clinician should assess for sexual maturity, or Tanner staging, while inspecting the genitalia. The sexual maturity rating for preadolescent and adolescent males uses a scale from 1 (prepubertal) to 5 (adult-like), based on changes in pubic hair distribution and growth of the penis and testes. The Tanner stages are:

- **Stage 1:** Testes are more than 2.5 cm, no change in penis size, no pubic hair
- **Stage 2:** Enlargement of testes, pigmentation of scrotal sac; no change in penis size; pubic hair is long, downy, and variable in pattern
- **Stage 3:** Further enlargement of testes; significant enlargement of penis, especially in diameter; increase in amount and curling of pubic hair
- **Stage 4:** Further enlargement of testes and penis, pubic hair is adult in type but not distribution, development of axillary and facial hair begins
- **Stage 5:** Testes and penis are adult in size, pubic hair is adult in distribution, body hair continues to grow; overall growth (height/weight/muscle) velocity peaks

## OLDER ADULTS

- The scrotal sac gets more pendulous with age.
- Testicular tissue mass decreases.
- The prostate gets larger with age. About 50% of men between the ages of 51 and 60 are affected by benign prostatic hyperplasia and up to 90% of men older than 80 are affected.

## OTHER CONSIDERATIONS

- Non-Hispanic Black males mature earlier than other races, although sexual development completes at approximately the same age.
- Sexual minority boys and men remain at highest risk for acquiring HIV/AIDS.
- 47% of transgender people have been sexually assaulted at some point in their lives. Sexual minority men are more likely than are heterosexual men to experience sexual violence victimization, such as childhood sexual abuse, sexual assault related to hate crimes, and intimate partner sexual assault.
- Pelvic inflammatory disease should be considered for all at-risk men with a uterus and fallopian tubes.
- Some men retain vaginas with or without reproductive organs after metoidioplasty but not all are safe to penetrate. A consultation with the patient's surgeon may be necessary.
- Metoidioplasty is a genital surgery that creates a microphallus with or without a neo-urethra. A vaginectomy may or may not be done at the time of the surgery.
- Phalloplasty is a genital surgery that creates a phallus using skin grafts from other sites and contains a neo-urethra. Vaginectomy is typically done at the time of the surgery.

## KEY DIFFERENTIALS IN MALE GENITALIA

- Epididymitis
- Balanitis
- Hydrocele
- Hypospadias
- Male genital *candidiasis*
- Orchitis
- Peyronie's disease
- Phimosis and paraphimosis
- Priapism
- Scrotal cellulitis
- Sexually transmitted infections
- Spermatocele
- Testicular cancer
- Testicular torsion
- Undescended testes
- Urethritis
- Varicocele

## KEY DIFFERENTIALS IN ANUS, RECTUM, AND PROSTATE

- Anal fissures
- Anorectal agenesis/imperforate anus
- Benign prostatic hyperplasia
- External and internal hemorrhoids
- Prostate cancer
- Pruritus ani
- Rectal polyps
- Rectal cancer
- Sexually transmitted infections

## KNOWLEDGE CHECK: MALE REPRODUCTIVE SYSTEM

1. A 3-month-old male infant is noted to have an undescended left testicle during his well-child check. The parents are very concerned. After acknowledging their concern, the advanced practice nurse should explain:

   **A.** As long as one testis is palpable, this is not a concern until the child is 5 years old

   **B.** The infant needs immediate referral for surgery for this emergent condition

   **C.** There is a high probability that the testicle will spontaneously descend before 1 year of age

   **D.** This is highly associated with a congenital disorder of sexual differentiation

2. A 28-year-old-male presents with acute onset of severe testicular pain. Physical examination reveals exquisite tenderness, acute swelling of the testicle, and absence of cremasteric reflex. These findings suggest:

   **A.** Femoral hernia

   **B.** Hydrocele

   **C.** Inguinal hernia

   **D.** Testicular torsion

3. Which statement is true regarding sexually transmitted infections?

   **A.** Chlamydial infection can be present without causing symptoms

   **B.** Gonorrhea is rarely found in the adolescent population

   **C.** Herpes is not a prevalent infection in any age group

   **D.** Screening for sexually transmitted infections should begin after 18 years of age

4. Which two are key risk factors for prostate cancer? (Select TWO.)

   **A.** Age, especially after age 50

   **B.** Being overweight

   **C.** History of genital infection

   **D.** History of genital trauma

   **E.** Race, especially African American men

5. What are the symptoms of benign prostatic hypertrophy? (Select all that apply.)

   **A.** Abdominal pain

   **B.** Dribbling post urination

   **C.** Nodular prostate

   **D.** Nocturia

   **E.** Weak urine stream

*(See answers next page.)*

**1. C) There is a high probability that the testicle will spontaneously descend before 1 year of age**

An undescended testicle is a failure of the testis to descend into the lower third of the scrotum by 4 months of age. The testicle may be located in the intra-abdominal space (cryptorchidism), the inguinal canal, or the upper third of the scrotum. There is no advantage to clinical observation of an undescended testicle longer than 12 months of age. Surgical correction is required prior to puberty to preserve fertility and decrease the risk of testicular cancer. The primary risk factor is prematurity.

**2. D) Testicular torsion**

Key signs and symptoms of testicular torsion include acute onset of testicular pain and swelling, transverse testicular lie, and a negative cremasteric reflex. Testicular torsion is a surgical emergency. In contrast, testicular swelling that occurs with hydrocele is painless, and it fluctuates. Femoral and inguinal hernias can cause pain if entrapped; however, the pain and palpable mass would be abdominal or in groin/inguinal areas.

**3. A) Chlamydial infection can be present without causing symptoms**

Most individuals who are infected with chlamydia are asymptomatic and lack abnormal exam findings. Screening is necessary to identify most sexually transmitted infections. Gonorrhea occurs most often in teens aged 15 to 19 years. The current prevalence of herpes in the United States is about one in every four or five adults. The United States Preventive Services Task Force (USPSTF) recommends that clinicians screen for HIV infection in all adolescents and adults aged 15 to 65 years; younger adolescents and older adults who are at increased risk of infection should also be screened.

**4. A and E) Age, especially after age 50; race, especially African American men**

Prostate cancer is rare in men younger than 40 and increases significantly after the age of 50. Prostate cancer develops more often in Black males, and they tend to be younger. The role of genetics, diet, sexually transmitted infection, smoking, and history of surgery/trauma on the development of prostate cancer is still unclear.

**5. B, D, and E) Dribbling post urination, nocturia, weak urine stream**

Benign prostatic hyperplasia (BPH) is an enlargement of the prostate gland. Key signs and symptoms include uncomfortable urinary symptoms: urinary frequency, impaired flow, weak urine stream, nocturia, and/or urinary dribbling post urination. Abdominal pain and penile discharge are more likely with prostatitis. A nodular prostate is more likely to indicate prostate cancer.

6. A urethral meatus that opens on the ventral surface of the penis is:

   A. Epispadias
   B. Hypospadias
   C. Normal placement
   D. Normal variation

7. Gender identity is determined by:

   A. Family and societal expectations
   B. Internal sense of self
   C. Reproductive organs
   D. Sexual orientation

8. Which of the following are effects of aging on the male reproductive system? (Select all that apply.)

   A. External genitalia remains unchanged
   B. Sexual responses may be slower
   C. Testicles stop producing sperm
   D. Testosterone levels decline

9. What is the first sign of puberty in males?

   A. Axillary hair
   B. Coarse dark pubic hair
   C. Lengthening of the penis
   D. Testicular enlargement

10. Which condition is an emergency?

    A. Hydrocele
    B. Varicocele
    C. Paraphimosis
    D. Phimosis

*(See answers next page.)*

**6. B) Hypospadias**

The urethra opens as a slit-like vertical opening, the urinary meatus, at the tip of the glans. Hypospadias is a congenital malformation of the male genitourinary tract in which the urethral opening is abnormally located on the ventral aspect of the penis. The condition varies in severity and may cause the urethral meatus to be located on the penile shaft, scrotum, or perineum. Similarly, but less commonly, epispadias is an abnormal dorsal placement of the urethral meatus. Surgical correction is required for both epispadias and hypospadias.

**7. B) Internal sense of self**

Gender identity is one's innermost concept of self as male, female, a blend of both, or neither. Gender expression is the appearance of one's identity as expressed through behavior, clothing, and voice, which may or may not conform to socially defined gender roles. Gender identity is distinguished from biological sexual characteristics, as not all individuals identify with the gender assigned at birth. Gender identity is distinct from sexual orientation, which is based on an individual's romantic and intimate relationships and attractions.

**8. B and D) Sexual responses may be slower, testosterone levels decline**

Physical age-related changes include prostate enlargement, testicular atrophy, thinning pubic hair, more pendulous scrotum, and slower sexual response (e.g., erection, orgasm, and ejaculation). Slowed sexual responsiveness may be related to declining testosterone levels. While fertility declines, males do continue to produce sperm and seminal fluid.

**9. D) Testicular enlargement**

Testicular growth is the first sign of puberty; normal onset is between the ages 9 to 14 years of age. After enlargement of the testicles, the penis also increases in size. Enlargement of the testicles and penis almost always occurs before the development of pubic hair. Growth of axillary hair occurs in Tanner stage 3, and height increases at peak rate during Tanner stage 4. In the final stage puberty, Tanner stage 5, facial hair develops, and mature testicular size and penis length is reached.

**10. C) Paraphimosis**

Paraphimosis is a condition that results from forcefully retracting tight foreskin back over the glans penis. The foreskin becomes entrapped behind the corona of the glans. Key findings include painful swelling of the distal glans penis with a constricted band of tissue proximal to the glans proximal to the corona. Paraphimosis is a medical emergency because it will eventually result in tissue ischemia and necrosis. Phimosis is a condition in which the foreskin of an uncircumcised penis cannot be retracted over the glans; this condition can be physiologic or pathologic and does not require emergent treatment. A varicocele is a collection of dilated twisted veins surrounding the spermatic cord that does not usually require intervention. A hydrocele is a collection of peritoneal fluid in the scrotal sac that results from a fascial defect in the inguinal canal; these are usually noted during infancy and most often resolve without intervention by 2 years of age.

14

# Mental Health and Substance Use

## KEY HISTORY CONSIDERATIONS

- Depressed mood
- Anhedonia
- Excessive worry
- Anger and irritability
- Panic attacks
- Fears or worries that the patient feels unable to control
- Episodes of increased energy, impulsivity, and risk-taking
- Trouble with the law or previous incarceration
- Insomnia or hypersomnia
- Isolation
- Presence of suicidal or homicidal ideation
- Hearing or seeing things that others do not
- History of hospitalizations, self-harm, or suicide attempts
- History of addiction or substance use
- History of trauma, abuse, or adverse childhood events
- Current nicotine, alcohol, or illegal drug use
- Taking medications not prescribed to the patient
- In children, chronic or recurrent abdominal pain, headaches, or chest pain

## MENTAL HEALTH ASSESSMENT: APPEARANCE, BEHAVIOR, COGNITION, AND SCREENINGS

A mental status assessment gives the clinician an understanding of the patient's cognitive, emotional, personality, and psychological functioning. This assessment can be done in the course of an individual's routine history and physical examination. With mental status assessment, there is overlap with subjective and objective assessments and findings. The mental status assessment is performed within the context of the patient's age, developmental level, and cultural norms. Assessments of a person's affect, mood, attention, judgment, and memory can be remembered using the mnemonic "ABC" as listed: **A**ppearance, **B**ehavior, and **C**ognition.

### APPEARANCE

- **Affect:** Appropriate for the situation, labile, pleasant, flat, nontoxic
- **Posture:** Lying, sitting, or standing; comfortable; obvious limitations or defects

- **Hygiene and grooming:** Appropriately dressed for the weather or situation, disheveled or neatly groomed
- **Body habitus:** Height, weight, waist circumference, body mass index (BMI), and comparison to previous measurements

## BEHAVIOR

- **Expressions:** Verbal or nonverbal expressions of pain, anxiety, illness, anger, fear, frustration, contentment, or sadness
- **Interactions:** Cooperative, guarded, aggressive, withdrawn
- **Activity level:** Calm, active, flat, restless, previous/recent/current impulsivity
- **Body movements and mobility:** Coordinated, limited, assistive devices, abnormal movements or involuntary tics present, slowed or very quick movements

## COGNITION

- **Orientation:** Oriented to time, person, and place; confused; disoriented; delirious
- **Attention and concentration:** Able to express coherent, organized thoughts, or rapidly shifting from one topic to next; any concerns with success in work, school, or at home
- **Speech pattern and pace:** Appropriate, rushed, slow, loud, or quiet; pressurized, garbled, or clear and articulate.
- **Judgment:** Thought content including irrational fears or overwhelming worry; thought patterns including negative patterns of all-or-nothing thinking, catastrophizing, overgeneralization, blaming, emotional reasoning, or always being right
- **Altered sensory perceptions:** Hearing voices or hallucinations, able to control impulses, insight into personal strengths
- **Memory:** Able to repeat three unrelated words and remember and repeat these words again in 5 minutes; concerns about memory loss
- **Mood:** Feelings of sadness, guilt, worry, fear, helplessness, or hopelessness; recent insomnia, hypersomnia, loss of appetite, increased appetite, or difficulty feeling enjoyment; feelings of elation, grandiosity, or mood instability; previous or current suicidal and/or homicidal thoughts and/or plan; agitated

## MENTAL HEALTH SCREENINGS

### PATIENT HEALTH QUESTIONNAIRE (PHQ-9 AND PHQ-2) DEPRESSION SCALES

- The PHQ-9 is a widely used, valid, and reliable nine-item tool for screening and monitoring the severity of depression. Question 9 of the tool screens for the presence and duration of suicidal ideation (SI). This screening tool and an instruction manual are available at no cost at www.phqscreeners.com.
- The brief PHQ-2 consists of the first two questions of the PHQ-9 and screens for core symptoms of major depressive disorder:

Over the *past 2 weeks*, how often have you been bothered by the following problems?

1. Little interest or pleasure in doing things
   - Not at all (0)
   - Several days (+1)
   - More than half the days (+2)
   - Nearly every day (+3)
2. Feeling down, depressed, or hopeless
   - Not at all (0)
   - Several days (+1)
   - More than half the days (+2)
   - Nearly every day (+3)

- The total scoring from the PHQ-2 ranges from 0 to 6. If the score is 3 or greater, depressive disorder is likely. Patients who screen positive should be further evaluated.

### GENERALIZED ANXIETY DISORDER SCALE (GAD-7 AND GAD-2)

- The 7-item Generalized Anxiety Disorder (GAD-7) is a validated screening tool for anxiety that includes a severity assessment scale. Free download is also available at www.phqscreeners.co.
- The abbreviated GAD-2 screening consists of the first two questions of the GAD-7:

Over the *past 2 weeks*, how often have you been bothered by the following problems?

1. Feeling nervous, anxious, or on edge
   - Not at all (0)
   - Several days (+1)
   - More than half the days (+2)
   - Nearly every day (+3)
2. Not being able to stop worrying
   - Not at all (0)
   - Several days (+1)
   - More than half the days (+2)
   - Nearly every day (+3)

- The scoring for the GAD-2 is similar to the PHQ-2, with a range from 0 to 6. The recommended cutpoint for a positive screening is a score of 3 or greater. The GAD-2 and PHQ-2 can be used together (referred to as the PHQ-4) to screen for depression and anxiety.

## SUBSTANCE USE ASSESSMENT

Similar to mental health disorders, when screening for substance use, it is appropriate to start with a short screening questionnaire and if positive, complete a longer questionnaire.

### SINGLE-QUESTION SCREENINGS FOR SUBSTANCE USE

The evidence suggests that single-screening questions can be effective tools to identify substance misuse. Note that screening negatively for the misuse of one substance does not negate the need to screen for misuse of other substances. Responses to these single questions serve as the foundation or basis for further dialogue and assessment. A response of one or more is considered a positive screen.

- Single-question screen to identify illicit substance use: "How many times in the past year have you used an illegal drug or used a prescription medication for nonmedical reasons?" If clarification of "nonmedical reasons" is needed, provide the explanation, "For instance, because of the experience or feeling it caused."
- Single-question screening for alcohol misuse: "How many times in the past year have you had *X* or more drinks in a day?" where *X* is five for men and four for women.

### CAGE QUESTIONNAIRE ADAPTED TO INCLUDE DRUG USE (CAGE-AID)

- Have you ever felt you ought to cut down on your drinking or drug use?
- Have people annoyed you by criticized your drinking or drug use?
- Have you ever felt bad or guilty about your drinking or drug use?
- Have you ever had a drink or used drugs first thing in the morning to steady your nerves or to get rid of a hangover (eye-opener)?

Items are scored 0 for "no" and 1 for "yes." A total score of two or greater is considered clinically significant. A score of "1" should warrant an additional follow-up.

### ABNORMAL PHYSICAL EXAMINATION FINDINGS IN SUBSTANCE USE DISORDERS

Specific health effects of substances to consider when determining components of the physical exam:

- Excessive alcohol consumption increases the risk of developing type 2 diabetes, pancreatitis, cancers, cardiomyopathy, dementia, hepatitis, and cirrhosis, in addition to the short-term intoxication, disinhibition, stupor, and potential for coma and death. Even moderate use of alcohol can interfere with sleep quality, lead to weight gain, and lead to impulsive behaviors and decisions.
- Tobacco use causes damage to nearly every organ in the body, often leading to lung cancer, heart disease, stroke, emphysema, and chronic bronchitis. Exposure to secondhand smoke also causes adverse health effects.
- Marijuana has not only immediate effects like distorted perception, difficulty problem-solving, and loss of motor coordination, but also effects with long-term use, including respiratory infections, impaired memory, and exposure to cancer-causing compounds.
- Opioids not only reduce the perception of pain but also produce drowsiness, mental confusion, euphoria, nausea, constipation, and respiratory depression. Most overdose deaths from substance use are attributable to opioids.

## RED FLAGS IN HISTORY AND PHYSICAL EXAM

- Threatening to hurt or kill themselves
- Seeking access to pills, weapons, or other means
- Talking or writing about death, dying, or suicide

- Feelings or statements of hopelessness
- Rage, anger, seeking revenge; feeling trapped
- Increased alcohol or other drug use
- Withdrawal from others
- Anxiety and agitation
- Sleep problems; insomnia or hypersomnia
- Dramatic mood changes
- Sudden and/or drastic change in behavior
- Feelings or statements that reflect not having a reason to live
- Substance use interfering with ability to function
- Legal trouble (driving under the influence of alcohol [DUI], incarceration, loss of job, difficulty with interpersonal relationships)
- Overdose
- Prostitution

## POPULATION HEALTH AND LIFE-SPAN CONSIDERATIONS

### INFANTS, CHILDREN, AND ADOLESCENTS

With children and adolescents, part of the assessment interview will be with parents or caregivers; if the young person can tolerate being separated from their parents, individual time spent with the child/teen is invaluable. In the individual time spent with the clinician (after confidentiality is made clear), the child/teen is often very forthcoming with their own concerns and experiences. The child/teen also can provide the clinician with best treatment options that fit with their values and preferences.

There are child/adolescent-specific screening tools that assess for mental health conditions. The PHQ-A is a derivative of the PHQ-9 that screens for depression in adolescents aged 11 to 17.

The Pediatric Symptom Checklist-17 is a broadly used questionnaire that is both valid and reliable. It is used to recognize psychosocial problems in children and assess changes in emotional and behavioral problems in children. This is appropriate for children aged 11 and older.

For adolescents, the HEADSS assessment can also be helpful in identifying mental health problems:

- **Home**: Where is the teen living? Who lives in the home? How is the teen getting along with people in the home? Has the teen ever run away or been incarcerated?
- **Education and/or Employment**: How is the teen functioning in school in terms of grades, performance in class, and teachers/peers? Any recent changes? Have there been any suspensions or missed school days? Any current or past employment? Any problems with work attendance?
- **Activities**: In which extracurricular and sports activities is the teen involved, if any? What do they do with their friends? What does the teen do for fun?

- **Drugs**: Which drugs, including alcohol, cigarettes, vaping, caffeine, stimulants, or pills, have been used by the teen, their family, and/or friends?
- **Sexuality**: How does the teen express their gender identity? How does the teen identify their sexual orientation? Has the adolescent been sexually active? Are they currently in a relationship? Does the teen use contraception and/or condoms? How many partners have they had? What is the teen's past history of sexually transmitted infections, pregnancy, abortion, and sexual abuse? Has the adolescent been a victim of trauma?
- **Suicide**: Is there a history of isolation or being withdrawn, emotional outbursts, or impulsive behavior? Has the teen had depression symptoms, including suicidal ideation (SI) or a past history of suicide attempts (SA)? If there has been SI, does the teen have a plan and access to the means to commit suicide?

## OLDER ADULTS

- Greater than 20% of adults aged 60 and over suffer from a mental or neurological disorder.
- Dementia and depression are the most common mental and neurological disorders in this age group. Anxiety disorders affect 3.8% of the older population, substance use problems affect almost 1%, and around a quarter of deaths from self-harm are among people aged 60 or over.
- Substance abuse problems among older people are often overlooked or misdiagnosed.
- Depression is associated with worse health in people with chronic conditions like heart disease, diabetes, and stroke.
- In older adults, depression may be disregarded as frailty, or it may be viewed as an inevitable result of life changes, chronic illness, and disability.
- The most common conditions include anxiety, severe cognitive impairment, and mood disorders (such as depression or bipolar disorder).
- Mental health issues are often implicated as a factor in cases of suicide. Older men have the highest suicide rate of any group.

## OTHER CONSIDERATIONS

- Postpartum depression (PPD) occurs between 10% and 20% of the population. It usually begins within the first month after having a baby but can occur up to 1 year following birth. The Edinburgh Postnatal Depression Scale is a commonly used, valid, and reliable instrument for detecting postpartum depression.
- Women who have had a major depressive episode are more likely to suffer from substance use disorder than those who have not had a major depressive episode.
- Black and Hispanic Americans are more likely to meet criteria for major depressive disorder (MDD).
- CDC statistics show that people with less education, less economic stability, and less insurance coverage are more likely to meet the criteria for MDD.
- Research also consistently shows that divorce increases the risk for depression symptoms.
- Major depression is most likely to affect people between the ages of 45 and 65. People in middle age are at the top of the bell curve for depression, but the people at each end of the curve—the very young and very old—may be at higher risk for severe depression.

## KEY DIFFERENTIALS

- Adjustment disorder
- Acute stress disorder
- Attention deficit disorder (ADD)
- Bipolar depression
- Borderline personality disorder
- Delusional disorder
- Dysthymia
- Generalized anxiety disorder (GAD)
- Major depressive disorder (MDD)
- Obsessive compulsive disorder (OCD)
- Panic disorder
- Phobias
- Posttraumatic stress disorder (PTSD)
- Postpartum depression (PPD)
- Psychotic disorder
- Schizophrenia
- Schizoaffective disorder
- Schizophreniform disorder
- Substance use disorder (SUD)

## KNOWLEDGE CHECK: MENTAL HEALTH AND SUBSTANCE USE

1. Manic or hypomanic episodes associated with bipolar mood disorder are likely to include:

   **A.** Fatigue and hypersomnia
   **B.** Feelings of worthlessness and slowed thinking
   **C.** Irritability and racing thoughts
   **D.** Memory loss and confusion

2. Which statement about depression screening and risk factors is true?

   **A.** Positive screening always requires urgent psychiatric mental health referral
   **B.** Risk factors to consider include chronic illnesses, gender, and socioeconomic factors
   **C.** Screening for mild depression is generally unnecessary unless a person has risk factors
   **D.** Screening tools are inaccurate for those over 65 years of age with chronic comorbidities

3. A parent mentions that her 16-year-old son is exhibiting symptoms of aggression at home and is engaging in risky behaviors and asks whether her son might be using drugs. Before responding, the advanced practice nurse correctly recalls that substance use disorder:

   **A.** Can begin but cannot be diagnosed during adolescence, as the disease is progressive
   **B.** Is often linked to stress and other comorbidities, such as ADHD or anxiety
   **C.** Occurs rarely in adolescence and usually is linked to poor parenting
   **D.** Requires a positive urine screen on more than one occasion for definitive diagnosis

4. What words summarize the five steps or strategies that can be implemented by clinicians to assess an individual's tobacco use and readiness to quit?

   **A.** Admit, assess, analyze, admonish, admire
   **B.** Ask, advise, assess, assist, arrange
   **C.** Seek, stop, solve, support, succeed
   **D.** Start, stop, strengthen, support, succeed

*(See answers next page.)*

**1. C) Irritability and racing thoughts**

Individuals with bipolar disorder will have unusual shifts in mood, energy, and activity levels. They may have a pattern of depressive episodes mixed with hypomanic or manic episodes. Mania and hypomania symptoms include grandiosity, racing thoughts, pressured speech, irritability, aggressive or angry outbursts, feelings of elation, and/or excessive involvement in reckless activities. Depressive symptoms include persistent sadness, hypersomnia (excessive sleepiness), fatigue, loss of interest in most or all normal activities, feelings of worthlessness or guilt, slowed thinking or trouble concentrating, and thoughts of suicide and/or death. Memory loss and confusion are more likely correlated with dementia or other comorbid disorders.

**2. B) Risk factors to consider include chronic illnesses, gender, and socioeconomic factors**

The USPSTF recommends screening in all adults regardless of risk factors. However, a number of factors are associated with increased risk of depression; prevalence rates vary by gender, age, race/ethnicity, education, marital status, geographic location, and employment status. Women, young and middle-aged adults, and nonwhite individuals have higher rates of depression. Others at increased risk include persons with chronic illnesses (e.g., cancer, diabetes, or cardiovascular disease), other mental health disorders (including substance misuse), or family history of psychiatric disorders. Among older adults, risk factors for depression include disability and poor health status related to medical illness, complicated grief, chronic sleep disturbance, loneliness, and a history of depression. Evidence-based screening tools include the Patient Health Questionnaire (PHQ) in various forms, the Geriatric Depression Scale in older adults, and the Edinburgh Postnatal Depression Scale in postpartum and pregnant women. All positive screening results should lead to additional assessments for severity of depression, comorbidities, and alternate diagnoses.

**3. B) Is often linked to stress and other comorbidities, such as ADHD or anxiety**

Studies have shown strong links between ADHD, substance use disorder, and anxiety. Clinicians who recognize that comorbidities, toxic stress, adverse childhood events, lack of social support, and intergenerational distress can add to an individual's vulnerability for substance use disorder are better able to implement screening, intervention, and referral. False assumptions that teens cannot develop substance use disorders, or that poor parenting underlies the diagnosis, are reflective of bias that delays treatment. Diagnostic criteria can be met during adolescence without lab testing.

**4. B) Ask, advise, assess, assist, arrange**

The five major steps to assess tobacco use and respond to an individual's readiness to quit are summarized as the "5 A's":

- **Ask:** Identify and document tobacco use status for every patient at every visit
- **Advise**: In a clear, strong, and personalized manner; urge every tobacco user to quit
- **Assess**: Determine readiness to make a quit attempt
- **Assist**: Support individuals in making a quit plan
- **Arrange**: Schedule follow up and refer if needed

5. In addition to feelings of sadness or depressed mood, characteristics of adult depression include:

   A. Disrupted sleep and slowed thinking
   B. Excessive involvement in reckless activities
   C. Hyperactivity and racing thoughts
   D. Memory loss and confusion

6. Which history is most consistent with a diagnosis of dysthymia, or persistent depressive disorder?

   A. 17-year-old male with a history of daily marijuana use for the past 6 months
   B. 35-year-old woman with fatigue and loss of interest in family or friends for 2 years
   C. 55-year-old male with a 2-year history of hypothyroidism and uncontrolled diabetes
   D. 55-year-old male with sadness and insomnia since his spouse's death 2 weeks ago

7. Which two individuals have the highest risk for suicide? (Select TWO.)

   A. 20-year-old male who was bullied as a teen
   B. 30-year-old female college graduate student
   C. 30-year-old male who recently became a father
   D. 60-year-old female nurse nearing retirement
   E. 80-year-old male who was widowed this year

8. A 50-year-old shares that they have been "worrying a lot." Which of the individual's additional statements MOST indicates need for mental health support or counseling?

   A. Believes themselves to be someone who over-analyzes situations
   B. Believes themselves to be very stressed and is not sleeping well
   C. Is having difficulty with adopting new routines despite attempts to do so
   D. Shares that symptoms interfere with their ability to function at work and home

9. Which is true about adolescent substance use?

   A. Rarely would an adolescent develop substance use disorder or addiction
   B. Rarely would an adolescent have changes in brain function from substance use
   C. Neuroadaptations from substance use can be dramatic during adolescence
   D. Neuroplasticity protects the adolescent brain from the effects of substance use

(*See answers next page.*)

### 5. A) Disrupted sleep and slowed thinking

Symptoms of depression include persistent sadness, depressed mood, sleep disturbances (insomnia or hypersomnia), fatigue, loss of interest in most or all normal activities, feelings of worthlessness or guilt, slowed thinking or trouble concentrating, change in appetite, and thoughts of suicide and/or death. While older adults can have memory difficulties, memory loss and confusion are more likely correlated with dementia or other disorders. Individuals with mood disorder can have symptoms of depression, and are also likely to present with grandiosity, racing thoughts, irritability, aggressive or angry outbursts, and/or excessive involvement in reckless activities.

### 6. B) 35-year-old woman with fatigue and loss of interest in family or friends for 2 years

Dysthymia, or persistent depressive disorder, is a chronic form of depression that interferes with normal daily activities and relationships. Physical and behavioral co-morbidities (diabetes, hypothyroidism, substance use) are not diagnostic criteria for persistent depressive disorder, although can be associated ones. Signs and symptoms of grief include sadness and difficulty sleeping; these are normal findings and are not consistent with a mental health diagnosis.

### 7. A and E) 20-year-old male who was bullied as a teen; 80-year-old male who was widowed this year

Risk factors for suicide include male gender, young adulthood, isolation, and history of trauma. While suicide rates have decreased for older adults, isolation associated with loss of a spouse is a significant risk factor. Stressors of education, parenthood, and retirement can be triggers, but these are not as highly associated with suicidality as a history of bullying and a history of loss of a spouse.

### 8. D) Shares that symptoms interfere with their ability to function at work and home

Interference with functioning is a key indicator of a mental health diagnosis. The diagnostic criteria for anxiety disorders include difficulty with managing work, home, school, or social situations, and these symptoms indicate need for mental health support and/or counseling. Being stressed, over-thinking, or having difficulties with adapting are not necessarily indicators of mental health disorders.

### 9. C) Neuroadaptations from substance use can be dramatic during adolescence

The American Academy of Pediatrics defines addiction as a developmental disorder and recommends screening for substance use disorder as a routine part of adolescent care. The rationale for this position is based on the understanding of neurobiology and the neuroadaptations that result from substance use, which can be more dramatic and happen more quickly during adolescence. The adolescent brain is particularly vulnerable to the toxic effects of substances. The neuroplasticity of the adolescent brain increases their risk of substance use disorder.

**10.** Having an empathetic approach to discussing substance misuse with patients implies that the advanced practice nurse:

**A.** Can treat individuals with tolerance despite their inability to change

**B.** Feels sorry for these individuals because they lack willpower

**C.** Has the ability to share emotions and consider patients' perceptions

**D.** Is justifiably angry at their choices but is able to treat them with sympathy

(*See answers next page.*)

**10. C) Has the ability to share emotions and consider patients' perceptions**
Empathy is the ability to recognize and share the emotions and perceptions of another. Empathy moves beyond tolerance and is not the same as sympathy (feeling sorrow or pity for someone). Empathy is an essential element of therapeutic communication. To have an empathetic approach to the individual misusing substances requires recognition that substance use disorder is a complex disease characterized by use despite consequences rather than a result of moral failing or personal weakness.

# Part III
# Evidence-Based Considerations for Population Health

15

# Determinants of Health and Wellness

## KEY HISTORY CONSIDERATIONS

Individuals seek visits with clinicians for primarily three reasons: to address episodic concerns, for wellness exams, and to manage chronic illnesses. At all these visits, clinicians assess a patient's history and obtain subjective information. One primary area of their history assessment that impacts and determines their level of health and wellness is their social history.

An individual's social history provides information regarding their health beliefs and behaviors, support systems, and safety, and allows a clinician to identify risk factors that may impact well-being. Note that the influence of culture on health beliefs, behaviors, practices, perceptions, and approaches is vast; this component of history requires a sensitive and humble approach that respects cultural, family, community, and personal values and norms.

Components of social history include: (1) substance use history; (2) relationships, including marital status, living arrangements, family dynamics, and support systems; and (3) safety of home, work, and/or school environments, which includes assessment for hazards, exposure to violence, trauma, or stressors, behaviors involving risk-taking, and social determinants of health.

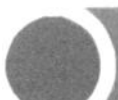

## ASSESSING DETERMINANTS OF HEALTH

Asking about the environments in which an individual resides, works, learns, plays, worships, and connects socially offers important insight into the determinants of their health. The following are key areas to consider related to the determinants that impact an individual's health:

- **Economic stability:** Access to employment, career counseling, and job training; access to high quality childcare; income and resources to meet daily needs, including food.
- **Neighborhood and built environments:** Access to safe, affordable housing in neighborhoods without exposure to violence, unsafe air or water, or other safety hazards.
- **Healthcare access and quality:** Availability of evidence-based healthcare services and preventive screenings; access to clinicians with linguistic and cultural competency; access to insurance coverage, and care meeting health literacy needs.
- **Social and community context:** Availability of resources and support within communities for recreation, worship, work, learning, and meeting basic needs; experiences of discrimination, isolation, violence, trauma, bullying, and loss.
- **Education access and quality:** Access to safe, quality education, including early childhood education; broadband access to internet, and emerging technologies.

An individual's understanding of health, experience of well-being, and ability to achieve wellness in all dimensions can change over time and is highly personal. Health literacy, the degree to which individuals have the capacity to obtain, process, and understand health information, significantly impacts wellness beliefs, behaviors, and overall well-being. Individuals with low health literacy experience barriers to care and are less likely to be able to navigate the complexity of the healthcare system.

Assessing an individual's determinants of health provides insight into their ability, readiness, and motivation to engage in behaviors to prevent disease and illness, including:

- Healthy lifestyle behaviors, including diet/nutrition, physical activity/exercise, and sleep
- Management of stress and coping with stressors
- Recent/needed health screenings (e.g., blood pressure, anxiety, depression, mammogram, colonoscopy, cholesterol, lead, sexually transmitted infections, and vision/hearing)

## ASSESSMENT OF HEALTH BEHAVIORS

Despite national goals for health and well-being, six in ten adults in the United States have a chronic disease, and four in ten adults have two or more. Some risk factors for chronic disease are non-modifiable, and include age, family health history, and ethnicity. The rising burden of chronic disease, however, is mostly linked to modifiable health behaviors, including physical inactivity, tobacco use or exposure, unhealthy diets, excessive alcohol intake, and lack of sleep.

Healthy lifestyle behaviors that are priorities:

- **Engage in regular physical activity.** Moving more and sitting less has tremendous health benefits, including decreased risk of heart disease, diabetes, some cancers, osteoporosis, depression, and anxiety. At least 150 minutes a week (30 minutes daily) of moderate-intensity exercise such as brisk walking is the recommendation for adults and older adults.
- **Maintain a healthy diet.** Recommendations include consuming five servings of fruits and vegetables daily; limiting saturated fats and added sugars to less than 10% of daily calories; including whole grains and a variety of proteins in one's diet; for infants, exclusively breastfeeding for the first 6 months of life. Good nutrition across the life span is key to avoiding heart disease, hypertension, stroke, cancers, mental health disorders, and obesity, and improving focus, mood, and the immune system. Nutritional choices and dietary patterns are linked to body weight.
- **Avoid smoking and use of tobacco products.** Tobacco use causes damage to nearly every organ in the body, often leading to lung cancer, heart disease, stroke, emphysema, and chronic bronchitis. Exposure to secondhand smoke also has adverse health effects.
- **Drink alcohol in moderation, if at all.** Excessive alcohol consumption increases the risk of developing diabetes, pancreatitis, cancers, cardiomyopathy, dementia, hepatitis, and cirrhosis, in addition to short-term intoxication, disinhibition, stupor, and potential for coma and death.
- **Sleep 7 to 9 hours each night.** Inadequate sleep (duration or quality) has been linked to hypertension, heart disease, diabetes, obesity, and suppressed immunity.

- **Reframe stressful situations.** Reframing allows an individual to view the current situation from a different perspective; relaxation, mindfulness, meditation, exercise, and laughter are positive strategies that allow stressful situations to be viewed differently. Unmanaged stress can lead to burnout, obesity, heart disease, and mental health disorders.

Participating in recommended health promotion strategies—for example, having recommended immunizations, dental visits, vision screening, and wellness exams—is associated with good health, and is especially important for children. Assessing growth, development, oral health, mental health, and risk factors, in an ongoing manner beginning in childhood, is essential to well-being across the life span.

Participating in health promotion strategies and developing healthy lifestyle behaviors are shaped by the opportunities that individuals have, and the choices they make according to these opportunities throughout life. Inequality in economic, cultural, health literacy, and social resources (social determinants of health) causes disparities in health and limits one's ability to participate in healthy lifestyle behaviors. These determinants also have an impact on beliefs that individuals have about themselves and their health and wellness.

## ASSESSMENT OF HEALTH DISPARITIES

When there are significant barriers to meeting wellness needs for individuals or families within a community, people experience health disparities or greater burden of illness, injury, disability, and/or mortality. Race, ethnicity, gender, sexual identity, age, disability, socioeconomic status, and geographic location all contribute positively or negatively to an individual's ability to achieve well-being. When individuals lack access to resources required for health and well-being (social determinants of health), they experience health disparities. Prevention of disparities in health requires access to high-quality education, nutritious food, decent and safe housing, reliable public transportation, culturally-sensitive healthcare providers (HCPs), health insurance, clean water, and nonpolluted air.

While population health has improved over time, disparities persist; for some populations, including minorities and indigenous people of color, low-income groups, women, children, older adults, individuals with disabilities, people who have experienced toxic stress or trauma, and individuals living in rural and inner-city areas, health disparities have persisted and, in some cases, widened.

Examples of health disparities in the United States include:

- About 10% of Navajo Nation on reservations in the southwestern United States live without electricity, and approximately 40% lack running water; this requires them to haul their water and use outhouses. Lack of resources leads to disparities. American Indians die at higher rates than any other Americans from liver disease, diabetes, injuries, and respiratory diseases.
- Evidence suggests that LGBTQ+ (lesbian, gay, bisexual, transgender, queer or questioning, and related communities) individuals face health disparities linked to societal stigma and more frequent experiences of violence, victimization, and discrimination. LGBTQ+ youth are two to three times more likely to commit suicide, and LGBTQ+ populations have the highest rates of tobacco, alcohol, and substance use.

- The rate of secondhand smoke exposure for children living in families with incomes below the poverty level is more than 4.5 times the rate for children in families with incomes significantly above the poverty threshold. This exposure increases risk of asthma, ear infections, respiratory infections, and sudden infant death syndrome.
- Significant racial and ethnic disparities persist in women's health and healthcare. These disparities are linked to broad structural, systemic, and societal inequities, including racism, implicit bias, economic factors, gender oppression, and unequal educational opportunities. Black American women have higher rates of poor health outcomes during and after pregnancy; they are more likely to have gestational diabetes, deliver preterm, and are three to four times more likely to die a pregnancy-related death.

Assessing and addressing the impact of systemic, structural, and societal inequities on individuals and populations requires the willingness of clinicians and healthcare systems to self-assess for implicit bias, and to recognize the impact of health determinants. Note that while implicit bias differs significantly from the conscious attitudes and behaviors of explicit or overt bias, either type of bias can exacerbate health disparities and create barriers to care. Reducing disparities requires national, state, local, and systems leadership to engage a diverse array of stakeholders; facilitate coordination and alignment among departments, agencies, offices, and partners; champion the implementation of effective policies and programs; and ensure accountability.

## WELLNESS EXAMS AND HEALTH PROMOTION

Assessing determinants of health, health literacy, and health beliefs and behaviors are important components of wellness exams. Wellness exams are a significant health promotion and disease prevention strategy, as the goals of the visit include early identification of health risks, and/or detection of health problems at an early stage when treatment is most likely to be effective. Sports physicals, well child exams, work physicals, and annual exams are examples of wellness exams; these clinician visits require age- and gender-appropriate history and physical exam.

Because the patient history taking during wellness exams is not problem-oriented, the history will not include a chief concern, although reason for the visit can be listed. In addition, there is not likely to be a need to collect HPI, or history of present illness. Rather, a wellness exam should include a comprehensive history and physical examination appropriate to the patient's age and gender, counseling and anticipatory guidance, risk reduction interventions, the ordering or administration of vaccine-appropriate immunizations, and the ordering of appropriate laboratory and/or diagnostic testing. The wellness exam differs from the episodic visit and chronic care management visit because the components of the wellness exam are based on age and risk factors, not a presenting problem.

Incorporating screenings for determinants of health within wellness exams is an evidence-based practice expectation. Social determinants of health have routinely been incorporated in the U.S. Preventive Services Task Force recommendations for assessing disease risk factors, screening, and management.

## COMPONENTS OF WELLNESS EXAMS

Across the life span:

- Comprehensive, culturally sensitive history and physical examination
- Anticipatory guidance regarding risks to health and well-being
- Recommendations for immunizations, screenings, and diagnostic testing
- Anticipatory guidance and support regarding reaching health and wellness goals

Additional life-span considerations:

- Assessment of growth and development are key priorities for well child exams
- Prenatal and postpartum exams are considered wellness exams and focus on well-being
- Preventive services for older adults include additional screenings for chronic diseases

# KNOWLEDGE CHECK: DETERMINANTS OF HEALTH AND WELLNESS

1. Which two statements are correct regarding the completion of wellness exams in a primary care office? (Select TWO.)

   A. Identifying disease risks related to health determinants are key to wellness visits

   B. These visits are focused on existing chronic disease processes

   C. These visits are focused on identifying signs and symptoms of disease

   D. Wellness exams or visits are rarely covered by insurance

   E. Wellness exams or visits in primary care include anticipatory guidance

2. Which statement is accurate about lifestyle-related diseases in the United States?

   A. Less than 5% of adults report tobacco use

   B. More than 50% of adults practice all key healthy lifestyle behaviors

   C. More than 50% of adults have at least one chronic illness

   D. Rarely is excessive alcohol use a factor in chronic disease

3. A 50-year-old male who emigrated to the United States from Cuba has type II diabetes and has been seen in the primary care office for the last year. The advanced practice nurse has given him many handouts designed to help him manage his diabetes. His last HbA1c was 9.2, and the patient says that he is trying to do his best. Which rationale for his uncontrolled diabetes is MOST LIKELY?

   A. He doesn't understand the potential negative outcomes

   B. He needs to experience negative outcomes to motivate change

   C. His health literacy level is lower than the materials given to him

   D. His spouse is not supportive of his needed dietary changes

4. Women of which race/ethnicity experience the highest rates of maternal mortality in the United States?

   A. Black American

   B. Asian American/Pacific Islander

   C. Hispanic/Latino

   D. White/Caucasian

5. The role of the advanced practice nurse in assessing health disparities includes:

   A. Asking each individual to explain their cultural beliefs and practices

   B. Completing physical assessments without regard to race or ethnicity

   C. Documenting advanced assessment without regard to race or ethnicity

   D. Recognizing barriers to care, and being sensitive to cultural influences

*(See answers next page.)*

**1. A, E) Identifying disease risks related to health determinants are key to wellness visits, wellness exams or visits in primary care include anticipatory guidance**

Wellness visits should include a comprehensive exam appropriate to an individual's determinants of health (economic stability, environment, healthcare access, community context, and education), counseling and anticipatory guidance, risk reduction interventions, and appropriate immunizations, lab and/or diagnostic testing. The wellness exam differs from the episodic visit or chronic care management visit because the components are based on risk factors, not a presenting problem.

**2. C) More than 50% of adults have at least one chronic illness**

Six in ten adults in the United States have a chronic illness, and four in ten have two or more. The rising burden of chronic disease is linked to modifiable health behaviors, including physical inactivity, tobacco use or exposure, unhealthy diets, excessive alcohol intake, and lack of sleep. Tobacco use continues to be the leading cause of preventable disease; approximately 15% of adults in the United States report use. Excessive alcohol consumption is a factor in the development of diabetes, pancreatitis, cancers, cardiomyopathy, dementia, hepatitis, and cirrhosis. Less than 7% of adults practice all key healthy lifestyle behaviors, i.e., exercise 150 minutes weekly, maintain a healthy diet, avoid tobacco use, drink alcohol in moderation if at all, and sleep 7 to 9 hours each night.

**3. C) His health literacy level is lower than the materials given to him**

Health literacy refers to how an individual has access to needed healthcare information; providing handouts to help manage diabetes is not likely to meet the needs of a recent immigrant. Assuming that the individual is noncompliant, not motivated, does not care, or isn't supported are all examples of implicit bias. Reevaluating patient education strategies is a requirement of evidence-based, culturally sensitive, quality care.

**4. A) Black American**

Significant racial and ethnic disparities persist in women's health and healthcare. Black American women have higher rates of poor health outcomes during and after pregnancy; they are more likely to have gestational diabetes, deliver preterm, and are three to four times more likely to die a pregnancy-related death.

**5. D) Recognizing barriers to care, and being sensitive to cultural influences**

An evidence-based approach to implementing assessment requires sensitivity to cultural norms. Learning to be culturally sensitive goes beyond asking an individual about their "cultural practices," as the majority of individuals are unable to articulate the inherent and significant influence of culture on their health and well-being. Instead, a culturally sensitive and humble approach to history taking and physical exam allows the individual to have the time and respect required to express their concerns and perspectives. Without a respectful approach, insensitivity to cultural perspectives (e.g., trying to be "color-blind," or implementing a paternalistic approach), can exacerbate health disparities and have a negative impact on the well-being of individuals, families, and communities.

6. Which measures BEST define healthcare disparities?

   A. Availability and training of primary care providers in the state or nation
   B. Incidence and prevalence of disease in the state or nation
   C. Mortality and morbidity rates of the entire population across time
   D. Variations in rates of disease occurrence between population groups

7. Which statement is TRUE about population health and determinants of health?

   A. Access to quality education is associated with improved health and well-being
   B. Genetics and family history have more impact on health than socioeconomic status
   C. Individuals diagnosed with chronic illnesses are unable to achieve a sense of well-being
   D. Individuals who are healthy are not likely to have consequences from family rejection

8. Patients with low health literacy are most satisfied with clinician visits when they:

   A. Are simply given a prescription when they request one
   B. Are told exactly what to do to manage or prevent illnesses
   C. Have an opportunity to teach back the information discussed
   D. Have not been given educational handouts or written information

9. Which statement is true about the significance of traumatic or adverse childhood experiences (ACEs)?

   A. Childhood is a timeframe characterized by happiness; fortunately ACEs are uncommon
   B. Children are resilient and are not likely to have long-term effects from ACEs
   C. Unfortunately, ACEs are not preventable; stress and toxic stress are part of life
   D. ACEs increase chronic disease risk in adulthood, including heart disease, diabetes, and cancer

10. What are the three most common causes of chronic illness in the United States? (Select THREE.)

    A. Environmental toxins
    B. Lack of exercise
    C. Poor diet or nutrition
    D. Tobacco use
    E. Vaccine hesitancy

*(See answers next page.)*

**6. D) Variations in rates of disease occurrence between population groups**

Health disparities are preventable differences in the burden of disease or injury between population groups. Populations can be defined by race, ethnicity, gender, age, income, disability, geographic location, or sexual orientation. While the availability of providers may have an impact on disparities and population health, access to care is not the only risk factor underlying disparities. Measures describing the progression of a disease over time for entire populations include morbidity (suffering from a disease) and mortality (death from a disease). Measures of disease frequency within populations include prevalence (existing cases) and incidence (new cases).

**7. A) Access to quality education is associated with improved health and well-being**

Access to safe, quality education, including early childhood education, has a significant impact on health and well-being. Key areas to consider related to the determinants that impact an individual's health: economic stability, housing, access to quality care, resources and support within communities, and experiences of bias, isolation, trauma, or loss. Rule of thumb: an individual's zip code matters more than their genetic code!

**8. C) Have an opportunity to teach back the information discussed**

Teach-Back is an evidence-based and highly effective communication technique to promote patient understanding; most patients retain very little of the information shared during a clinical encounter, and teaching back the information helps individuals to solidify the steps they need to take for good self-care. Avoiding written information is not the solution; providing management without effective communication decreases patient satisfaction and leads to poorer patient outcomes.

**9. D) ACEs increase chronic disease risk in adulthood, including heart disease, diabetes, and cancer**

ACEs are common. More than half of adults report having experienced at least one type of ACE, and nearly one in six reports experiencing four or more. ACEs are preventable; the consequences of toxic stress from ACEs are linked to chronic diseases in adulthood, including heart disease, diabetes, cancer, depression, anxiety, substance use disorder, and learning disabilities.

**10. B, C, D) Lack of exercise, poor diet or nutrition, tobacco use**

Six in ten adults in the United States have a chronic disease, and four in ten adults have two or more. The rising burden of chronic disease is linked to modifiable health behaviors, including physical inactivity, tobacco use or exposure, unhealthy diet, excessive alcohol intake, and lack of sleep. While environmental toxins and vaccine-preventable illnesses have significant impact on health, the most common causes for the overall population are healthy lifestyle behaviors. Participating in health promotion strategies and developing healthy lifestyle behaviors are shaped by the opportunities that individuals have, and the choices they make according to these opportunities throughout life.

# Pediatric and Adolescent Populations*

16

## INTRODUCTION

The steps of the pediatric/adolescent exam are the same as an adult: inspection, palpation, and auscultation. However, pediatric and adolescent populations experience dynamic periods of accelerated physical growth—particularly in infancy and adolescence—and periods of progressively developing cognitive, language, social-emotional, and gross- and fine-motor skills. Assessment and diagnosis in this population require a developmental approach that incorporates growth and development assessments and considerations.

## DEVELOPMENTAL APPROACH TO HISTORY TAKING

A caregiver or legal guardian is often the primary historian for an infant or young child. Most children will gradually provide more of their own health history as they mature and develop. However, some children (or adolescents) may have a developmental disorder that affects communication. History taking should be tailored to the caregiver, young child, or adolescent accordingly.

### CAREGIVERS AS HISTORIANS

- Caregivers report their *perception* of the child's signs and symptoms.
- Give thorough consideration to the differential diagnoses that occur most commonly in the child's age group. For example, a caregiver might report a concern of "belly pain" in a toddler due to an acute onset of fussiness and refusal to eat. In addition to causes of abdominal pain, consider other causes of "acute onset of fussiness and refusal to eat" in a toddler, like painful lesions of the oropharynx associated with common viral infections (e.g., herpangina, herpetic gingivostomatitis, hand-foot-and-mouth disease).
- Assessing severity of symptoms is an important aspect of assessment and diagnosis; infants and young children are unable to articulate the extent and severity of their symptoms. The more severe the symptoms of illness or injury, the more likely the child will experience interruptions in appetite, sleep, elimination, or activity (i.e., "eating, sleeping, peeing, pooping, and playing"). For example, "Is she still sleeping through the night?" or "Is he playing as much as he normally does?"

*This chapter is coauthored by Rosie Zeno, DNP, APRN-CNP, CPNP-PC, Assistant Professor of Clinical Practice, College of Nursing, The Ohio State University, Columbus, Ohio.

- Likewise, changes in appetite, sleep, elimination, or activity patterns can help to further guide the focused assessment by pointing to specific or concomitant conditions the child cannot articulate. For example, certain changes in elimination may increase suspicion for conditions like urinary tract infection, constipation, dehydration, or diabetes mellitus.

## SCHOOL-AGE CHILDREN

- By age 4 to 5 years, children can usually provide some of their own health history. It is important to ask age-appropriate questions according to the child's level of development (Table 16.1).

**Table 16.1 Developmentally Rephrased History Questions**

| | |
|---|---|
| "Do you have painful bowel movements?" | "Does it hurt when you poop?" |
| "Is the pain persistent or does it come and go?" | "Does it hurt all the time or just sometimes?" |
| "Do you have a history of abdominal pain?" | "Has your belly hurt like this before?" |
| "Have you had any nausea or vomiting?" | "Have you felt like throwing up? |

- Pay attention to non-verbal cues of comprehension and adjust terminology and questions as needed. It is particularly important to avoid using medical jargon and complex phrasing when interviewing children. Some children will give a yes or no answer, even if they do not understand the question. History questions should be rephrased to ensure comprehension and accurate history collection.

## ADOLESCENTS

Adolescence is the transition from childhood to adulthood. Teens are prone to high-risk behaviors that can cause substantial morbidity and mortality, like substance use or unprotected sex. In adolescents aged 10to 19 years, the leading cause of death is accidental injury followed by suicide. While caregivers can provide useful past medical and family history, it is also crucial to prioritize time for a one-on-one conversation with the adolescent.

- Ensuring time for confidential conversations between adolescent and clinician increases the number of adolescents willing to seek health care and the number willing disclose necessary information for an accurate assessment.
- Begin by telling the adolescent that information they share is confidential unless they report concerns about hurting themselves or hurting someone else. Immediate risks to safety must be disclosed.
- Be aware of federal and state laws regarding adolescent consent and confidentiality as these laws can vary from state to state.

Establishing a trusting rapport and straightforward dialogue aids in obtaining the most accurate health history. Adopt a respectful, nonjudgmental attitude when establishing rapport with adolescents.

- Do not assume to know the adolescent's sexual orientation or gender identity.
- Ask direct questions with genuine interest and allow for open-ended dialogue.

- Limit use of medical jargon and use terminology that is common and direct.
- Phrase questions in a manner that normalizes adolescent behavior without assigning judgment (Box 16.1).

**Box 16.1 Examples of Phrasing for Adolescent History Questions**

| |
|---|
| Some teens try smoking or vaping. Do you know anyone who vapes? Have you tried it?" |
| "What do you consider sex?" "Do you have sex with males, females, or both?" |
| "What percentage of the time do you use condoms?" |
| "Have you ever had sex when you didn't want to? Tell me more about that." |

## KEY HISTORY CONSIDERATIONS

**Birth history:** For children aged 0 to 2 years, it is particularly important to inquire about birth history especially when the child presents with a concern for poor growth, delay in development, respiratory illness, or infectious disease in the newborn.

- Prenatal care? Planned or unplanned pregnancy?
- Maternal health during pregnancy (e.g., infections, hypertension, diabetes, trauma, medications, depression/anxiety, substance use, smoking)?
- Gestation at delivery and birth weight?
- Labor and delivery complications (e.g., premature labor, breech position, fetal distress, birth injuries, hypoxia)?
- Type of delivery (e.g., vaginal, cesarean, induction, instrumentation)?
- Apgar scores?
- Newborn infections or respiratory distress? Respiratory support required?
- Prolonged hospital stay or neonatal intensive care unit (NICU) stay?
- Hyperbilirubinemia, hypoglycemia, feeding problems?
- Universal hearing screen passed?
- Vitamin K administration? Hepatitis B vaccination?
- Newborn screening results? (varies by state)

**Immunization status:** Children typically receive the majority of their lifetime immunizations in the first 1.5 years of life. Therefore, infants and young children are particularly vulnerable to vaccine-preventable diseases. When evaluating children for infectious diseases, it is important to ask whether the child's vaccines are up to date, delayed, or behind. Vaccine schedules can be found on the CDC's Advisory Committee on Immunization Practice's (ACIP) website.

**Social history:** Children do not exist independently of their caregivers or their family context. They rely on caregivers to meet their needs and ensure their health and safety. The environment in which children grow and develop is critical to their health and wellness. It is imperative for the clinician to have a proper understanding of a child's psychosocial environment by investigating the following factors:

- **Living conditions:** Single-family home, multi-generational family home, apartment?
- Who lives in the home?
- Composition of the family?
- Occupation of the caregivers?

- Daycare, attending school, homeschooling?
- Extracurricular, intramural activities?
- Family violence?
- Substance use, smoking?
- Relationships, bullying?

## DEVELOPMENTAL HISTORY

- *Developmental surveillance* refers to the process of recognizing children who may be at risk for developmental delays. Surveillance is performed at every routine health encounter through direct observation of the child's development and by questioning the caregiver whether the child is meeting age-appropriate developmental milestones (Table 16.2).

**Table 16.2 Developmental Milestones**

| Age | Social/ Emotional | Language/ Communication | Cognitive | Motor |
|---|---|---|---|---|
| 2 months | Smiles<br>Makes eye contact with caregiver<br>Self-soothes briefly | Coos, makes gurgling sounds<br>Turns head toward sounds | Pays attention to faces and follows with eyes | Develops head control and smoother movement in arms and legs |
| 4 months | Smiles spontaneously at people; copies some facial expressions | Begins to babble<br>Copies sounds<br>Cries in different ways when hungry, tired, or in pain | Responds to affection<br>Reaches for things<br>Follows movement<br>Recognizes familiar people from a distance | Holds head steady<br>Rolls front to back<br>Brings hands to mouth; uses hands and eyes together |
| 6 months | Knows familiar faces<br>Recognizes strangers<br>Responds to others' emotions; likes to look at self in mirror | Responds to sounds by making sounds<br>Responds to own name | Brings things to mouth<br>Shows curiosity about things out of reach<br>Passes things from one hand to another | Rolls back to front<br>Begins to sit without support; when standing, supports weight on legs |
| 9 months | May have stranger anxiety<br>Has favorite toys | Understands "no"<br>Copies sounds and gestures<br>Uses finger to point | Plays peek-a-boo<br>Develops object permanence (looks for things out of sight) | Stands, holding on<br>Sits without support<br>Pulls to standing<br>Crawls |

*(continued)*

Table 16.2 Developmental Milestones (*continued*)

| Age | Social/ Emotional | Language/ Communication | Cognitive | Motor |
|---|---|---|---|---|
| 1 year | Cries when caregiver leaves<br>Has favorite things and people<br>Plays games such as pat-a-cake | Responds to simple requests<br>Waves bye-bye<br>Shakes head "no"<br>Says words like "mama," "dada," "uh oh!" | Copies gestures<br>Puts things in a container and takes things out of it<br>Explores things by shaking, banging, throwing | Pulls up to standing<br>Cruises (walks while holding on)<br>May stand alone<br>May take a few steps |
| 18 months | Plays simple pretend, like feeding a doll<br>May have temper tantrums<br>Shows affection to familiar people | Says several single words<br>Points to show someone what they want, points to pictures in a book | Knows what ordinary things are, like brush, spoon, phone<br>Points to one body part; scribbles<br>Follows command like "sit down" | Walks alone<br>Drinks from a cup<br>Eats with a spoon<br>Pulls toys or carries toys while walking; may walk up stairs |
| 2 years | Imitates others<br>Gets excited when with other children and begins to involve them in games and play<br>Shows more independence and defiance | Says sentences of 2–4 words<br>Points to things in a book<br>Follows simple commands<br>Knows names of familiar people and body parts | Begins to sort shapes and colors<br>Plays simple make-believe games<br>Builds a tower of 4 cubes; finds things when hidden | Stands on tiptoe<br>Kicks a ball<br>Begins to run<br>Climbs onto and down from furniture without help<br>Walks up and down stairs while holding on |
| 3 years | Copies adults and friends<br>Shares, cooperates, shows concern and affection without prompting<br>Dresses and undresses self | Follows instructions with 2 or 3 steps<br>Understands prepositions (on, in, under); words are 75% understandable to strangers | Can button, complete puzzles with 3 or 4 pieces, copy a circle<br>Turns book pages one at a time<br>Builds towers of more than 6 blocks | Climbs well<br>Runs easily<br>Jumps forward<br>Pedals a tricycle<br>Walks up and down stairs, one foot on each step |

(*continued*)

**Table 16.2 Developmental Milestones (*continued*)**

| Age | Social/ Emotional | Language/ Communication | Cognitive | Motor |
|---|---|---|---|---|
| 4 years | Enjoys doing new things, remembers parts of stories, uses scissors, starts to understand time<br><br>Brushes teeth | Can say first and last names, uses pronouns correctly; can sing a song or recite a nursery rhyme from memory | Names some colors, numbers; draws a person with 2–4 body parts; plays board games, card games<br><br>Can print some letters | Hops, stands on one leg for 2 seconds, catches a bounced ball most of the time<br><br>Climbs stairs, alternating feet |
| 5 years | Likes to sing, dance, act, participate in imaginative play<br><br>Knows the difference between real and make-believe | Speaks clearly<br><br>Tells a simple story with complete sentences; uses future tense<br><br>Says name and address | Prints letters and numbers; copies a triangle and shapes<br><br>Knows about everyday things (e.g., food, money)<br><br>Draws a person with at least 6 body parts | Stands on one foot for 10 seconds or longer; may be able to skip, somersault<br><br>Uses toilet on own<br><br>Swings, climbs |

*Source:* Adapted from Centers for Disease Control and Prevention. (2019). *Milestone checklist*. Retrieved from https://www.cdc.gov/ncbddd/actearly/pdf/checklists/Checklists-with-Tips_Reader-2019_508.pdf

- *Developmental screening* refers to the use of standardized tools to identify children at risk for delays in the developmental domains of motor (gross and fine), language, cognitive, emotional, and psychosocial. Standardized developmental screening should be performed with a valid and reliable screening tool at ages 9, 18, and 24 or 30 months. See Table 16.3 for commonly used valid and reliable developmental screening tools.

**Table 16.3 Developmental Screening Tools**

| Screening Tool | Ages | Type of Screening |
|---|---|---|
| Ages & Stages Questionnaires® (ASQ®-3)<br><br>**(Squires & Bricker, 2009)** | 1–66 months | Developmental screening: communication, gross/ fine motor, problem-solving, and personal/ social skills |
| Ages & Stages Questionnaire—Social Emotional (ASQ:SE-2)<br><br>**(Squires, Bricker, & Twombly, 2015)** | 1–72 months | Social/emotional screening: self-regulation, compliance, social communication, adaptive functioning, autonomy, affect, and interaction with people |
| Parents' Evaluation of Developmental Status (PEDS©)<br><br>**(Glascoe, 2016)** | 0–8 years | Surveillance and screening of development, behavior, and mental health |

(*continued*)

**Table 16.3 Developmental Screening Tools (*continued*)**

| Screening Tool | Ages | Type of Screening |
|---|---|---|
| Parents' Evaluation of Developmental Status—Developmental Milestones (PEDS: DM) (Glascoe & Robertshaw, 2016) | 0–8 years | Surveillance and screening of development and mental health: expressive/receptive language, fine/gross motor skills, self-help, academics, and social/emotional skills |
| The Modified Checklist for Autism in Toddlers, Revised, with Follow-Up™ (M-CHAT-R/F) (Robins, Fein, & Barton, 2009) | 16–30 months | Risk of autism spectrum disorder (ASD) |

- When a child is not developing skills in one or more domains according to the expected timeframe, the child has a *developmental delay*. When a child exhibits mental or physical impairment (or a combination of both) that results in functional limitations of the activities of daily living, the child has a *developmental disorder* or *developmental disability*.
- A developmental delay should prompt referral for further diagnostic evaluation. Children aged 0 to 3 years have greater neuroplasticity and therefore higher capacity for improved outcomes the earlier services are established.

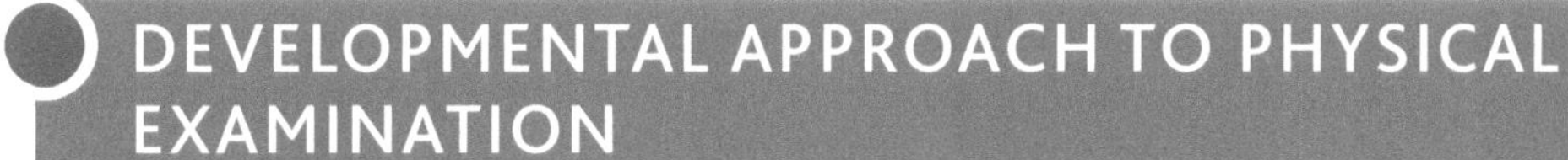

# DEVELOPMENTAL APPROACH TO PHYSICAL EXAMINATION

## VITAL SIGNS

Vital signs for infants and children can vary greatly in comparison to the normal range for adults. See Table 16.4.

**Table 16.4 Pediatric Vital Signs**

| Age | Heart Rate (Beats/Minute) | Blood Pressure (mmHg) | Respiratory Rate (Breaths/Minute) |
|---|---|---|---|
| Premature | 110–170 | SBP 55–75 DBP 35–45 | 40–70 |
| 0–3 months | 110–160 | SBP 65–85 DBP 45–55 | 35–55 |
| 3–6 months | 110–160 | SBP 70–90 DBP 50–65 | 30–45 |
| 6–12 months | 90–160 | SBP 80–100 DBP 55–65 | 22–38 |
| 1–3 years | 80–150 | SBP 90–105 DBP 55–70 | 22–30 |
| 3–6 years | 70–120 | SBP 95–110 DBP 60–75 | 20–24 |
| 6–12 years | 60–110 | SBP 100–120 DBP 60–75 | 16–22 |
| >12 years | 60–100 | SBP 110–135 DBP 65–85 | 12–20 |

DBP, diastolic blood pressure; SBP, systolic blood pressure.

## TEMPERATURE

- Assessment of temperature in newborns is a priority. Infants, especially those with low birthweight, can have difficulty maintaining body temperature. Infants have less subcutaneous fat, thus have less insulation. Their small size, increased ratio of body surface to body weight, and inability to shiver impair the infant's ability to conserve heat. Cold stress in a newborn can lead to hypoglycemia, hypoxia, and hypothermia. Fever in an infant under 6 weeks of age can be a sign of sepsis and requires immediate further evaluation.
- Rectal temperature is preferred as the standard reference for core body temperature in infants and young children.
- Oral temperature can be obtained when children are developmentally able to maintain the oral thermometer under the tongue.

## PULSE

- In children under the age of 2 years, assessment of pulse rate is best assessed by auscultating the apical pulse. The apical pulse is located just left of the midclavicular line at the fifth intercostal space in children younger than 7 years and at the left midclavicular line at the fifth intercostal space in children over 7 years. In children over the age of 2 years, pulse rate can be determined by palpating the temporal, carotid, femoral, apical, brachial, popliteal, radial, posterior tibial, and dorsalis pedis pulses.
- Causes of abnormal pulse rates or rhythms in children should be noted prior to assessing the pulse rate; these include changes in body temperature, hypoxia, anxiety, sepsis, pain, medications, and/or crying. Further investigation is warranted if a child has an irregular heart rhythm, and the child should be assessed for signs of disruption in cardiac output, such as weak, thready pulse, increased rate, cyanosis, tachypnea, fussiness, decreased activity, and poor feeding. Infants and young children commonly have sinus arrhythmia (i.e., the heart rate varies with respiration, which is not associated with heart problems).

## RESPIRATORY RATE

- Respiratory rate is most accurately assessed for a full minute while the infant or young child is calm or sleeping.

## BLOOD PRESSURE

- Routine blood pressure (BP) measurements are performed annually beginning at 3 years old. Prior to age 3, consider BP for any child suspected of having an underlying cardiac or renal disease.
- Use the proper BP cuff size to obtain an accurate measurement. The cuff should cover approximately two-thirds of the upper arm. Using a cuff too large will result in a lower than actual BP reading, and too small of a cuff will result in a higher than actual BP reading.
- Infants with suspected cardiovascular or renal abnormalities can be assessed for blood pressure using a neonatal-sized cuff. For non-critical infants, it is best practice to use an oscillometer device, at least 1.5 hours after a feeding or medical intervention, taken in the supine or prone position, using the proper size cuff on the right upper arm, and taken while the infant is asleep or in a quiet awake state. Normal blood pressure is determined by post-conceptual age in weeks.

## PHYSICAL ASSESSMENT

Physical assessment is typically performed in systematic manner. With children, it is important to modify the order of the exam according to the child's comfort or cooperation level, which will vary from child to child. In general, the best approach is to proceed from the "least distressing" (e.g., heart, lungs) to "most distressing" (e.g., ears, throat) aspects of the exam. Any aspect of the physical exam that necessitates the most cooperation, or may be potentially uncomfortable, should be performed last.

### INFANTS AND CHILDREN

- Newborns (0 to 1 month) and young infants (1 to 6 months) prefer to stay warm and secure. Perform as much of the exam as possible prior to removing blankets, clothes, or diapers. Any exam technique that might make the infant cry should be postponed until the end. Once an infant is distressed and crying, it is very difficult to auscultate heart and lung sounds or perform an eye exam.
- Much of the exam can initially be performed while the caregiver is holding the infant. When the infant is content, it is an ideal time to auscultate heart and lung sounds. Certain aspects of the exam are best performed with the infant lying supine on the exam table: otoscopic ear exam, oropharynx, abdomen, genitalia, and hips. If the infant begins crying, seize the opportunity to perform an effective exam of the mouth, dentition, and posterior oropharynx.
- Stranger anxiety peaks between 6 to 12 months and generally resolves around age 2, but children of any age may be apprehensive. If a child appears fearful or nervous, begin the encounter at a physical distance from the child while gathering history from the caregiver. Often, once a child realizes that the parent is comfortable, the child is apt to relax too. Young children frequently look to their caregivers for social cues.
- For older infants (6 to 12 months) and young children (1 to 4 years), the most worrisome aspects are the otoscopic ear exam; the oral exam with tongue depressor; and/or, lying down for abdominal palpation or anogenital exam. Plan to reserve these exam aspects for last.
- Transform the physical exam into *play* for the child to increase cooperation. Ask, "Can you open your mouth big like an alligator?" "Can you show me how you climb up on this table?" Give positive reinforcement when the child plays along.
- Demystify the equipment (otoscope, stethoscope). Even though not invasive, some older infants and toddlers are fearful of the stethoscope. Demonstrate assessment techniques on the child's stuffed animal or a sibling/caregiver before using with the child to promote trust and confidence. Let children touch the otoscope speculum to see that it does not hurt. Describe the equipment in familiar terms: "Do you want to see my flashlight? I use this to look in ears."
- Do not give the child choices for things that are not optional. For example, do not ask "Can I look in your ears?" Instead ask, "Should I look in your ears or your mouth first?" This approach gives the child some control and can generate cooperation.
- Safety is paramount. Whether cooperative or not, the child must be secured and properly positioned for the exam. Safe positioning may require assistance from a caregiver or another provider. Children cry and become combative when they are afraid or upset about being restrained. If the exam is being performed with the child safely secured, it should not cause pain.

### ADOLESCENTS

- Pubertal changes mark the beginning of adolescence. The mean age of pubertal onset is approximately 10.5 years in females and 11.5 years in males. Providing privacy and preserving modesty is paramount. Keep all parts of the body covered when not being assessed. Adolescents often have concerns or feel self-conscious regarding their developing bodies. It is important to reassure the adolescent when everything is normal.
- If an adolescent requires an exam of the genitalia or female breasts (for system-specific concerns or assessing Tanner stage), the use of a chaperone is recommended. Some states have mandatory chaperone laws, so it is important to be aware of respective state laws. A chaperone can be a caregiver or another health care provider, but it should be the adolescent's choice.

## GROWTH ASSESSMENT

Accurate and reliable growth measures are essential. Deviations in growth trajectories may be indicative of neglect, chronic illness, malnutrition, hormonal conditions, or congenital syndromes. Growth measurements are interpreted differently than adults because children are continuously growing. Trends in height (or length), weight, head circumference, and body mass index (BMI) or weight-for-length are compared to a reference population of children of the same age and natal sex and *reported as a percentile*. The Centers for Disease Control and Prevention (CDC; 2010) recommends using the World Health Organization (WHO) international growth charts for children aged 0 to 23 months; and the 2002 CDC growth charts for children and adolescents aged 2 to 18 years.

### INFANTS AND YOUNG CHILDREN

- Measure length with infant/child lying supine on a recumbent infant length board or examining table.
- Weigh infant wearing a clean, dry diaper (or nude) on an accurately calibrated scale.
- Obtain head circumference for children aged 0 to 3 years. Use a flexible, but non-elastic measuring tape placed just above the brow line anteriorly and over the occipital prominence posteriorly.
- Average newborns weigh 3 to 3.5 kg (5lb. 9oz. to 7lb. 11oz.) and measure 18 to 22 inches long.
- Newborns may lose up to 10% of their birth weight in the first few days of life. A loss of >10% warrants prompt evaluation.
- Newborns should gain 15 to 30 g/day (0.5 to 1oz. per day). It is normal for breastfed infants to gain weight on the lower end of the range. Most newborns recover birth their weight by 10 to 14 days.
- Average infants double their birth weight by 6 months of age and triple their birth weight by 1 year of age.
- Linear growth velocity averages 2.5 cm/month from birth to 6 months, 1.3 cm/month from 7 to 12 months, and about 7.6 cm/year after 12 months old.
- Failure to thrive (FTT) describes a condition of inadequate growth and undernourishment. Infants or children with poor weight gain, deceleration in growth, or growth measures that drop below the third percentile should be evaluated

further. If neglect, organic disease, or severe malnutrition is suspected, the child should be hospitalized for evaluation.

- A head circumference that trends upward may indicate an intracranial pathology, like hydrocephalus. A head circumference that stalls in growth may indicate a premature fusion of sutures or a congenital syndrome associated with microcephaly.

### OLDER CHILDREN AND ADOLESCENTS

- Children and adolescents who can stand steadily without assistance should be weighed with a calibrated electronic- or beam-balance scale. Obtain height using a portable or wall-mount stadiometer with the child standing erect, facing forward, with heels and occiput against the wall. Height and weight should be obtained without shoes.
- Prior to the accelerated growth period in adolescence, school-aged typically grow an average 2.5 inches and gain an average of 5 to 7 pounds per year.
- Assess BMI annually beginning at 2 years of age.
- In contrast to adults, BMI is assessed by comparing the measurement to an age-and sex-specific reference population and reported as a percentile.
  - **Normal:** BMI between the fifth and 85th percentile
  - **Overweight:** BMI between the 85th to 95th percentile
  - **Obesity:** BMI greater than or equal to the 95th percentile
- A progressive decrease in weight or BMI below the third percentile may warrant further investigation. Older children and adolescents should be asked about intentional weight loss and evaluated for an eating disorder if indicated.
- Specialized growth charts provide growth references for special populations of children whose growth might vary from typically developing children like those with history of prematurity or Down Syndrome.

## NUTRITION ASSESSMENT

The Academy of Nutrition and Dietetics (the Academy) and the American Society for Parenteral and Enteral Nutrition (ASPEN) have developed a set of evidence-based diagnostic criteria to identify and document pediatric undernutrition in routine clinical practice. These criteria are outlined in Table 16.5. These criteria are intended for use in children and adolescents aged 1 month to 18 years and can be used across multiple populations including primary care, inpatient, and residential care settings.

**Table 16.5 Indicators for Identification of Pediatric Undernutrition**

| | Mild Malnutrion | Moderate Malnutrion | Severe Malnutrion |
|---|---|---|---|
| Single Data Point Available | | | |
| Weight-for-height z score | –1 to –1.9 z score | –2 to –2.9 z score | –3 or greater z score |
| BMI-for-age z score | –1 to –1.9 z score | –2 to –2.9 z score | –3 or greater z score |
| Length/ height-for-age z score | No data | No data | –3 z score |
| Mid-upper arm circumference | Greater than or equal to –1 to –1.9 z score | Greater than or equal to –2 to –2.9 z score | Greater than or equal to –3 z score |

*(continued)*

**Table 16.5 Indicators for Identification of Pediatric Undernutrition (*continued*)**

| | Mild Malnutrion | Moderate Malnutrion | Severe Malnutrion |
|---|---|---|---|
| Two or More Data Points | | | |
| Weight gain velocity (<2 years of age) | Less than 75% of the norm for expected weight gain | Less than 50% of the norm for expected weight gain | Less than 25% of the norm for expected weight gain |
| Weight loss (2–20 years of age) | 5% usual body weight | 7.5% usual body weight | 10% usual body weight |
| Deceleration in weight for length/ height *z* score | Decline of 1 *z* score | Decline of 2 *z* score | Decline of 3 *z* score |
| Inadequate nutrient intake | 51%–75% estimated energy/protein need | 26%–50% estimated energy/protein need | ≤25% estimated energy/ protein need |

*Source:* Republished with permission of John Wiley and Sons, Inc., from Becker, P., Carney, L. N., Corkins, M. R., Monczka, J., Smith, E., Smith, S. E., ... White, J. V. (2015). Consensus statement of the Academy of Nutrition and Dietetics/American Society for Parenteral and Enteral Nutrition: Indicators recommended for the identification and documentation of pediatric malnutrition (undernutrition). *Nutrition in Clinical Practice, 30*(1), 147–161. doi:10.1177/0884533614557642. Permission conveyed through Copyright Clearance Center, Inc.

## MENTAL HEALTH ASSESSMENT

- If a child is presenting with a mental health or behavioral issue, the use of a screening tool along with the history can be useful with caregivers. For example, the Pediatric Symptom Checklist (PSC) is a valid and reliable 35-item instrument that assesses a variety of mental health/behavioral issues (e.g., internalizing and externalizing disorders) in children and youth between 4 and 18 years of age. There is a 17-item valid and reliable short version of the scale as well. The PSC has been adapted for young children, 18 to 60 months of age, and for children who are younger than 18 months (Sheldrick, Hensen & Merchant, 2012; Sheldrick, Hensen & Neger, 2013). The scales are freely downloadable and available in multiple languages at https://www.massgeneral.org/psychiatry/services/treatmentprograms.aspx?id=2088.
- Clinicians should take a thorough psychosocial history at each adolescent health supervision visit. The HEEADSS (or HE²ADS²) instrument asks questions in the following psychosocial domains: Home, Education/Employment, Eating, Activities, Drugs, Sexuality, and Suicide/depression (Smith & McGuinness, 2017). This is reviewed in Chapter 15, "Determinants of Health and Wellness."
- The U. S. Preventive Services Task Force (USPSTF) recommends screening for major depressive disorder (MDD) in adolescents aged 12 to 18 years. The clinician should use a standardized depression-screening tool for depression, such as the Patient Health Questionnaire for Adolescents (PHQ-A). The 9-item PHQ-A has the highest positive predictive value for depression in children and adolescents compared to other available depression screens (USPSTF, 2016).
- If the adolescent is depressed, a suicidal risk assessment should be performed, including whether he/she has a plan and means to commit suicide. The adolescent also should be assessed for bipolar disorder and other mental health disorders, such as anxiety and substance abuse.
- The Guidelines for Adolescent Preventive Services (GAPS) also is a well-established, self-report tool for assessing the special needs of adolescents (Elster & Kuznets, 1994). In addition, the AAP recommends screening all adolescents for tobacco, drugs, and

alcohol use with the CRAFFT (Car, Relax, Alone, Forget, Friends, Trouble) tool. This screening tool takes less than 2 minutes to administer, has good sensitivity and specificity, and can help clinicians identify those adolescents that may be experiencing the consequence of substance use or abuse (USPSTF, 2014).

- The CRAFFT is freely available at www.projectcork.org/clinical_tools/pdf/CRAFFT.pdf.Clinicians should be prepared to provide the necessary counseling and referrals when particular concerns are identified.

## RED FLAGS IN HISTORY AND PHYSICAL EXAM

### INFANTS

- Inability to keep down fluids or irretraceable vomiting
- Difficulty feeding
- Decreased or absence of wet diapers
- Decreased movement on one side of the body
- Stiffness or floppiness
- Shrill cry or cry that cannot be soothed
- Lethargy and/or hypersomnia
- Not achieving developmental milestones
- Loss of previously mastered developmental skills
- Bulging fontanelles
- Petechiae rash
- Fever under the age of 3 months
- Poor growth patterns
- Signs of neglect

### SCHOOL-AGED CHILDREN

- Poor school performance
- Behavioral problems
- Frequent outbursts or tantrums
- Socially withdrawn
- Aggressive, frequently fights with other children
- Disruptive
- Loss of skills
- Has difficulty with simple assignments, directions, and schoolwork
- Inappropriate interest in sexuality or knowledge of sexuality that is beyond the child's developmental level
- Signs of physical, sexual, or emotional abuse
- Bedwetting
- Frequent somatic complaints
- Poor growth patterns (e.g., underweight, overweight, or drastic change from current trajectory)
- Signs of neglect

## ADOLESCENTS

- Withdrawal from family or peer group
- Change in behavior (e.g., more aggressive, angry, loss of interest in activities)
- Sudden drop in grades or change in academic performance
- Change in eating habits
- Change in sleeping habits (e.g., hypersomnia or insomnia)
- Depressed mood
- Self-mutilation
- Suicidality
- Drug or alcohol paraphernalia
- High-risk behaviors including sexual promiscuity and substance use
- Skipping school or poor school attendance
- Appears fearful, anxious, paranoid
- Getting into trouble at school or with the legal system
- Homelessness or running away from home
- Underweight or overweight

## KNOWLEDGE CHECK: PEDIATRIC AND ADOLESCENT POPULATIONS

1. Which approaches to completing a physical exam can increase a younger child's cooperation? (Select all that apply.)

   A. Ask the child if it is okay to begin their physical exam
   B. Examine only the physical systems that the child permits
   C. Find ways to transform the physical exam into a play activity
   D. Modify the order of the exam based on the child's cooperation
   E. Perform the most distressing parts of the exam first

2. According to the American Academy of Pediatrics, well child exams from birth to 18 months of age should occur at birth, during the first week of life, and:

   A. Every 2 months until the child is 18 months old
   B. Every 3 months until the child is 18 months old
   C. At ages 1 month, 2 months, 4 months, 6 months, 9 months, 12 months, 15 months, and 18 months
   D. At ages 1 month, 3 months, 6 months, 9 to 10 months, 12 to 15 months, and 18 months

3. Which developmental milestone should be expected for a 9 month old?

   A. Passes objects from one hand to another
   B. Points to two pictures upon request
   C. Speaks three to five words clearly
   D. Waves bye-bye

4. Which is true regarding an infant's weight?

   A. Babies should double their birth weight by 12 months
   B. Babies should triple their birth weight by 12 months
   C. Infants commonly have weight measurements that fall below the third percentile
   D. Newborn infants should maintain their birth weight through the first 2 weeks of life

5. An advanced practice nurse notes that a 4-year-old male has enlargement of his calf muscles, which are soft and pliable on palpation. The child's mother is concerned because he is unable to raise himself from the floor without bracing his knees with his hands. Which diagnosis is MOST LIKELY?

   A. Cerebral palsy
   B. Cystic fibrosis
   C. Duchenne muscular dystrophy
   D. Legg-Calve-Perthes

*(See answers next page.)* 

**1. C and D) Find ways to transform the physical exam into a play activity; Modify the order of the exam based on the child's cooperation**

To increase cooperation, begin with the least distressing components of the exam and postpone any exam technique that will potentially cause the child to cry. (Once a child is crying, it is very difficult to complete the exam effectively.) Modify the order of the exam according to the child's comfort or cooperation level. While children may have the option of choosing the order of the exam, be cautious about asking permission or giving choices for exam components that are not actually optional. Use toys, games, or distractions to demystify the equipment and facilitate physical exam.

**2. C) 1 month, 2 months, 4 months, 6 months, 9 months, 12 months, 15 months, and 18 months**

The recommended periodicity of well child exams is specific to growth and developmental milestones, vaccine guidelines, and needed screenings. Timely well child visits ensure necessary preventive care.

**3. A) Passes objects from one hand to another**

Infants begin to transfer objects from hand to hand at about 6-months-old; this developmental milestone would be expected of a 9-month-old. Waving bye-bye and shaking head "no" is a milestone for 1-year-olds. Children begin to say words at 1 year of age and can say several single words clearly by 18 months. Pointing to indicate wants is an expectation at 18 months of age and pointing to pictures in a book is language milestone typical of 2-year-olds.

**4. B) Babies should triple their birth weight by 12 months**

The average infant will double his birth weight by 6 months of age and triple his birth weight by 12 months. Newborns are expected to lose up to 10% of their birth weight in the first few days of life and should recover their birth weight by at least 2 weeks of age. Infants with poor weight gain or growth measurements that trend downward or fall below the third percentile may have a failure to thrive, and the cause should be explored.

**5. C) Duchenne muscular dystrophy**

Duchene muscular dystrophy (DMD) most commonly affects boys between the ages of 2 and 5; physical signs include "pseudo-hypertrophy" of calf muscles because of tissue abnormalities. Symptoms include clumsy movements and frequent falls. Gower sign, using the hands against the thighs while trying to stand, is characteristic of DMD. Individuals with cerebral palsy will have disordered movements, muscle tone, and posture; however, they will not present with calf muscle enlargement or Gower sign. Cystic fibrosis primarily impacts the lungs and digestive system. Legg-Calve-Perthes is a bone disorder that affects the hip and leads to limping and leg pain.

6. Which is a common clinical manifestation of congenital heart disease in children not yet diagnosed?

   A. Bruising
   B. Hyperglycemia
   C. Obesity
   D. Poor weight gain

7. Which is a developmental red flag in early childhood?

   A. Failure to turn to sound or voice at 6 months
   B. Failure to say single words by 9 months
   C. Inability to walk without holding on by 12 months
   D. Inability to follow simple commands by 15 months

8. Which statement is correct about head circumference measurement in children?

   A. Head circumference is plotted on the growth curve specific for age but not gender
   B. Measuring head circumference is a routine part of growth assessment until 18 months of age
   C. Measurements that trend upward or that stall in growth over time should be further evaluated
   D. The measuring tape encircles from the base of skull (right above the neck) to mid-forehead

9. According to the American Academy of Pediatrics (AAP), at what ages should all children be screened for autism spectrum disorders?

   A. 9 months old and 3 years old
   B. 12 months old and 4 years old
   C. 18 months and 24 months old
   D. 3 and 5 years old

10. Which statement about confidentiality when assessing adolescents is MOST accurate?

    A. Adolescents are not likely to share personal information, even if offered confidentiality
    B. State and federal laws prohibit teens from receiving any type of confidential care
    C. Teens are not entitled to confidentiality without parental consent
    D. Teens are more willing to seek care when clinicians offer confidentiality

(*See answers next page.*)

**6. D) Poor weight gain**

Congenital heart disease in pediatric populations presents as cyanotic events, poor feeding or weight gain, tachypnea, heart murmurs, shortness of breath, and/or easy fatigability. Bruising is common and most often normal in children, although it can indicate abnormal platelet function. Hyperglycemia is associated with diabetes and endocrine disorders. Obesity would be unusual in children with congenital heart disease.

**7. A) Failure to turn to sound or voice at 6 months**

Infants turn their head towards sound at 2 months of age; failure to respond normally by 6 months is a red flag, or marker for further evaluation. Other developmental red flags include no babbling by 9 months, no first words by 15 months, inability to walk by 18 months, and inability to follow simple command (one-step instructions) by 24 months.

**8. C) Measurements that trend upward or that stall in growth over time should be further evaluated**

Weight, height/length, BMI, weight for length, and head circumference trends are compared to a reference population of children of the same age and gender and is reported as a percentile. These measures should be assessed and documented to allow the clinician to monitor changes over time. Head circumference should be measured for all children up to age 3. This measurement should be obtained with a flexible but non-elastic measuring tape. The measuring tape should be placed just above the brow line anteriorly and over the occipital prominence posteriorly. An upward-trending head circumference may indicate hydrocephalus or other intracranial pathology. A head circumference that stalls in growth may indicate a premature fusion of sutures/ fontanels or a congenital syndrome associated with microcephaly.

**9. C) 18 months and 24 months old**

The AAP recommends that all children be screened for autism spectrum disorders at ages 18 and 24 months, along with regular developmental surveillance.

**10. D) Teens are more willing to seek care when clinicians offer confidentiality**

Discussing confidentiality not only increases the number of teens willing to divulge private information but also increases the number of adolescents willing to seek healthcare. Although adolescents under age 18 are still minors, they are entitled by law to consent to reproductive healthcare and to have confidential conversations with the clinician. Laws can differ from state to state about what is allowable, so it is important for clinicians to have an understanding of their respective state laws. All states and the District of Columbia allow minors to consent to sexually transmitted infection (STI) testing and treatment without parental permission; some states have consent laws addressing confidential substance misuse treatment, pregnancy prevention and care, mental health care, and emergency care.

# 17

# Pregnant Populations

## KEY HISTORY CONSIDERATIONS

- First day of last normal menstrual period
- Planned or unexpected pregnancy
- Desired or undesired pregnancy; options if undesired
- Form of contraception at the time of pregnancy (if applicable)
- History of hypertension, diabetes, autoimmune conditions, cancer, depression, posttraumatic stress disorder (PTSD), trauma
- History of gestational hypertension, gestational diabetes, preeclampsia, eclampsia, HELLP syndrome, postpartum hemorrhage, postpartum depression, shoulder dystocia, retained placenta, third- or fourth-degree perineal laceration, issues with infant's health
- GTPAL (Gravida [number of pregnancies], Term [number of full-term births], Preterm [number of pre-term births, after 20 weeks gestation], Abortions [number of elective terminations and/or miscarriages, including births prior to 20 weeks gestation], Living [number of living children]
- Method of previous births, ectopic pregnancies, miscarriages, and history of fetal/neonatal demise
- History of sexually transmitted infections (STIs)
- Recent signs/symptoms or exposure to COVID-19
- Vaccination status
- History of gynecological surgeries
- Family history of genetic conditions, preeclampsia, diabetes
- Smoking, alcohol, recreational drug use (current/past/presence of addiction)
- History of exposure to secondhand smoke
- Intimate partner violence (current/past)
- Recent travel for patient and/or partner to areas with Zika virus and timing of that travel
- Pets in the home
- Access to care, nutritious food, stable housing, support system, or lack of access thereof

# PHYSICAL EXAMINATION: INSPECTION, PALPATION, AND AUSCULTATION

## GENERAL SURVEY AND VITAL SIGNS

1. The clinician should start the physical exam by noting the patient's vital signs. Blood pressure is especially important and needs to be taken at every visit. If maternal blood pressure is elevated at the initial prenatal visit, the clinician should attempt to find pre-pregnancy records to determine if chronic hypertension exists. Trends should be noted. If diastolic blood pressure increases 15 degrees or more and/or systolic blood pressure increases 30 degrees or more over their baseline, this is clinically significant, even if they do not meet the criteria for hypertension.
2. Height, weight (current and pre-pregnancy), and body mass index (BMI) should be obtained and compared to past metrics. Trends and trajectories should be noted. Maternal BMI should be calculated at the initial prenatal visit using the pre-pregnancy weight to guide weight gain recommendations during pregnancy as well as to assess for risk for comorbid conditions. See Table 17.1.

**Table 17.1 Institute of Medicine Weight Gain Recommendations for Pregnancy**

| Prepregnancy Weight Category | Body Mass Index* | Recommended Range of Total Weight (lb) | Recommended Rates of Weight Gain† in the Second and Third Trimesters (lb; Mean Range [lb/week]) |
|---|---|---|---|
| Underweight | <18.5 | 28–40 | 1 (1.0–1.3) |
| Normal weight | 18.5–24.9 | 25–35 | 1 (0.8–1.0) |
| Overweight | 25–29.9 | 15–25 | 0.6 (0.5–0.7) |
| Obese (includes all classes) | 30 and greater | 11–20 | 0.5 (0.4–0.6) |

*Body mass index is calculated as weight in kilograms divided by height in meters squared, or as weight in pounds multiplied by 703, divided by height in inches.

†Calculations assume a 1.1–4.4 lb weight gain in the first trimester.

*Source:* Modified from Institute of Medicine. (2009). *Weight gain during pregnancy: Reexamining the guidelines*. Washington, DC. National Academies Press. © 2009 National Academy of Sciences.

3. Note if the patient appears in distress, toxic, or in active labor.
4. A mental health assessment and safety/violence screening should be routinely conducted during pregnancy and postpartum.

## INSPECTION

1. Note the patient's affect, demeanor, and overall appearance.
2. Note if the patient appears visibly pregnant (fundus above the symphysis pubis) and how the size of the fundus compares to the number of weeks pregnant.
3. Note if the breasts are symmetric and if the nipples are everted, flat, or inverted.

4. Note any changes to the skin of the breasts, including dimpling, peau d'orange appearance, erythema, or edema. (For more information on breast examinations, please refer to Chapter 11, "Breasts and Axillae.")
5. Complete a comprehensive skin exam.
6. A complete visual inspection of the external genitals should be performed.
   - In early pregnancy, Chadwick's sign may be observed during a speculum exam—the cervix appears bluish-purplish in color or cyanotic.
   - The skin on and around the genitals should be free from lesions, edema, or erythema.
   - Discharge increases during pregnancy and continues to increase as the pregnancy gets further along. This normal discharge is called "leukorrhea" and is typically thin, white, milky, and has a mild odor. Leukorrhea will be the heaviest during the last weeks of pregnancy. The mucous plug is a protective collection of mucus that accumulates in the cervical canal that acts as a barrier for unwanted bacteria and infection. When the body is getting ready for labor, the mucous plug is expelled. This can happen in one piece or gradually in small pieces over time. It is typically clear, or slightly pink/blood tinged in color but usually indicates the beginning signs of labor.
   - The cervical os has a different appearance and feel in nulliparous women versus multiparous women. In the nulliparous woman, the cervical os is pinpoint in size and rounded. In the multiparous woman, the os has the appearance of a slit. When labor gets closer, the cervix softens, shortens, and thins.

## INSPECTION ABNORMAL FINDINGS

- Obesity carries risks during pregnancy. There is an increased risk of spontaneous abortion, recurrent miscarriage, neural tube defects, hydrocephaly, and cardiovascular, orofacial, and limb reduction anomalies. There is also an increased risk of cardiac dysfunction, proteinuria, sleep apnea, nonalcoholic fatty liver disease, gestational diabetes mellitus, and preeclampsia. The risk of stillbirth increases with class of obesity. Obese mothers also face an increased risk of cesarean birth, failed trial of labor, endometritis, wound rupture or dehiscence, and venous thrombosis.
- Melasma, acne, and striae gravidarum (stretch marks) are common during pregnancy and are often due to hormonal changes. Pregnancy-specific skin conditions include pruritic urticarial papules and plaques of pregnancy, prurigo of pregnancy, intrahepatic cholestasis of pregnancy, pemphigoid gestationis, impetigo herpetiformis, and pruritic folliculitis of pregnancy.
- The presence of any lesions, erythema, edema, discharge, or bleeding in the genital region, inside the vaginal vault, or at the cervix is abnormal.
- The presence of lesions on the skin or in the vaginal canal can indicate a sexually transmitted infection such as herpes simplex or genital warts and requires further attention.
- Abnormal discharge during pregnancy is any discharge that has a green, yellow, or thick, clumpy white appearance. It is also abnormal for the discharge to have a strong odor and/or is accompanied by erythema or pruritus. Green or yellow discharge can indicate the presence of an STI such as chlamydia, trichomoniasis, or gonorrhea. A thick white, cottage cheese-like discharge can indicate a vulvovaginal candidiasis infection. A greyish discharge can indicate a bacterial vaginosis infection. Red, pink,

or brown discharge can indicate bleeding and requires immediate follow-up when seen during pregnancy. A watery discharge that causes either an obvious gush or a continuous trickle may indicate a patient's amniotic sac breaking. Malodorous discharge can be due to bacterial vaginosis, trichomoniasis, a retained tampon or other foreign body, or vulvovaginal candidiasis.

- A small amount of bleeding in early pregnancy can be normal especially following intercourse or following an internal speculum exam. If bleeding is heavier with or without other symptoms, it could be due to something more serious like infection, early pregnancy loss, or ectopic pregnancy.
- Bleeding in later pregnancy is usually more serious and could signal preterm labor or a problem with the placenta. Placental abruption, placenta previa, and placenta accrete can all cause bleeding during pregnancy.

## PALPATION

1. If greater than 12 weeks gestation or if dates are unknown, an abdominal exam to assess if the fundus is palpable in the abdomen is useful.
   - At 12 weeks gestation, the fundus should be palpable just caudally to the symphysis pubis.
   - At 16 weeks gestation, the fundus should be palpable midway between the symphysis pubis and the umbilicus.
   - At 20 weeks gestation, the fundus should be palpable at the umbilicus.
2. As pregnancy progresses past 20 weeks gestation, the clinician will measure the fundal height at each visit. This is the measurement in centimeters from the top of the symphysis pubis to the fundus. The measurement approximately correlates with the current number of weeks gestation. Clinicians will also assess the fetal presentation by utilizing Leopold's maneuvers after approximately 28 weeks gestation.
   - Leopard's maneuvers are typically done in four steps and are used to determine the fetal position.
   - Identify the fetal part in the uterine fundus.
   - Use the palmar surface of both hands to identify which side of the uterus contains the fetal back and which contains "small parts" such as hands and feet.
   - Use the thumb and third finger to identify the fetal presenting part.
   - Use both hands to outline the fetal presenting part. (Figure 17.1)
3. In full-term pregnancy or for concerns prior to term, clinicians may again need to perform a cervical exam to evaluate for labor or preterm labor. There are five main findings from a cervical exam: dilation, effacement, fetal station, position of the cervix, and consistency of the cervix. These five metrics together make up the Bishop's Score. The Bishop's Score is a tool used to determine how likely it is that the patient will go into labor and whether induction should be considered. Each of the five metrics is scored on the scale of 0 to 3. The higher the Bishop's score, the more likely induction will be successful. If the Bishop score is 7 or less, induction will likely not be successful.

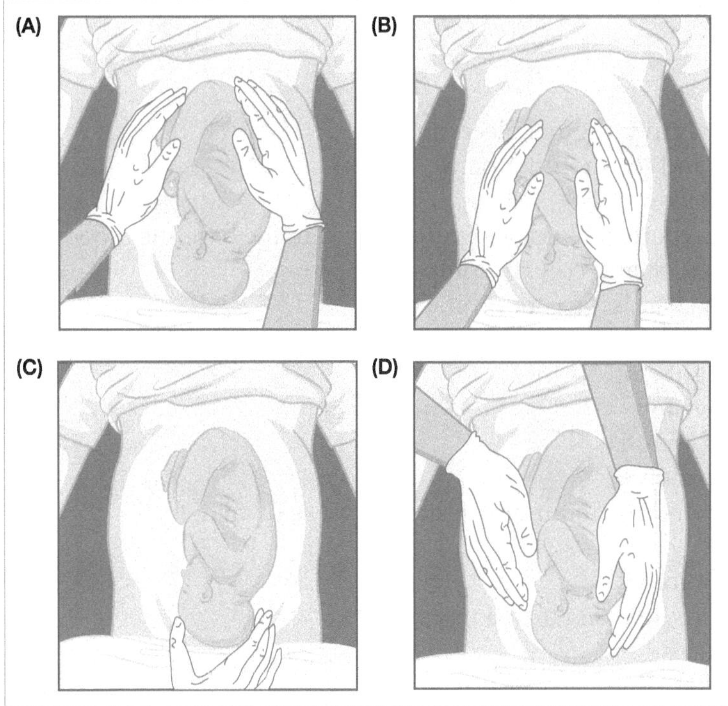


**Figure 17.1** Performing Leopold's maneuvers.

## AUSCULTATION

1. The clinician may auscultate maternal heart and lungs during an initial physical exam. Fetal heart tones are auscultated at each visit, typically with a Doppler. Fetal heart tones can be heard with a Doppler after 10 to 12 weeks gestation, depending on the strength of the Doppler. A fetoscope may also be used to auscultate fetal heart tones, however, this requires an experienced clinician, and the patient must typically be at least 24 weeks' gestation. The average fetal heart rate is between 110 to 160 beats per minute.

### AUSCULTATIONS ABNORMAL FINDINGS

- Fetal bradycardia or tachycardia is a cause for concern and could indicate fetal distress or impending fetal demise. This finding requires prompt assessment and intervention.

## SPECIAL TESTS

- Lab work, ultrasounds, fetal stress tests, and screening tests can also provide additional information in which to help the clinician determine the health of the mother and the health of the fetus. Guidelines, patient preferences, and individualized considerations need to be taken into account with each patient encounter.

## RED FLAGS IN HISTORY AND PHYSICAL EXAM

- Moderate to heavy vaginal bleeding
- Abdominal and/or shoulder pain
- Fever and chills
- New-onset hypertension or a significant rise in the baseline blood pressure
- Proteinuria or decreased urine output
- Edema of the hands, face, or orbital areas
- Severe headache(s)
- Sudden weight gain
- Changes in vision
- Shortness of breath
- Mental confusion
- Sense of impending doom or heightened sense of anxiety
- Seizures
- Suicidal ideation
- Hallucinations, delusions, or a manic mood
- Elevated glucose
- History of diabetes

## SPECIAL POPULATION CONSIDERATIONS

- Women who will be age 35 or older at their estimated due date are considered to be advanced maternal age (AMA). There are increased risks with AMA pregnancies, including an increased risk of chromosomal abnormalities, fetal growth restriction, gestational diabetes, gestational hypertension, preeclampsia, placental insufficiency, preterm birth, and stillbirth.
- Pregnant adolescents have unique needs. This population needs regular screening for alcohol and substance use, depression and mood disorders, safety and violence, and nutritional screenings. STI and bacterial vaginosis screening should be completed upon presentation of the pregnancy, during the third trimester, with any symptoms, and postpartum.
- Pregnant patients who are obese should be counseled on their risks for the pregnancy, labor, and birth. Some of the effects of obesity on pregnancy include an increased risk of spontaneous abortion and recurrent miscarriage. Additional risks associated with obesity during pregnancy are increased findings of neural tube defects; hydrocephaly; and cardiovascular, orofacial, and limb reduction anomalies. There is also an increased risk of cardiac dysfunction, proteinuria, sleep apnea, nonalcoholic fatty liver disease, gestational diabetes mellitus, and preeclampsia. The risk of stillbirth increases with class of obesity. Mothers with obesity also face an increased risk of cesarean birth, failed trial of labor, endometritis, wound rupture or dehiscence, and venous thrombosis.

- Maternal mortality is 3.3 times as high among black mothers as among white mothers. To improve the maternal health of this population, a multi-faceted approach should be employed. Screening for social determinants of health, including access to high-quality care across the life span, should be part of every visit.

## KEY DIFFERENTIALS

- Anemia of pregnancy
- Asymptomatic bacteriuria
- Eclampsia
- Ectopic pregnancy
- Gestational diabetes
- Gestational hypertension
- Hyperemesis gravidarum
- Leukorrhea
- Normal pregnancy
- Placental abruption
- Placenta previa
- Placenta accrete
- Preeclampsia
- Spontaneous abortion

# KNOWLEDGE CHECK: PREGNANT POPULATIONS

1. What does the Institute of Medicine (IOM) recommend regarding weight gain during pregnancy for obese women (BMI >30)?

   **A.** 0 weight gain
   **B.** 5- to 10-pound weight loss
   **C.** 11- to 20-pound weight gain
   **D.** 25- to 35-pound weight gain

2. Complications for an infant related to maternal gestational diabetes include:

   **A.** Intrauterine growth retardation
   **B.** Macrosomia and shoulder dystocia
   **C.** Precipitous vaginal delivery
   **D.** Postnatal hypertension and hyperglycemia

3. Which is an effective strategy for decreasing the incidence of neural tube defects in neonates?

   **A.** Eliminating alcohol intake before and during pregnancy
   **B.** Eliminating exposure to secondhand smoke for all women, infants, and children
   **C.** Increasing intake of folic acid before and during pregnancy
   **D.** Increasing iron supplementation for all individuals with anemia

4. A 30-year-old pregnant woman presents with chief concern of "bleeding" during the first trimester. Which additional history would be most concerning?

   **A.** Light spotting for 2 days that resolved
   **B.** No abdominal cramping associated
   **C.** Recent sexual activity including intercourse
   **D.** Sudden decrease in pregnancy symptoms

5. When the uterine fundus is at the level of the umbilicus during pregnancy, the gestational age of the fetus is:

   **A.** 16 weeks
   **B.** 20 weeks
   **C.** 28 weeks
   **D.** 34 weeks

*(See answers next page.)*

**1. C) 11- to 20-pound weight gain**

The IOM recommends weight gain of 11 to 20 pounds for all obese women and does not differentiate between Class I (BMI 30–34.9), Class II (BMI 35–39.9), and Class III (BMI 40 or greater). The recommendations balance the risks of having large-for-gestational-age infants, small-for-gestational-age infants, and preterm births and postpartum weight retention. Recommended weight gain during pregnancy for an individual with normal BMI is 25 to 35 pounds. Weight loss is not recommended, related to the risk of negative health consequences.

**2. B) Macrosomia and shoulder dystocia**

Patients with gestational diabetes mellitus (GDM) have a greater risk of preeclampsia and cesarean delivery, as well as an increased risk of developing type 2 diabetes later in life. Infants born to mothers with GDM have an increased incidence of macrosomia or excessive birth weight, neonatal hypoglycemia, hyperbilirubinemia, shoulder dystocia, and birth trauma.

**3. C) Increasing intake of folic acid before and during pregnancy**

While avoiding exposure to secondhand smoke, eliminating alcohol intake, and treating anemia during pregnancy are all recommended, the only strategy listed that prevents neural tube defects is increasing the intake of folic acid during both preconception and pregnancy. Folic acid intake can be increased through vitamin supplementation and fortified foods.

**4. D) Sudden decrease in pregnancy symptoms**

Bleeding or spotting during the first trimester occurs in approximately 25% of pregnancy. Light bleeding can occur during implantation, after sexual intercourse, and with pelvic exams. Sudden decrease in pregnancy symptoms, back pain, mild to moderate pelvic pain or cramping, passage of tissue, and persistent or heavy bleeding are all signs of miscarriage. Severe shoulder, back, rectal or pelvic pain, vomiting, and lightheadedness or fainting in addition to bleeding may indicate ectopic pregnancy and requires emergency care.

**5. B) 20 weeks**

At 12 weeks gestation, the fundus of the uterus is palpable just superior to the symphysis pubis. At 16 weeks gestation, the fundus is palpable midway between the symphysis pubis and the umbilicus. At 20 weeks gestation, the fundus is in line with the umbilicus. At approximately 28 weeks gestation, the fundus is palpable midway between the umbilicus and xiphoid process; the examiner should be able to determine fetal presentation. At 34 weeks gestation, the fundus is palpable just below the xiphoid process.

6. Which three pregnant individuals have the HIGHEST risk for prenatal complications? (Select THREE)

   A. 30-year-old with first pregnancy
   B. 31-year-old pregnant with twins
   C. 31-year-old who had a previous C-section delivery
   D. 36-year-old with mild preeclampsia and ketonuria
   E. 36-year-old with type 1 diabetes controlled by insulin

7. Physical examination during the first trimester of pregnancy characteristically reveals:

   A. Bluish-discoloration and softening of the cervix
   B. Breast engorgement with distinct, non-tender masses
   C. Dilation and effacement of the cervix
   D. Hypopigmentation of the abdomen, face, and hands

8. For a healthy woman with a normal pre-pregnancy BMI, how many additional daily calories are recommended during lactation?

   A. 250
   B. 500
   C. 750
   D. 1000

9. When discussing postpartum adjustment to motherhood, a woman confides to the advanced practice nurse that she is feeling worthless, tired, and sad. What is the nurse's BEST response?

   A. Postpartum blues are normal after having a baby, especially if you are breastfeeding
   B. You need to talk to your spouse about sharing more of the baby's care
   C. Your symptoms are a concern. Tell me how long have you been feeling this way?
   D. While these symptoms are to be expected, I think that you need to see a counselor

10. Signs and symptoms of preeclampsia include:

   A. Glucosuria, urinary frequency, and leukorrhea
   B. Nausea, abdominal pain, and blurry vision
   C. Recurrent urinary tract infections and fatigue
   D. Seizure activity and loss of consciousness

(*See answers next page.*)

**6. B, D, and E) 31-year-old pregnant with twins, 36-year-old with mild preeclampsia and ketonuria, 36-year-old with type 1 diabetes controlled by insulin**

Conditions that increase risk for prenatal complications include pregnancies of multiple gestation, preeclampsia, gestational diabetes, previous preterm birth, substance use, young age (adolescence), over 35 years of age, and maternal health conditions (e.g., hypertension, thyroid disease, diabetes, or renal disease.) Those who are pregnant for the first time or who have had a previous C-section delivery are not considered high risk for prenatal complications.

**7. A) Bluish-discoloration and softening of the cervix**

Early signs of pregnancy include bluish discoloration of the cervix and vagina (Chadwick's sign) and softening of the cervix (Goodell's sign). Breast engorgement and tenderness would be expected without palpable, distinct, non-tender masses. Darkening of the skin (melasma/chloasma) is associated with pregnancy. Cervical dilation and effacement occur during the first stages of labor.

**8. B) 500**

An additional 500 calories per day is recommended for well-nourished breastfeeding mothers; this is approximately 2300 to 2500 calories/day to sustain lactation. Good nutrition for the mother during breastfeeding is important to support the health of both mother and baby.

**9. C) Your symptoms are a concern. Tell me how long have you been feeling this way?**

Symptoms of postpartum depression include feelings of sadness, fatigue, worthlessness, guilt, hopelessness, and/or irritability. While these symptoms can also be associated with hormonal fluctuations during the postpartum period, key to differentiating postpartum depression is the length of time that symptoms have persisted, the intensity of the symptoms, and the person's ability to function. Evidence-based assessment and management require recognition of the symptoms, listening carefully to the individual's history, and avoiding assumptions and implicit bias.

**10. B) Nausea, abdominal pain, and blurry vision**

Preeclampsia a significant cause of maternal and fetal morbidity and mortality. Signs and symptoms of preeclampsia headache, changes in vision, upper abdominal pain, nausea or vomiting, edema, weight gain, proteinuria, and elevated blood pressure. Glycosuria and urinary frequency are more likely associated with diabetes in pregnancy. Recurrent urinary tract infections indicate disease processes unrelated to preeclampsia. Preeclampsia-eclampsia may develop before, during, or after delivery; seizures related to eclampsia can occur more than 48 hours after delivery.

# Older Adult Populations

## INTRODUCTION

Older adults are at an increased risk for certain conditions and injuries. This population has special needs and considerations. Prevention should be priority. Targeted assessments are important to identify and predict older adults who may be at risk for adverse outcomes. This chapter reviews specific assessments for older adults and additional considerations for clinicians when evaluating this population.

## KEY HISTORY CONSIDERATIONS

- Hearing loss; access to hearing aids
- Vision problems, changes
- Constipation
- Confusion, forgetfulness
- Grief
- Incontinence
- Problems with eating
- Skin breakdown
- Pain (location, acute, chronic)
- Fatigue, lethargy
- Frailty
- Unexplained weight loss
- Frequent infections
- Loss of ability to complete activities of daily living and instrumental activities of daily living
- Loss of function
- Quality of life
- Social support
- Living arrangements
- History of falls
- Transportation
- Nutritional intake and access to food
- Medications, side effects, polypharmacy
- Chronic conditions (controlled, uncontrolled)
- Physical activity
- Sexual activity

- Nicotine use
- Alcohol intake
- Immunization status
- Advanced directives

# VITAL SIGNS

## FEVER

- With advanced age, the body's thermoregulatory measures are less effective. Older adults are less capable to adapt to extreme environmental temperatures, putting them at risk for both hypothermia and heat-related illness. Older adults are also less likely to develop a fever with infection, making body temperature a less reliable indicator of their health status.

## PULSE

- Because the older adult's heart takes longer to recover from activity and stress, if an older adult presents with tachycardia, the clinician should review the activities that preceded the assessment to determine whether they are related to the elevated pulse rate. Allow an older adult to rest after a period of activity that may have increased their pulse rate and reassess.

## BLOOD PRESSURE

- Geriatric patients have risks for both hypertension and hypotension. The elevated blood pressure associated with hypertension remains a leading risk factor for ischemic heart disease and stroke and has a prevalence rate of 60 to 80% in the geriatric population. Although strict or aggressive blood pressure management does reduce the overall mortality rate, this population may have adverse effects from treatment which led the Eighth Joint National Commission (JNC 8) to change the target blood pressure for those ≥60 years old to a SBP <150 mm Hg and DBP <90 mm Hg. Systolic hypertension with a widened pulse pressure is also more common in the older population due to atherosclerosis and a stiff aorta.
- Orthostatic hypotension is more common in the geriatric population (20%) in part due to diminished baroreceptor sensitivity. Studies have shown that antihypertensive medications may also play a role in postural hypotension, which demonstrates the need to discuss risks, benefits, and patient preference when managing hypertension in this population. Orthostatic blood pressure should be assessed in older adults on blood pressure medications and especially in patients who screen positive for fall risk.

# MENTAL HEALTH ASSESSMENT

## APPEARANCE

1. **Affect:** Appropriate for the situation, labile, pleasant, flat, nontoxic
2. **Posture:** Many older adults have kyphosis. This can be due to conditions such as compression fractures, osteoporosis, and degenerative disk disease.
3. **Hygiene and grooming:** Personal hygiene in the older adult can deteriorate over time due to such things as loss of function, neglect, depression, and dementia.
4. **Body habitus:** Review the patient's height, weight, body mass index (BMI), and compare them to previous measurements. Older adults are at risk for malnutrition due to such things as impaired ability to eat; social isolation; changes in smell, taste, and appetite; dementia; medications; and alcoholism. An older adult losing weight without intention could also mean another condition such as malignancy or Alzheimer's and it should be closely monitored.

## BEHAVIOR

1. Watch the patient for any verbal or nonverbal expressions of pain, anxiety, illness, anger, fear, frustration, contentment, or sadness.
2. Note the patient's interactions with caregivers, family members, or spouses. Patients with dementia or cognitive impairment may exhibit agitation, apathy, or aggressiveness. They may say inappropriate things or exhibit impulsivity. Depressed older adults may appear flat and speak slowly.
3. Observe the patient's body movements and mobility. Older adults often use assistive devices to help improve functional mobility. Ensure their comfort and proper use of these devices.
4. Observe for the presence of any abnormal movements or involuntary tics or tremors, which could signify a movement disorder or other underlying condition.

# COGNITION ASSESSMENT

1. Ask the patient to tell you who they are, the time, and place. Note any confusion, disorientation, or delirium.
2. Observe the older adult's speech pattern and pace. The speech should be coherent and organized in thought and content. When possible, the patient should speak for themselves.
3. Test the patient's memory by saying three unrelated words to the patient, asking them to repeat those words immediately and again in 5 minutes.
4. Complete the clock test by asking the patient to draw a clock. This screens for moderate to severe dementia. The clock drawing interpretation scale (CDIS) is the tool used to evaluate and score the picture and is based on a 20 point quantitative scoring system. The Mini-Cog is another screening test for dementia that is based on a memory test (the ability to recall three words from memory), and the ability to

draw a clock. A score of <3 has been validated for a positive dementia screening. A score of <4 also requires additional evaluation.

5. Observe the patient's mood. Note if the patient appears to have sadness, guilt, worry, fear, helplessness, or hopelessness.
   - Older adults are at an increased risk for depression due to such causes as other serious comorbidities, disability, life changes, and loneliness/social isolation.
   - Sometimes depression in older adults can present as grumpiness, irritability, insomnia, attention problems, confusion, or fatigue.
   - The five-item Geriatric Depression Scale (GDS) is a valid and reliable tool for screening for depression in the older adult. A score >5 is suggestive of depression and >10 is almost always indicative of depression.

## SYSTEMS-SPECIFIC DIFFERENCES

Each chapter of this text includes an older adult section. Please review each of these sections to learn differences and considerations in the older adult population within each body system.

## ILLNESS PRESENTATION IN THE OLDER ADULT

It is important to consider the differences in the presentation of illness in the older adult. Older adults often do not have classic symptoms of illness. For example, an older adult who has a urinary tract infection may present with confusion, social withdrawal, hallucinations, or agitation in lieu of the typical dysuria and urinary frequency seen in the younger adult population. These differences can be subtle and are often disregarded as "normal aging" or depression. It is imperative that the clinician be aware of these age-specific differences in disease presentation.

## HEARING, VISION, AND ORAL HEALTH ASSESSMENT

- Hearing, vision, and oral health need to be regular assessed with the older adult. Both hearing and vision decline with aging and can significantly impact quality of life if not identified and corrected. Oral health often declines with age which puts the older adult at higher risk for dental caries, tooth loss, and periodontal disease. Twenty-five percent of people over the age of 65 have no natural teeth. Refer to Chapter 5, "Eyes, Ears, Nose, and Throat," for more information on these assessments. Referrals to specialists including optometrists, dentists, and audiologists are important for maintaining health and function in these areas.

## FUNCTIONAL MOBILITY ASSESSMENT

- The Timed Up and Go (TUAG) is a test used to assess a patient's mobility and their risk for falls. Ask the patient to get out of their seat, walk three meters across the room, do a 180-degree turn, return to their chair, and sit back down. If the patient is able to do this in less than 12 seconds, no further testing is needed. If it takes longer than 12 seconds, functional impairment likely exists. This test has been shown to help predict falls, fractures, and mortality.
- The handgrip strength is also used to test functional mobility in the older adult. This can be assessed using a handgrip dynamometer. Poor handgrip strength predicts accelerated dependency in activities of daily living (ADLs) and cognitive decline. Grip strength should be measured three times in a row with a rest period between each of between 20 second and 1 minute. No encouragement should be provided during the assessment. The strongest grip should be recorded.

## ACTIVITIES OF DAILY LIVING (ADL) ASSESSMENT

ADLs are the basic self-care tasks that are considered fundamental in caring for oneself and maintaining independence. Measuring ADLs an additional way to monitor a patient's functional status and helps to objectively predict future decline and/or improvement. As a person ages, these gradually take more time to complete.

- A widely used tool to assess ADLs is the Katz Index of Independence in Activities of Daily Living. This tool asks about ability to independently bathe, dress, toilet, transfer, feed, and have self-control over urination and defecation. It is rated 0 to 6, with a score of 0 indicating that a patient is very dependent and a score of 6 indicating that a patient is very independent.

## INSTRUMENTAL ACTIVITIES OF DAILY LIVING (IADL) ASSESSMENT

IADLs are another measure of a patient's ability to independently live in the community. These are more complex and are often lost before the basic "activities of daily living." These are essential for independent, safe living and include meal preparation, money management, shopping for groceries and personal items, doing housework, using a telephone, medication management, and having a reliable means of transportation.

- The Lawton-Brody Instrumental Activities of Daily Living (IADL) Scale is a valid, reliable tool that is scored 0 to 8 for females and 0 to 5 for males. 0 indicates low function and dependence and 5 (for males) or 8 (for females) indicates high functioning and independence.

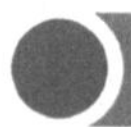

## NUTRITION ASSESSMENT

- The older adult is at high risk for malnutrition, so nutrition assessments should be part of routine older adult assessments. Nutritional decline often occurs due to preventable factors. Identification and intervention of these underlying factors can make a significant difference in outcomes. Asking the older adult about things like dysphagia, problems with dentition or dentures, medication side effects that cause anorexia or nausea, and difficulty handling silverware are important to early identification and intervention.
- There are many valid and reliable nutritional assessment tools available to screen for malnutrition in adults and are typically used in the nursing home and rehabilitation settings. The Malnutrition Screening Tool (MST) and the Mini Nutritional Assessment® (MNA) are two screening tools that are well known and should be considered if a patient presents with recent weight loss, recent poor intake/appetite, and/or a low BMI. Both tools have a high sensitivity and specificity (MST sensitivity 93%, specificity 93% and MNA® sensitivity 97.9%, specificity 100%). The MST can be found in Table 18.1. The MNA can be found at www.mna-elderly.com/forms/mini/mna_mini_english.pdf.

**Table 18.1 Malnutrition Screening Tool**

| | **Answer** | **Points** |
|---|---|---|
| Have you recently lost weight without trying? | No | 0 |
| | Unsure | 1 |
| If yes, how much weight have you lost? (Answer this question only if *unsure* was marked on above question) | 2–13 lb | 1 |
| | 14–23 lb | 2 |
| | 24–33 lb | 3 |
| | 34 lb or more | 4 |
| | Unsure | 2 |
| Have you been eating poorly due to a decreased appetite? | No | 0 |
| | Yes | 1 |
| **Total Points** | | |

**Interpretation of Score for Malnutrition Screening Tool**

| **Risk Category** | **Total Score** |
|---|---|
| Not at risk | 0 or 1 |
| At risk | 2+ |

*Source:* From Ferguson, M., Capra, S., Bauer, J., & Banks, M. (1999). Development of a valid and reliable malnutrition screening tool for adult acute hospital patients. *Nutrition, 15*, 458–464. doi:10.1016/S0899-9007(99)00084-2, with permission from Elsevier.

## FALLS RISK ASSESSMENT

Falls are a significant cause of morbidity and loss of independence in the older adult population. Falling once doubles the chances of falling again. Older adults are at higher risk for falls due to a variety of factors including, but not limited to, lower body weakness, vision problems, home hazards, osteoporosis, difficulties with balance and walking, and vitamin D deficiency.

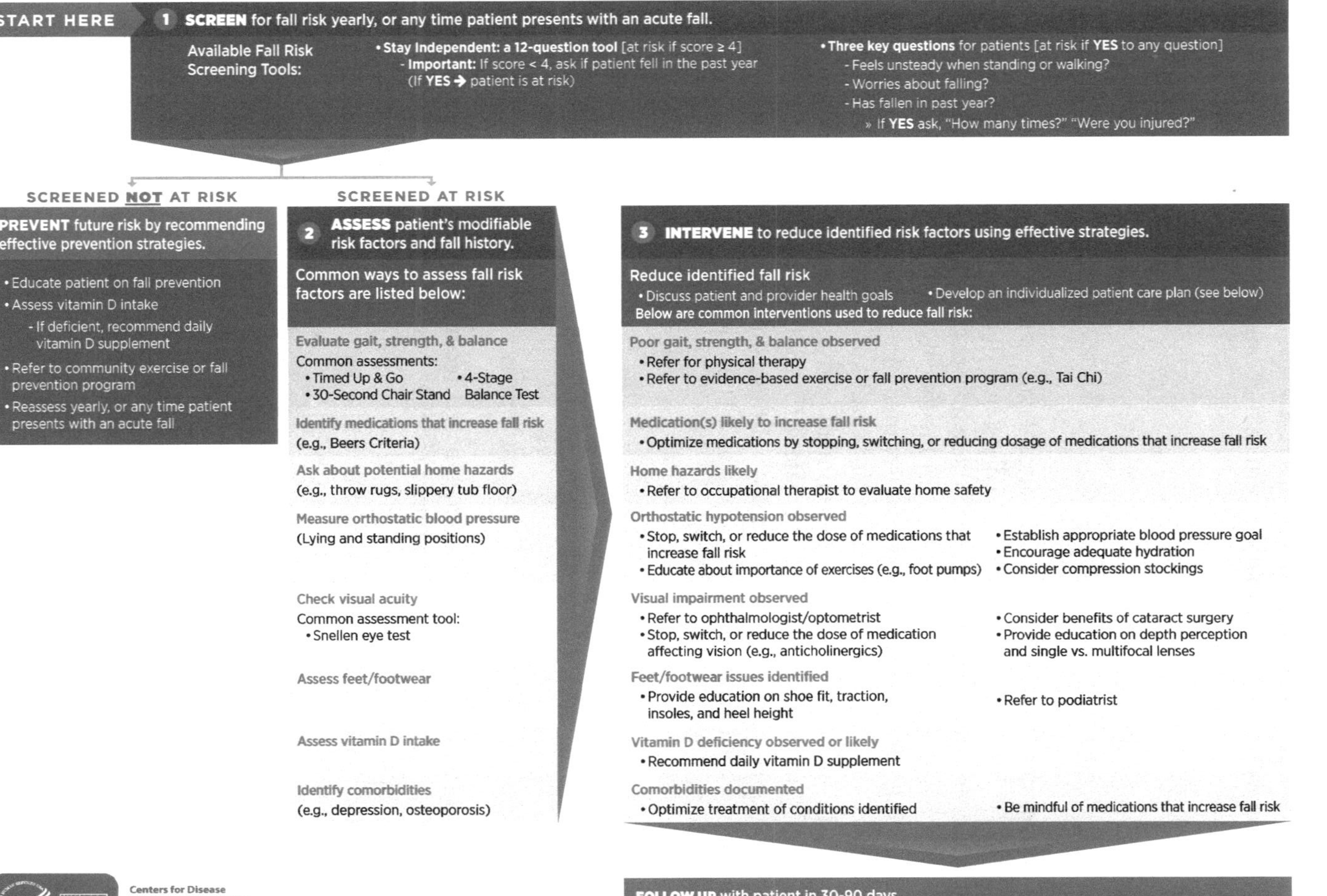


**Figure 18.1** STEADI Algorithm for Fall Risk Screening, Assessment, and Intervention Among Community-Dwelling Adults 65 Years or Older

- The STEADI Algorithm for Fall Risk Screening, Assessment, and Intervention is an evidence-based tool designed to reduce fall risk. It is based on the three–step process of screening, assessing, and intervening where appropriate (Figure 18.1). This algorithm can also be found at www.cdc.gov/steadi/pdf/STEADI-Algorithm-508.pdf.
- There are many other valid and reliable falls risk assessment tools, both for the inpatient setting as well as for the outpatient setting that can be used with the older adult population.

## ENVIRONMENTAL ASSESSMENT

As noted above, home hazards are a significant fall risk for older adults. Between 20% and 55% of all unintentional falls and fall-related injuries in older adults happen inside the home, and approximately 75% of these falls occur while performing routine daily activities. Reducing home hazards is an inexpensive intervention to reduce the risk of falls. The goal of completing an environmental assessment is to develop and implement effective strategies to reduce hazards and fall risks and maintain the older adult's ability to function in a safe environment. An assessment can also improve the older adult's accessibility. The Home Safety Checklist assessment ten domains: housekeeping, floors, bathroom, traffic lanes, lighting, stairways, ladders/step stools, outdoor areas, footwear, and personal precautions. This checklist can be found at www.acsu.buffalo.edu/~drstall/homesafe.html.

## AMERICAN GERIATRICS SOCIETY'S BEERS CRITERIA® MEDICATION LIST

The American Geriatric Society has evidence-based recommendations on potentially inappropriate use of certain medications in the older adult population. This medication list is periodically updated and is accompanied with the rationale as to why these medications should be avoided and the strength of evidence to support these recommendations. This can be accessed at American Geriatrics Society Updated Beers Criteria for Potentially Inappropriate Medication Use in Older Adults (geriatricscareonline.org).

## RED FLAGS IN HISTORY AND PHYSICAL EXAM

- Unintended weight loss
- History of falls
- Loss of function or disability
- Inability to care for self or complete ADLs
- Memory loss that disrupts daily life

- Challenges in planning or solving problems
- Difficulty completing familiar tasks
- Confusion with time or place
- Sudden behavior and/or personality changes
- Signs of elder abuse (physical, sexual, emotional, financial, neglect)

## KEY DIFFERENTIALS

- Alzheimer's disease
- Cachexia
- Dementia
- Elder abuse
- Falls
- Frailty
- Incontinence
- Major depressive disorder (MDD)
- Malignancy
- Malnutrition
- Osteoarthritis
- Osteoporosis
- Polypharmacy
- Poverty
- Social isolation
- Substance use disorder
- Presbycusis

## KNOWLEDGE CHECK: OLDER ADULT POPULATIONS

1. Older adults are MOST at risk for adverse drug events because they:
   - **A.** Are less able to be compliant
   - **B.** Are prescribed more medications
   - **C.** Compensate too rapidly to medications
   - **D.** Have increased body size and metabolism

2. What are the warning signs of elder abuse? (Select all that apply.)
   - **A.** Asks for help with managing activities of daily living
   - **B.** Expresses frustration with declining health
   - **C.** Lack of cleanliness, poor hygiene
   - **D.** Refuses to speak, uncommunicative
   - **E.** Significant withdrawals from financial accounts

3. In the United States, the majority of older adults:
   - **A.** Are medically disabled
   - **B.** Live in long-term care facilities
   - **C.** Live independently in the community
   - **D.** Require assistance with activities of daily living

4. Which signs and symptoms are commonly seen in the early stages of Alzheimer's disease?
   - **A.** Delirium and disorientation
   - **B.** Dysphagia and weight loss
   - **C.** Dystonia, bradykinesia, and tremor
   - **D.** Loss of spontaneity and mood changes

5. Which statements are true regarding the nutritional status of older adults? (Select all that apply.)
   - **A.** Inadequate micronutrient intake is uncommon in older adults
   - **B.** Medical conditions can predispose older adults to vitamin and mineral deficiencies
   - **C.** Obtaining a nutritional history for an older adult is likely to be inaccurate or unreliable
   - **D.** Physical exam findings are unlikely to reveal signs of malnutrition in the elderly
   - **E.** Social isolation, ill-fitting dentures, and lack of resources for food are common risk factors

*(See answers next page.)* 

**1. B) Are prescribed more medications**

Older adults are primarily at risk for adverse drug events because they are prescribed more medications, which increases the likelihood of drug–drug interactions, toxic levels of medications, and side effects. Older adults generally weigh less, although they do have an increased proportion of fat and less water composition than younger adults. Renal and liver metabolism decline with age, which increases medication sensitivity. Older adults compensate more slowly to medications and are especially sensitive to anticholinergic side effects. Age is not a risk factor for medication noncompliance.

**2. C, D, and E) Lack of cleanliness, poor hygiene; refuses to speak, uncommunicative; significant withdrawals from financial accounts**

Approximately one out of every ten individuals over the age of 60 is estimated to have been affected by some form of elder abuse, most commonly emotional, financial, and physical abuse. Warning signs include unexplained physical injuries, weight loss, poor hygiene, changes in mental status, refusal to speak, signs of dehydration, significant withdrawals from bank accounts, belongings or money missing from home, unpaid bills, and/or unsafe living conditions. Assess interactions with caregivers, as caregiver burnout is a risk factor. Effectively communicating emotions, asking for help, and expressing frustrations, are not likely when an older adult is experiencing abuse.

**3. C) Live independently in the community**

Most Americans over the age of 65 live in the community, not in nursing homes or other institutions. Only 4.5 percent of older adults live in nursing homes and 2 percent in assisted living facilities. The majority of older adults (93.5%, or 33.4 million) live in the community independently. While older adults have increasing rates of chronic illnesses, more than 95% of all older adults are non-disabled.

**4. D) Loss of spontaneity and mood changes**

In early stages, Alzheimer's dementia presents with mild cognitive impairment, mood changes, and loss of responsiveness to one's environment. Alzheimer's disease is irreversible and progressive, and leads to worsening cognition; problems include wandering, personality changes, disorientation, and hallucinations or delusions. Tremors, bradykinesia, and dystonia are more likely with Parkinson's disease. While dysphagia, weight loss, and disorientation can be seen in individuals who have neurocognitive disorders, these symptoms are not commonly present in early stages of Alzheimer's dementia and would require further evaluation.

**5. B and E) Medical conditions can predispose older adults to vitamin and mineral deficiencies; social isolation, ill-fitting dentures, and lack of resources for food are common risk factors**

Assessing the nutritional status of older adults is important because inadequate micronutrient intake and vitamin and mineral deficiencies are common; these are exacerbated by age-related medical conditions and social determinants. Determinants of health that commonly impact older adults include social isolation, lack of access to dental care despite increased need, and lack of resources for food. Assessment of the nutritional status of older adults should include nutritional history, usual food intake based on 24-hour dietary recall, physical exam with particular attention to signs associated with inadequate nutrition, and select lab tests, if needed.

6. Which assessment is associated with the normal physiologic changes of aging?

A. Arthritic pain
B. Decreased kidney function
C. Inadequate nutrition
D. Injuries related to falls

7. What is the most common source of bacteremia in older adults?

A. Bronchitis
B. Pharyngitis
C. Skin infections
D. Urinary tract infections

8. Identify consequences associated with polypharmacy for older adults (select all that apply):

A. Cognitive impairment
B. Decreased medical costs
C. Improved functional capacity
D. Increased risk of adverse side effects
E. Medication non-adherence

9. A 75-year-old male is brought into the office by his wife, who states that within the past 2 days he has become unusually agitated and incoherent. He slept very poorly last night. Which differential diagnosis is MOST LIKELY from this history?

A. Anxiety
B. Delirium
C. Dementia
D. Depression

10. When completing a mental status assessment for a 75-year-old man who is having no health problems, the advanced practice nurse should expect that this individual:

A. Is likely to have some early signs of Alzheimer dementia
B. Is likely to have declines in cognition and mild depression
C. May take a little longer to respond, but his cognition will be intact
D. Will have some losses in language comprehension and ability to communicate

*(See answers next page.)*

**6. B) Decreased kidney function**

Normal physiologic changes associated with aging include progressive structural and functional deterioration of the kidney, resulting in decreased creatinine clearance, renal blood flow, and glomerular filtration rate. While changes may be noted in physical health, functional ability, or cognition, resultant diseases, disorders, or injuries are not the result of normal physiologic processes. In other words, an older adult with pain, inadequate nutrition, injuries, and/or comorbid disease processes is experiencing abnormalities in health and wellness that can be treated and resolved.

**7. D) Urinary tract infections**

Urinary tract infections are the most common cause of bacteremia in older adults, and can present without symptoms, or with few symptoms. A change in mental status or decline in function may be the only presenting problem in an older patient with an infection. Bronchitis and pharyngitis are less likely to be the underlying cause of bacteremia; assess for pneumonia or influenza when an older adult presents with respiratory infection. Skin infections can occur but are not as common.

**8. A, D, and E) Cognitive impairment, increased risk of adverse side effects, medication non-adherence**

Polypharmacy, the use of five or more medications daily by an individual for one or more than one condition, is correlated with negative consequences, including cognitive impairment, increased risk of adverse side effects and drug-drug interactions, functional decline, and non-adherence related to the complexity and cost of care. Assessing for polypharmacy in older adults is imperative, as the consequences of potential disease progression, treatment failure, and adverse drug events can be life-threatening.

**9. B) Delirium**

Delirium is an acute change in attention, cognition, and consciousness; causes include dehydration, infection, and medications. Mental health disorders, including anxiety disorders, depression, and dementia, cause persistent symptoms over time. Delirium is more common among older adults, who are particularly vulnerable to stress and impaired cholinergic function.

**10. C) May take a little longer to respond, but his cognition will be intact**

An older adult without health problems should have a normal mental status assessment. Although they may respond more slowly, their consciousness, behavior, speech, affect, mood, and cognition should all be intact. Declining cognition, dementia, depression, or loss of ability to communicate would all be considered abnormalities.

# Part IV
# Practice Tests

# Practice Test I: Assessment and Diagnosis of Patients Across the Life Span

1. Body mass index (BMI) is a direct measurement of an individual's:

   A. Risk of cardiovascular disease and/or stroke
   B. Body mass divided by the square of their height
   C. Health status reflecting their lifestyle behaviors
   D. Genetic risk factors for diabetes and/or hypertension

2. In reviewing the evidence about the accuracy of a specific screening test, the clinician found that the test has a specificity of 80%. Which interpretation of this finding is accurate?

   A. The test correctly identifies 80% of individuals who do not have the disease (true negatives)
   B. The test correctly identifies 80% of individuals who have the disease (true positives)
   C. 80% of individuals without the disease are likely to test positive (false positives)
   D. 80% of individuals with the disease are likely to test negative (false negatives)

3. Which statement is TRUE in regard to asking individuals with depression about suicidal ideation?

   A. Asking about suicidal thoughts or plan is not associated with higher likelihood for suicide
   B. Asking about suicidal thoughts is likely to increase the risk for suicide in depressed individuals
   C. Individuals considering suicide will very rarely share their thoughts or imminent plans
   D. Individuals considering suicide are not likely to be influenced by a clinician's concern

4. A 50-year-old male presents to the office for evaluation with cough and shortness of breath. When the advanced practice nurse enters the room, they observe that the patient is sitting forward in the chair in a tripod position and has pale pink mucosa. What should be the clinician's next step?

   A. Listen to his lungs
   B. Listen to his heart
   C. Introduce themselves
   D. Request collaboration

5. An older adult with several chronic illnesses presents to the office for a wellness exam. When the clinician assesses the individual's use of medications, which component of the wellness visit is being addressed?

   **A.** Health history including past medical history
   **B.** Patient education and anticipatory guidance
   **C.** Primary preventive measures
   **D.** Review of systems including pertinent negatives

6. Which statement is true regarding the risks and protective factors for individuals with suicidal ideation?

   **A.** An individual who has only mild anxiety or mild depression does not need to be screened for suicidal ideation
   **B.** Individuals are not likely to be influenced by a family member's suicide if they are isolated from them
   **C.** Evidence-based strategies can help individuals to self-identify protective factors and improve their safety
   **D.** The period immediately following discharge from a psychiatric hospitalization is the safest time for individuals who have had suicidal ideation

7. Screening for breast cancer through use of mammography is considered which level of prevention?

   **A.** Preliminary
   **B.** Primary
   **C.** Secondary
   **D.** Tertiary

8. When using the Generalized Anxiety Disorder-2 (GAD-2) screening tool, what are the first questions an advanced practice nurse should ask to screen for anxiety? Over the last 2 weeks, how often have you been bothered by: (Select all that apply)

   **A.** Feeling nervous, anxious, or on edge
   **B.** Not being able to stop or control worrying
   **C.** Using alcohol to relax, feel better, or fit in
   **D.** Feeling hopeless, helpless, and suicidal

9. Which of the following statements is an example of objective information?

   **A.** Leg pain after an injury from a fall
   **B.** Experiencing sharp pain with movement
   **C.** Limps and grimaces with ambulation
   **D.** Unable to work due to pain and vertigo

**10.** Romberg's test is positive if an individual:

**A.** Is unable to maintain an upright stance with eyes closed
**B.** Maintains an upright stance with eyes closed
**C.** Has nystagmus with position change from seated to supine
**D.** Has nausea with position change from seated to supine

**11.** Which deep tendon reflex score appropriately documents the finding of clonus?

**A.** 1+
**B.** 2+
**C.** 3+
**D.** 4+

**12.** Vibratory sensation is often diminished in:

**A.** Adolescents with depression
**B.** Children who are blind or deaf
**C.** Adults during pregnancy and postpartum
**D.** Older adults with neuropathy

**13.** Over the course of a few days, a 40-year-old female has noticed increasing facial weakness around her left eye, forehead, and mouth. Her physical exam reveals weakness in raising her left eyebrow, asymmetry in facial expressions, and an inability to completely close her left eye. She is not experiencing pain and has not had recent exposures or trauma. Which diagnosis is MOST LIKELY?

**A.** Allergic reaction
**B.** Bell's palsy
**C.** Ischemic stroke
**D.** Atypical migraine

**14.** A 6-year-old is brought to the clinic because they are having behavior problems at school. Which finding must be present to diagnose attention deficit hyperactivity disorder (ADHD)?

**A.** Compulsivity
**B.** Inattention
**C.** Poor social skills
**D.** School failures

**15.** An individual with 20/50 visual acuity as determined by screening with a Snellen chart can clearly see:

**A.** At 20 feet what a person with normal vision can see clearly from 50 feet
**B.** At 50 feet what a person with normal vision can see clearly from 20 feet
**C.** 50% of what the average person sees at 20 feet
**D.** 50% of what the average person sees at 50 feet

**16.** Which is true about diabetic peripheral neuropathy?

**A.** This rare complication occurs only in those not immunized
**B.** The associated burning pain typically appears first in the hands
**C.** Distal muscle weakness and loss of coordination are common signs
**D.** Muscle cramping and spasticity are the usual presenting symptoms

**17.** Which assessment is a priority for the young child who presents after being treated for bacterial meningitis?

**A.** Screening for asthma
**B.** Hepatosplenomegaly
**C.** Cardiac function
**D.** Hearing screening

**18.** A 40-year-old male who works in construction reports low back pain. He has had similar pain before; this episode of pain has persistent for 3 weeks. The pain worsens with heavy lifting and with any twisting movement and does not radiate down the leg or thigh. The MOST LIKELY diagnosis is:

**A.** Lumbosacral strain
**B.** Nerve root compression
**C.** Ruptured or herniated disc
**D.** Compression fracture

**19.** Using a valgus stress test, applying inward pressure at the lateral thigh and outward pressure from the medial ankle, assesses the knee for integrity of the:

**A.** Lateral collateral ligament (LCL)
**B.** Medial collateral ligament (MCL)
**C.** Anterior cruciate ligament (ACL)
**D.** Posterior cruciate ligament (PCL)

**20.** MATCH the musculoskeletal test to assess upper extremities with the diagnosis indicated when findings are positive:

| | |
|---|---|
| **A.** Cozen's test | 1. de Quervain's tenosynovitis |
| **B.** Empty can test | 2. Medial epicondylitis |
| **C.** Finkelstein test | 3. Carpal tunnel syndrome |
| **D.** Reverse Mill's test | 4. Lateral epicondylitis |
| **E.** Tinel's test | 5. Supraspinatus |

**21.** Which patient is MOST at risk for developing gout?

**A.** A 30-year-old female with ulcerative colitis
**B.** A 40-year-old female with rheumatoid arthritis
**C.** A 50-year-old male who drinks two to six beers daily
**D.** A 60-year-old male who follows a plant-based diet

**22.** A mother calls to report that her 15-year-old son has been unusually irritable, agitated, and unable to sleep for more than a few hours each night. The adolescent was recently diagnosed with major depressive disorder and has been taking a selective serotonin reuptake inhibitor (SSRI) for 6 weeks. The advance practice nurse is MOST concerned because:

**A.** A therapeutic level of the drug has not been reached
**B.** Antipsychotic medication is warranted to treat probable substance abuse
**C.** The adolescent may be experiencing mania associated with mood disorder
**D.** The mom is reporting expected and common side effects

**23.** Which diagnosis is MOST LIKELY for an individual with symptoms of hypersomnia, fatigue, impaired concentration, helpless feelings, self-blame, and decreased appetite for the past 4 weeks?

**A.** Anorexia nervosa
**B.** Concussion
**C.** Depression
**D.** Psychosis

**24.** When assessing an individual for exposure to intimate partner violence, the advanced practice nurse is aware that:

**A.** Screening increases the desperation felt by the victim
**B.** Physical violence perpetrated by intimate partners is often associated with controlling behaviors
**C.** Pregnant individuals and parents of newborns have less risk of experiencing physical violence
**D.** Victims should avoid reporting injuries for their own safety

**25.** Which statement BEST describes posttraumatic stress disorder?

**A.** Characterized by reoccurring, intense, distressing dreams
**B.** Not likely to cause feelings of shame, guilt, or detachment
**C.** Rare phenomenon of war, combat, or violence
**D.** Symptoms include little reactivity to internal cues or triggers

**26.** Which history statement is LEAST likely to be associated with risk of substance use disorder?

**A.** Adverse childhood events
**B.** Lack of physical activity
**C.** Undiagnosed attention deficit disorder
**D.** Untreated mental illness

**27.** Which answer BEST summarizes who should be screened for unhealthy alcohol use, according to the U.S. Preventive Services Task Force (USPSTF)?

**A.** Adults who have had one or more motor vehicle crashes, regardless of cause
**B.** All adults regardless of gender, socioeconomic status, or comorbid conditions
**C.** Any individual who is high risk for substance abuse based on family history
**D.** Those individuals who are being counseled for other mental health disorders

**28.** Use of which substance is the single greatest cause of preventable deaths globally?

**A.** Tobacco
**B.** Opioids
**C.** Alcohol
**D.** Marijuana

**29.** A 40-year-old female presents to the primary care office for a work physical. Which approach is BEST to address her past history of opioid abuse and chronic back pain?

**A.** Be sure that anyone interacting with the patient is aware of her addiction history
**B.** Recognize that nothing needs to be said, as the substance abuse is past history
**C.** Screen for substance use at this visit and assess her management of pain
**D.** Tell the patient that she will have to find another health care provider if she relapses

**30.** Depletion of which neurotransmitter is MOST associated with substance use disorder?

**A.** Dopamine
**B.** Epinephrine
**C.** Norepinephrine
**D.** Serotonin

**31.** Match each primary skin lesion with the example to which it most closely aligns:

| | |
|---|---|
| **A.** Macules | **1.** Lipomas |
| **B.** Papules | **2.** Impetigo |
| **C.** Pustules | **3.** Insect bites |
| **D.** Vesicles | **4.** Psoriasis |
| **E.** Nodules | **5.** Freckles |
| **F.** Plaque | **6.** Shingles |

**32.** Which diagnosis is BEST described as a deep-seated infection of the pilosebaceous unit, which includes the hair shaft, hair follicle, erector pili muscle, and sebaceous gland?

**A.** Folliculitis
**B.** Cellulitis
**C.** Furuncle
**D.** Acrochordon

**33.** Testing visual fields by confrontation assesses for the function of which cranial nerve?

**A.** II optic
**B.** III oculomotor
**C.** IV trochlear
**D.** VI abducens

**34.** Placing a familiar object in an individual's hand for identification by sensation rather than by sight is called:

**A.** Graphesthesia
**B.** Extinction phenomenon
**C.** Point localization
**D.** Stereognosis

**35.** Which of the following is a true statement regarding proteinuria?

**A.** Protein in the urine always indicates ongoing, chronic kidney damage
**B.** Mild to moderate proteinuria during pregnancy is an expected finding
**C.** Individuals with diabetes and hypertension are expected to have proteinuria
**D.** Proteinuria can be benign and transient, or may indicate renal disease

**36.** Signs and symptoms associated with the diagnosis of interstitial cystitis include:

**A.** Asymptomatic urinary tract infections
**B.** Dysuria and recurrent pyelonephritis
**C.** Hesitancy and urge incontinence
**D.** Urinary frequency and pelvic pain

**37.** A 25-year-old with type 1 diabetes mellitus (T1DM) presents with symptoms of acute gastroenteritis, resulting in significantly decreased oral intake. Which findings should the advanced practice nurse expect as a result?

**A.** Decreased blood glucose and pale pink mucosa
**B.** Increased blood glucose and dry mucous membranes
**C.** Poorly concentrated urine with low specific gravity
**D.** Normal blood glucose with no changes in physical exam

**38.** A 22-year-old male with a BMI of 30 presents for a sports physical with a blood pressure of 142/102 mmHg. Physical exam reveals a continuous systolic-diastolic bruit present over the right mid-abdomen without palpable masses. Which differential diagnosis is MOST LIKELY?

**A.** Essential hypertension
**B.** Renovascular hypertension
**C.** Substance use disorder
**D.** White coat syndrome

**39.** A 50-year-old female with a history of osteoarthritis presents with epigastric pain that began 1 month ago. She describes her discomfort as gnawing pain, worse when her "stomach is empty," and improved with eating. She has not had fever; however, she does have nausea and bloating. What is the likely cause of her pain?

**A.** Cholelithiasis
**B.** *Escherichia coli* (*E. coli*)
**C.** *Helicobacter pylori* (*H. pylori*)
**D.** Ischemic colitis

**40.** The most common cause of acute and persistent diarrhea in adults is:

**A.** Long-term use of medications
**B.** Food allergies or intolerances
**C.** Irritable bowel syndrome
**D.** Viral, bacterial, or parasitic infections

**41.** The advanced practice nurse is teaching a student how to assess the spleen. Which statement made by the student MOST indicates the need for further teaching and clarification?

**A.** I may be able to palpate the spleen in my patient with mononucleosis
**B.** If the spleen is palpable, the likelihood of splenomegaly is significantly increased
**C.** Splenic dullness can be percussed just posterior to the left mid-axillary line
**D.** The spleen that is normal in size, shape, and contour is easy to palpate and percuss

**42.** Which nutritional choices INCREASE the risks of colorectal cancer?

**A.** High fiber and low saturated fat
**B.** Limited processed foods and sugar
**C.** Low fiber and limited calcium
**D.** Plant-based or vegetarian diets

**43.** A young adult presents for follow-up after being treated for lead poisoning. The individual shares that their abdominal pain and constipation have resolved and asks whether they are still anemic. Because lead can interfere with red blood cell production, which anemia are they MOST LIKELY to have had?

**A.** Microcytic anemia
**B.** Mild hemolytic anemia
**C.** Mild macrocytic anemia
**D.** Thrombocytopenia

**44.** Which type of incontinence is characterized by spasms of the detrusor muscle?

**A.** Overflow incontinence
**B.** Painful bladder syndrome
**C.** Stress incontinence
**D.** Urge incontinence

**45.** A pregnant individual is screened for hepatitis B and has the following lab results: HBsAg (-), anti-HBs (-), anti-HBc (-). The lab results indicate that the individual:

**A.** Could have had hepatitis B
**B.** Currently has acute hepatitis B
**C.** Is not immune to hepatitis B
**D.** Has had hepatitis B immunization

**46.** MATCH the assessment sign indicating possible abdominal abnormality with its description.

| | |
|---|---|
| **A.** Obturator sign | **1.** Bruising at flank |
| **B.** Psoas or iliopsoas sign | **2.** Bruising around umbilicus |
| **C.** Cullen sign | **3.** Palpation of left lower quadrant causes right sided pain |
| **D.** Gray-Turners sign | **4.** Pain on passive extension of the right thigh |
| **E.** Rovsing's sign | **5.** Referred pain to the left shoulder |
| **F.** Kehr's sign | **6.** Pain on passive internal rotation of flexed hip |

**47.** Beyond mammogram screening, which evidence-based strategies are recommended to support early detection of breast malignancy in asymptomatic women at average risk for breast cancer?

**A.** Education to support breast cancer awareness
**B.** Monthly self-breast examinations (SBE)
**C.** Annual clinical breast examination (CBE)
**D.** Genetic testing

**48.** Which infant's presentation is MOST concerning?

**A.** 4-week-old with rectal temperature of 100.8°F
**B.** 4-month-old with rectal temperature of 102°F
**C.** 9-month-old with a rash that blanches after fever of 102°F resolved
**D.** 12-month-old with temporal temperature of 100.8°F for 2 days

**49.** At what average age can a child print letters and numbers, draw a person with six body parts, name colors, hop, jump, skip, run, swing, and climb?

**A.** 2 years old
**B.** 3 years old
**C.** 4 years old
**D.** 5 years old

**50.** Which child's assessment indicates that they are MOST contagious?

**A.** A 15-month-old diagnosed with bilateral acute otitis media
**B.** A 2-year-old who was exposed to influenza approximately 12 hours ago
**C.** A 5-year-old with vesicular rash from varicella whose fever has resolved
**D.** A 12-year-old who received vaccinations last month for COVID-19 and influenza

**51.** Which disease commonly presents in an atypical manner in older adults?

**A.** Acute myocardial infarction
**B.** Osteoporosis
**C.** Resistant hypertension
**D.** Urinary incontinence

**52.** The advanced practice nurse assesses an 83-year-old male who presented with abdominal pain. Which assessment is most concerning?

**A.** Constipation
**B.** Fever
**C.** Recent laxative use
**D.** Loss of appetite

**53.** An older adult presents with a history of rheumatoid arthritis and has been taking ibuprofen for many years. Which of their organ systems would be most at risk for damage from chronic non-steroidal anti-inflammatory drug (NSAID) use? (Select all that apply.)

**A.** Cardiovascular
**B.** Gastrointestinal
**C.** Neurologic
**D.** Respiratory
**E.** Renal

**54.** Damage to which cranial nerve causes an inability to rotate the head and weakness in shrugging the shoulders?

**A.** V trigeminal
**B.** VI abducens
**C.** XI spinal accessory
**D.** XII hypoglossal

**55.** Which breast assessment finding is MOST concerning?

**A.** Asymmetry in size without palpable masses
**B.** Axillary lymphadenopathy without skin changes
**C.** Bilateral nipple depression below the areolar surface
**D.** Symmetric breast tissue density without distinct masses

**56.** Which breast assessment in a female is associated with precocious puberty?

**A.** An 8-year-old with elevation of the nipple; no palpable glandular tissue or areolar pigmentation
**B.** An 8-year-old with glandular tissue in sub-areolar region; breast and nipple project as single mound
**C.** A 12-year-old with enlargement of the areola and increased areolar pigmentation
**D.** A 12-year-old with completed breast development; smooth contour bilaterally

**57.** Which statement BEST reflects evidence-based recommendations for assessing an individual's plan for pregnancy or parenthood?

**A.** Ask all individuals of reproductive age about their intentions for pregnancy or parenthood
**B.** Ask all individuals not using contraception about their readiness for pregnancy or parenthood
**C.** Remind all adolescents and perimenopausal women that they are at risk for pregnancy
**D.** Remind all individuals of reproductive age that 75% of all pregnancies are unplanned

**58.** Chronic, recurring, vulvovaginal candidiasis may indicate undiagnosed:

**A.** Anxiety disorder
**B.** Bacterial vaginosis
**C.** Diabetes mellitus
**D.** Postmenopausal stage

**59.** Characteristics of polycystic ovarian syndrome include:

**A.** Dysmenorrhea, constipation, and chronic pelvic pain
**B.** Excessive androgen, insulin resistance, and unopposed estrogen
**C.** Excessive FSH and LH and premature ovarian failure
**D.** Ovarian insufficiency, vasomotor instability, and early menopause

**60.** A complication of pelvic inflammatory disease is:

**A.** Adenomyosis
**B.** Endometriosis
**C.** Infertility
**D.** Pyelonephritis

**61.** When examining the cervix of a 21-year-old nulliparous female, the advanced practice nurse notes that the cervix is pink, and the external os is small and round, with a small ring of dark-red tissue surrounding the os. The dark-red tissue is:

**A.** An endocervical polyp
**B.** Concerning for chlamydia
**C.** Concerning for HPV infection
**D.** The squamocolumnar junction

**62.** A 25-year-old female presents with 2 days of abdominal pain and vaginal discharge after sexual intercourse with a new male partner. She uses a hormonal intrauterine device (IUD) for contraception and has a negative pregnancy test. On exam, the IUD strings are visible, uterus is normal in size and contour, the cervix is friable, and cervical motion tenderness is present. Which diagnosis has the highest priority for this visit?

**A.** Pelvic inflammatory disease
**B.** Pregnancy
**C.** Contraceptive need
**D.** Bleeding disorder

**63.** In general, postmenopausal women are at greatest risk for:

**A.** Alzheimer's dementia
**B.** Breast cancer
**C.** Heart disease
**D.** Osteoporosis

**64.** When completing the history and physical exam for a 70-year-old woman with vaginal bleeding, the advanced practice nurse recognizes the priority concern is:

**A.** Endometrial cancer
**B.** Endometrial polyps
**C.** Uterine fibroids
**D.** Uterine lining atrophy

**65.** A 30-year-old male is concerned about HIV exposure and presents to primary care for screening. In completing his assessment, the advanced practice nurse is aware that the MOST common signs of acute retroviral syndrome are:

**A.** Abdominal pain, weight loss, and insomnia
**B.** Fever, fatigue, rash, and pharyngitis
**C.** Productive, persistent cough and headache
**D.** Chest pain, nausea, and generalized pruritus

**66.** Which assessment is consistent with a diagnosis of plaque psoriasis?

**A.** Reddish pink, well-demarcated macules, papules, and plaques with a silvery scale
**B.** Dry, sensitive, inflamed itchy skin that began during infancy or early childhood
**C.** Rash appears as linear vesicular lesions on an erythematous base
**D.** Flares may result from exposure to allergens, including laundry detergents

**67.** Bony overgrowths of the distal interphalangeal (DIP) joints are called:

**A.** Bouchard nodes
**B.** Ganglion cysts
**C.** Heberden nodes
**D.** Swan-neck deformities

**68.** A 60-year-old female has persistent, aching right shoulder pain that began 3 weeks ago after a fall on the ice. Which physical assessment findings indicate the likelihood of a torn rotator cuff?

**A.** Decreased grip strength
**B.** Pain over lateral epicondyle of humerus
**C.** Pain and edema over radial styloid
**D.** Inability to actively resist adduction

**69.** A 70-year-old male has a history of morning stiffness and pain that is most acute in his right knee on awakening. He feels some relief as the day progresses; prolonged gardening exacerbates his knee pain. Which disease process is MOST LIKELY?

**A.** Osteoarthritis
**B.** Osteoporosis
**C.** Meniscal tear
**D.** Rheumatoid arthritis

**70.** Petechial lesions are typically:

**A.** Papular and pustular
**B.** Ecchymotic patches
**C.** Flat pinpoint lesions
**D.** Blanching macules

**71.** What type or pattern of a rash begins and becomes concentrated on the trunk, then spreads with fewer lesions to the extremities?

**A.** Confluent
**B.** Centrifugal
**C.** Centripetal
**D.** Dermatomal

**72.** Which condition is commonly co-occurring with atopic dermatitis?

**A.** Clubbing
**B.** Asthma
**C.** Cellulitis
**D.** Impetigo

**73.** An adolescent male presents with concern about a rash that appeared suddenly after showering. Physical exam reveals wheals that are scattered across his trunk, arms, and legs. What question asked by the advanced practice nurse is likely to be MOST important for determining the cause of this rash?

**A.** Have you recently been hiking in the woods or working outside in the yard?
**B.** Did you use any type of new product, shampoo, or soap, in the shower?
**C.** Are you feeling ill, nauseated, fatigued, or feverish?
**D.** Has anyone in your family traveled outside of the country?

**74.** A 50-year-old has concerns about whether several scattered lesions could be melanoma. Which presentation is MOST concerning for the possibility of skin cancer?

**A.** Diameter of each is less than 5 mm
**B.** Lesions are palpable, smooth
**C.** Several are irregular in shape and color
**D.** Small scattered brown nevi are macular

**75.** A 60-year-old female with a history of obesity and tobacco use has concerns about the yellow discoloration of her toenails, which are thickened and brittle. She explains that sometimes it seems that there are "white crumbs" under the nails. The advanced practice nurse knows the likely diagnosis is:

**A.** Actinic keratosis
**B.** Onychomycosis
**C.** Psoriasis
**D.** Tinea corporis

**76.** The most common form of skin cancer is:

**A.** Basal cell carcinoma
**B.** Cutaneous T-cell lymphoma
**C.** Malignant melanoma
**D.** Squamous cell carcinoma

**77.** A 71-year-old female presents with burning pain on the left side of her back that began 2 days ago. Her physical exam reveals a vesicular rash with a band-like presentation. The advanced practice nurse is aware that effective management is required urgently to prevent:

**A.** Cellulitis
**B.** Opioid dependence
**C.** Post-herpetic neuralgia
**D.** Varicella

**78.** A 40-year-old female has used high-potency topical corticosteroids for 6 months to treat intertrigo in her axillary region, unaware of potential side effects. Which assessment would the advanced practice nurse likely find as a consequence of prolonged use of the corticosteroid?

**A.** Discoloration of the skin, or vitiligo
**B.** Scarring or epidermal scars
**C.** Thickening of the skin or lichenification
**D.** Thinning of the skin or cutaneous atrophy

**79.** Which positive immunoglobulin (Ig) serological test indicates an acute hepatitis?

**A.** IgA
**B.** IgE
**C.** IgG
**D.** IgM

**80.** MATCH the description of the location to the name of the lymph nodes located in the area:

| | |
|---|---|
| **A.** Just above the clavicle | **1.** Anterior cervical |
| **B.** At the base of the skull | **2.** Submandibular |
| **C.** In front of the tragus | **3.** Supraclavicular |
| **D.** Below the jaw line | **4.** Occipital |
| **E.** In front of the sternocleidomastoid muscle | **5.** Preauricular |

**81.** A 15-year-old who presented 5 days ago with rhinosinusitis returned today because of worsening symptoms. The teen has a fever of 102°F and complains of a stiff neck, mild confusion, and headache. Which of the following statements is MOST accurate?

**A.** The patient was misdiagnosed when seen 5 days ago, and likely has influenza
**B.** The patient was incorrectly managed 5 days ago, and needs treatment for pneumonia
**C.** This is not unexpected; rhinosinusitis usually takes more than 10 days to resolve
**D.** This is concerning; the adolescent should be evaluated for meningeal irritation

**82.** Which assessment is NOT indicative of strep pharyngitis?

**A.** Tonsillar exudate
**B.** Fever
**C.** Cough
**D.** Lymphadenopathy

**83.** Which diagnosis is most consistent with an individual's history of "sinus infection symptoms" that persisted for 2 months before resolving?

**A.** Acute sinusitis
**B.** Subacute sinusitis
**C.** Recurrent sinusitis
**D.** Chronic sinusitis

**84.** Which of the following is essential to the diagnosis of chronic obstructive pulmonary disease (COPD)?

**A.** Chest x-ray that shows a flattened diaphragm
**B.** Chest x-ray that shows hyperinflation
**C.** Pulmonary function study results show FEV1/FVC ratio of <70%
**D.** Pulmonary function study results show FVC of <30%

**85.** A child has suspected scarlet fever. He likely has a sandpaper rash and:

**A.** Coryza
**B.** Cough
**C.** Conjunctivitis
**D.** Strep pharyngitis

**86.** An advanced practice nurse notes the bluish-green areas of skin discoloration over the sacral area and buttocks of an infant as pictured in the image. The infant's mother is an adolescent from Taiwan who thinks that the child has always had this but is unsure. Which diagnosis is MOST LIKELY?

**A.** Acrocyanosis
**B.** Ecchymosis
**C.** Congenital melanocytosis
**D.** Purpura

**87.** A 60-year-old female presents with what she considers to be "adult acne," but wonders if this might be something other than acne, as the redness flares with stress, exercise, spicy foods, and alcohol. Based on the findings and image, which diagnosis is MOST LIKELY?

**A.** Cystic acne
**B.** Cellulitis
**C.** Rosacea
**D.** Senile keratosis

**88.** A 40-year-old who "never gets headaches" presents to the office after having had a severe and debilitating headache associated with intense vomiting, blurry vision, and pain described as the "worst headache of my life." The headache had a sudden onset and lasted about 5 minutes. Which term BEST describes this headache?

**A.** Migraine with aura
**B.** Rebound headache
**C.** Tension-type
**D.** Thunderclap

**89.** Which migraine symptom is MOST commonly experienced by adults and adolescents?

**A.** Aura
**B.** Unilateral pain
**C.** Dizziness
**D.** Photophobia

**90.** Which is an expected finding with assessment of lymph nodes?

**A.** Cluster of matted lymph nodes
**B.** Small, mobile, soft anterior cervical nodes
**C.** Small, fixed, non-tender supraclavicular nodes
**D.** Unilateral lymphadenopathy

**91.** A patient arrives at the Emergency Department after they fell on their stairs at home. While interviewing the patient, the advanced practice nurse notices that the individual seems to have a hard time understanding directions and responding to questions appropriately. The clinician correctly suspects that the patient may have experienced trauma to which lobe or area of their brain?

**A.** Temporal
**B.** Parietal
**C.** Frontal
**D.** Occipital

**92.** Which type of malignancy begins in the plasma cells of the immune system, leading to damage to the bone marrow?

**A.** Carcinoma
**B.** Sarcoma
**C.** Leukemia
**D.** Multiple myeloma

**93.** As a component of assessing wellness, clinicians should ask individuals who are immunocompromised about:

**A.** Daily use of industrial-strength, antibacterial cleansers
**B.** Handwashing, food safety, and travel precautions
**C.** Their ability to abstain from sexual intimacy and intercourse
**D.** Their ability to remain isolated from children and older adults

**94.** When assessing the abdomen of an 18-year-old college student who has been experiencing fatigue, the advanced practice nurse notes the presence of dullness to percussion and tenderness to light palpation in the left upper quadrant just below the costal margin. Which anatomic structure is MOST LIKELY to be the cause of this tenderness?

**A.** Kidney
**B.** Liver
**C.** Spleen
**D.** Thymus

**95.** Both pleural effusion and lobar pneumonia are characterized by which assessments?

**A.** Dullness to percussion and decreased breath sounds to auscultation
**B.** Hyperresonance to percussion and crackles to auscultation
**C.** Resonance to percussion and wheezes to auscultation
**D.** Tympany to percussion and decreased tactile fremitus

**96.** Which sexually transmitted infection can be detected using nucleic acid amplification testing (NAAT) of urine?

**A.** Human immunodeficiency virus
**B.** Hepatitis B virus
**C.** Herpes simplex type 2
**D.** Chlamydia trachomatis

**97.** Soft, low-pitched breath sounds normally heard over most lung fields are BEST described as:

**A.** Vesicular
**B.** Bronchovesicular
**C.** Bronchial
**D.** Tracheal

**98.** A 75-year-old male, non smoker, previously diagnosed with congestive heart failure, is currently experiencing increasing dyspnea and cough. If his symptoms are related to exacerbation of his heart failure, which adventitious breath sounds are likely to be heard with his physical exam?

**A.** Discontinuous crackles on inspiration that do not clear with coughing
**B.** Scattered inspiratory and expiratory wheezes in the bases of the lungs
**C.** Upper airway inspiratory stridor audible without a stethoscope
**D.** Unilateral, continuous, sonorous, or rumbling breath sounds

**99.** Which statement is true regarding spirometry?

**A.** Airflow measurements with spirometry indicate whether a disease is viral or bacterial
**B.** Spirometry measures the ability of a person to inhale and exhale air respective to time
**C.** Spirometry is most useful post-surgery as a means of preventing atelectasis and pneumonia
**D.** The test is done by individuals with asthma at home to determine airway obstruction

**100.** Which differential diagnosis is associated with INCREASED tactile fremitus?

**A.** Asthma
**B.** Chronic bronchitis
**C.** Pneumonia
**D.** Pneumothorax

**101.** Which history is MOST consistent with the diagnosis of acute bronchitis?

**A.** Child who has wheezing associated with a respiratory infection every autumn
**B.** Young adult with 3 days of cough, chest discomfort, sore throat, and malaise
**C.** Adult who recently quit smoking but continues to have a persistent morning cough
**D.** Older adult with cough, increased respiratory rate, fatigue, and fever for 2 days

**102.** Where is the middle lobe of the right lung BEST auscultated?

**A.** Anterior chest
**B.** Supraclavicular area
**C.** Midaxillary area
**D.** Posterior chest

**103.** The chest x-ray of an 85-year-old shows a significant pleural effusion. Which symptom is MOST LIKELY associated with this finding?

**A.** Bradycardia
**B.** Bradypnea
**C.** Dyspnea
**D.** High fever

**104.** Which individual has the highest risk for severe pertussis?

**A.** A 6-month-old who is healthy and unvaccinated
**B.** An 18-month-old in daycare who has received all recommended vaccines
**C.** A college student who lives in a dorm and is up to date on vaccines
**D.** An unvaccinated individual who is in the third trimester of pregnancy

**105.** Which of the following is a symptom of undiagnosed obstructive sleep apnea?

**A.** Exercise intolerance
**B.** Unable to arouse easily from sleep
**C.** Unexplained daytime sleepiness
**D.** Weight loss

**106.** The overall goal of the preparticipation physical evaluation is:

**A.** Identifying athletes who have mental health or substance use disorders
**B.** Excluding athletes from sports participation when there are risks
**C.** Maintaining the health of athletes, including their safe participation in sports
**D.** Preventing morbidity and mortality associated with sports participation

**107.** A 14-year-old female presents for a pre-participation physical. Her physical exam reveals unequal shoulder height. Forward flexion at the waist reveals asymmetrical scapulae and a unilateral rib hump. The advanced practice nurse correctly suspects:

**A.** Kyphosis
**B.** Lordosis
**C.** Scoliosis
**D.** Spondylolysis

**108.** A 2-year-old female presents with decreased use of the left arm; her mother believes this started when an older sibling pulled her up onto a chair. The child's physical exam reveals guarding of the extremity with a slightly flexed, pronated arm and focal tenderness. Which statement by the advanced practice nurse is MOST accurate?

**A.** To heal this injury, your daughter is likely to need a cast
**B.** This injury is very common in young children
**C.** Your daughter may have an underlying serious illness
**D.** Your older child may have inadvertently caused this wrist sprain

**109.** A 70-year-old male presents with low back pain. Which of his assessments are "red flags" indicating the need for immediate evaluation and treatment?

**A.** New onset of urinary incontinence
**B.** Pain with straight leg raising at 90 degrees
**C.** Previous history of paraspinal muscle spasm
**D.** Weakness with dorsiflexion of the great toe

**110.** Which blood pressure reading meets the American Heart Association/American College of Cardiology (AHA/ACC) guidelines for Stage 1 hypertension?

**A.** 128/78 mm/Hg
**B.** 128/88 mm/Hg
**C.** 132/92 mm/Hg
**D.** 142/88 mm/Hg

**111.** Which assessment is consistent with a Grade 2 ankle sprain?

**A.** Minimal swelling, significant tenderness
**B.** Significant swelling, minimal tenderness
**C.** Moderate pain and swelling, decreased range of motion
**D.** Severely impaired function, unable to bear weight or ambulate

**112.** Risk factors for osteoporosis include female gender, age, certain medications, smoking, and:

**A.** Elevated vitamin D levels
**B.** Elevated calcium levels
**C.** Lack of weight-bearing exercise
**D.** Strenuous exercise

**113.** Physical manifestations of Marfan syndrome include myopia, mitral valve prolapse, pectus deformities, scoliosis, and

**A.** Exaggerated kyphosis
**B.** Increased limb length
**C.** Joint stiffness
**D.** Webbed neck deformities

**114.** Pain at the bony prominence where the patellar tendon attaches to the tibia indicates:

**A.** Genu varum
**B.** Metatarsus adductus
**C.** Osgood-Schlatter disease
**D.** Tibial torsion

**115.** Which condition is MOST LIKELY to cause significant hearing loss, ear pain, vertigo, and mastoiditis?

**A.** Cholesteatoma
**B.** External otitis
**C.** Cerumen impaction
**D.** Otitis media with effusion

**116.** A pterygium is more common in people exposed to:

**A.** Contact lenses and contact lens solutions
**B.** Elevated blood glucose and lipid levels
**C.** Secondhand cigarette smoke
**D.** Ultraviolet light, dust, and wind

**117.** Identify the auscultatory sites labeled in the diagram by matching the colored dot with the name of the site:

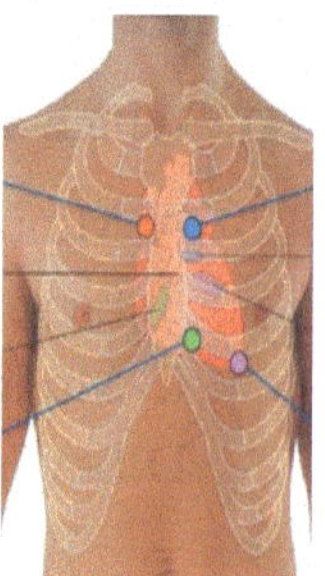

| | |
|---|---|
| **A.** Red dot | **1.** Tricuspid |
| **B.** Blue dot | **2.** Mitral |
| **C.** Green dot | **3.** Aortic |
| **D.** Purple dot | **4.** Pulmonic |

**118.** A patient presents with eye pain, severe headache, seeing halos around lights, and nausea/vomiting. Which emergent condition is of primary concern?

**A.** Open angle glaucoma
**B.** Subconjunctival hemorrhage
**C.** Macular degeneration
**D.** Narrow angle glaucoma

**119.** An asymmetric corneal light reflex is indicative of:

**A.** Nystagmus
**B.** Strabismus
**C.** Cataracts
**D.** Exophthalmia

**120.** Within a normal physical exam, the point of maximal impulse (PMI) is BEST palpated at the:

**A.** Right sternal border, 2nd intercostal space
**B.** Left sternal border, 2nd intercostal space
**C.** Left sternal border, 4th intercostal space
**D.** Left midclavicular line, 5th intercostal space

**121.** Absence of the red reflex in a newborn:

**A.** Can indicate a serious diagnosis like retinoblastoma or cataracts
**B.** Indicates inexperience of the examiner
**C.** Is not significant as the reflex is not present until 4 to 6 months of age
**D.** Indicates that the infant should be reexamined at the 2 month well baby check

**122.** An 18-year-old presents with a chief concern of earache. Physical exam reveals the left tympanic membrane to be erythematous and bulging; bony landmarks of the ear are not able to be visualized. There is no tenderness to palpation of the pinna or tragus, and no ear drainage. The adolescent states that the pain started abruptly and is interfering with sleep. Which diagnosis is most appropriate?

**A.** Acute otitis media
**B.** Otitis externa
**C.** Otitis media with effusion
**D.** Eustachian tube dysfunction

**123.** Peripheral pulses are graded on a 3-point scale according to the strength or force of the pulse. Documentation of a normal pulse would be:

**A.** 0
**B.** 1+
**C.** 2+
**D.** 3+

**124.** When assessing pupil response and eye movement in response to light and shifting vision, which assessment is an expectation of a normal exam?

**A.** Convergence of the eyes when shifting focus to objects that are near
**B.** Constriction of the pupil when shifting focus to objects that are far
**C.** Dilation of the pupil when shifting focus to objects that are near
**D.** Divergence of the eyes when shifting focus to objects that are near

**125.** A young adult presents with a small, erythematous, swollen, tender lump near the edge of their lower eyelid. Which differential diagnosis should be the FIRST consideration?

**A.** Blepharitis
**B.** Chalazion
**C.** Hordeolum
**D.** Xanthelasma

**126.** How are accurate blood pressure readings obtained? (Select all that apply.)

**A.** Obtain the blood pressure reading while the person is seated
**B.** Rest the individual's arm at the level of their heart
**C.** Place an electronic BP cuff on their arm over a thin layer of clothing
**D.** Have the individual uncross their legs and place feet flat on the floor
**E.** Talk with the person while taking the reading to keep them comfortable

**127.** A 70-year-old female who has a history of diabetes and hypertension presents to the office with sore throat, rhinorrhea, and congestion for 3 days. She has no known exposures, and is up to date with immunizations, including influenza, pneumonia, and COVID-19 vaccines. Which diagnosis is MOST LIKELY?

**A.** Acute bronchitis
**B.** Upper respiratory infection
**C.** Acute bacterial rhinosinusitis
**D.** Early-stage heart failure

**128.** The advanced practice nurse is concerned that a 19-year-old may have a peritonsillar abscess, as the teen is having fever, malaise, otalgia, and a muffled voice. The patient presents to the urgent care unable to open their mouth, a finding known as:

**A.** Trismus
**B.** Torticollis
**C.** Tetanus
**D.** Dysphagia

**129.** Which statement is true regarding the characteristics of inguinal hernias in older adults?

**A.** Inguinal hernias are painful, persistent, and require urgent surgical consultation
**B.** These hernias are always asymptomatic in older adults, and rarely require repair
**C.** Most inguinal hernias cause a dull ache and fullness that worsens with straining
**D.** Incarcerated inguinal hernias can be reduced manually through the fascial defect

**130.** Abnormal findings with a prostate exam include asymmetry; the posterior lobe is palpated as hard and nodular. The nodularity is painless with palpation; the sulcus is not palpable. These assessment findings are MOST consistent with:

**A.** Acute prostatitis
**B.** Benign prostatic hypertrophy
**C.** Chronic bacterial prostatitis
**D.** Malignancy or carcinoma

**131.** Expected physical findings during pregnancy include all of the following, EXCEPT:

**A.** Hyperpigmentation of the skin on the face
**B.** Diffuse redness of the palms of the hands
**C.** Dark pigmented line at the midline of the abdomen
**D.** Hypopigmentation of the nipples and areolae

**132.** A pregnant woman confides that her father had hemophilia, and she is worried about her child inheriting the disease. Knowing that hemophilia is an X-linked recessive disorder, the advanced practice nurse responds accurately by saying:

**A.** If your child is a boy, he is not at risk for having hemophilia
**B.** If your child is a boy, there is a 50% risk that he will have hemophilia
**C.** Whether your child is a boy or a girl, your baby will inherit hemophilia
**D.** You cannot transmit hemophilia to your baby if you do not have it yourself

**133.** Which statement is true regarding urinary tract infections (UTIs) in women during pregnancy?

**A.** UTI symptoms during pregnancy are the same as they would be if not pregnant
**B.** Physical assessment is only required if the individual is symptomatic
**C.** Pyelonephritis can result if UTIs are not diagnosed and adequately treated
**D.** No physical exam or lab testing is required to diagnose UTI during pregnancy

**134.** The leading causes of death in the United States for all ages are:

**A.** Unintended injuries or accidents
**B.** Heart disease and cancer
**C.** Kidney disease and viral illnesses
**D.** Acute and chronic respiratory diseases

**135.** Which statement is true regarding populations experiencing health disparities?

**A.** Access to care has little impact on the prevalence of health disparities
**B.** Historical experiences of bias have little impact on current health status
**C.** Individuals who have experienced trauma have greater health risks
**D.** Individuals who have survived violence develop higher levels of coping

**136.** Which statement regarding cancer health disparities is accurate?

**A.** Black men have the highest incidence and mortality rates of prostate cancer
**B.** Hispanic women are more likely to die from colorectal cancer than any other cancer
**C.** Caucasian men are more likely to die from colorectal cancer than any other cancer
**D.** Lung cancer has the lowest associated mortality rates of all cancers regardless of ethnicity

**137.** Which statement regarding wellness is accurate?

**A.** No medications have proven significantly effective for smoking cessation
**B.** Sitting more than 8 hours daily is associated with obesity, hypertension, and diabetes
**C.** Spending 1 hour in the gym each week will offset health risks related to poor diet
**D.** To have any impact on health, an overweight individual must lose more than 25kg

**138.** Which question or statement made by the advanced practice nurse is LEAST consistent with effective communication?

**A.** Do you mind if we spend a few minutes talking about your smoking?
**B.** How would your life be different if you were not a smoker?
**C.** What I hear you say is that you tried to quit smoking and have failed in the past.
**D.** Why do you continue to smoke knowing that your health will deteriorate?

**139.** Best practice for the advance practice nurse who is assessing an individual using telehealth technologies includes:

**A.** Being attentive to verbal and non-verbal communication
**B.** Knowing that telehealth is not reimbursed by any insurers
**C.** Recognizing that virtual care cannot be confidential
**D.** Telling individuals that their assessment will be very limited

**140.** A 70-year-old female with chronic hypertension presents to primary care for follow up. Auscultation of her heart sounds reveals a harsh, crescendo-decrescendo murmur during systole, at the right sternal border, second intercostal space. The murmur is heard best when she is seated and leaning forward. Which diagnosis is MOST LIKELY?

**A.** Aortic stenosis
**B.** Aortic regurgitation
**C.** Mitral stenosis
**D.** Mitral regurgitation

**141.** Which condition allows the backflow of blood into the heart, which causes a medium/high-pitched, harsh murmur that can be heard continuously between S1 and S2, and is auscultated best at the apex of the heart?

**A.** Aortic stenosis
**B.** Mitral stenosis
**C.** Aortic regurgitation
**D.** Mitral regurgitation

**142.** Which assessment MOST LIKELY indicates mitral stenosis?

**A.** Rumbling diastolic murmur heard best at the apex using the bell of the stethoscope
**B.** Harsh mid-systolic murmur heard best at the right second and third intercostal spaces
**C.** High-pitched blowing diastolic murmur best heard at the left second to fourth intercostal spaces
**D.** Harsh medium/high pitched holosystolic murmur heard best at the apex

**143.** When assessing a patient's lower extremities for pitting edema, the advanced practice nurse documents "deep pitting edema; lower legs and ankles are noticeably swollen." This assessment can also be documented as pitting edema that is:

**A.** 1+
**B.** 2+
**C.** 3+
**D.** 4+

**144.** Which assessment would NOT be indicated during a thorough cardiovascular and peripheral vascular physical exam?

**A.** Assess the radial pulse in conjunction with auscultation of the apical pulse
**B.** Auscultate the apical pulse while gently palpating the carotid artery
**C.** Palpate the left and right carotid arteries simultaneously at the carotid sinus
**D.** Palpate over the heart region to determine any thrills, lifts, or heaves

**145.** Which heart sound, described as a "ventricular gallop," occurs as a result of early ventricular filling associated with decreased compliance of the left ventricle and volume overload?

**A.** S1
**B.** S2
**C.** S3
**D.** S4

**146.** In which individual would auscultation of an S3 heart sound be MOST concerning?

**A.** A 25-year-old in the third trimester of pregnancy
**B.** A 65-year-old who recently quit smoking
**C.** A 5-year-old who was just playing tag
**D.** A 15-year-old athlete who presents for sports physical

**147.** A peripheral vascular exam includes the inspection of the hands for specific signs of abnormalities. MATCH the abnormality with its description.

| | |
|---|---|
| **A.** Clubbing | **1.** Painful, erythematous, raised lesions |
| **B.** Janeway lesions | **2.** Dark-red, linear lesions in the nailbeds |
| **C.** Osler's nodes | **3.** Reddening at the thenar and hypothenar eminences |
| **D.** Splinter hemorrhages | **4.** Deformity that changes angle of nailbed |
| **E.** Palmar erythema | **5.** Nontender maculae on the palms and soles |

**148.** Low calcium levels can result in ECG changes that include:

**A.** ST segment elevation
**B.** ST segment depression
**C.** Prolonged QT interval
**D.** Prominent Q waves

**149.** Which finding BEST supports a diagnosis of pectus excavatum?

**A.** Sternal depression causing abnormal contour of the chest wall
**B.** Increased anteroposterior diameter of the chest
**C.** Sternal protrusion deformity of the anterior chest wall
**D.** Paradoxical movement of the chest wall during respiration

**150.** An individual presents with productive cough, fatigue, and weight loss. Which additional subjective findings increase the likelihood that the person has pulmonary tuberculosis?

**A.** Increased thirst and hunger, despite weight loss
**B.** Homeless, currently staying in local shelter
**C.** Spouse has noticed that breath seems "fruity"
**D.** Symptoms began acutely less than 1 week ago

# Practice Test I: Answers and Rationales

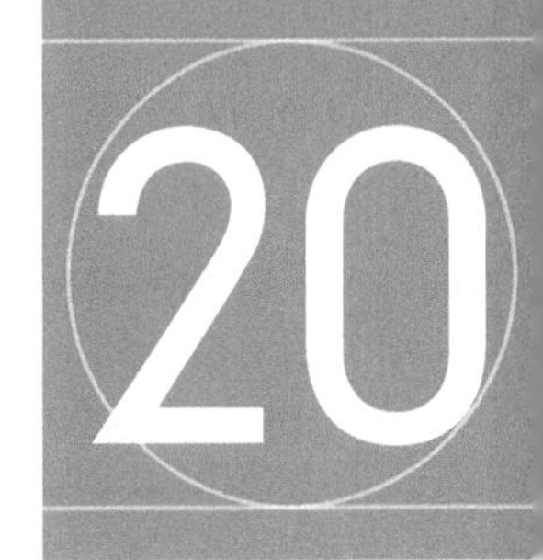


**1. B) Body mass divided by the square of their height**

Body mass index (BMI) is an expression of the relationship between weight and height and is calculated by body mass (kg) divided by the square of the body height. Health status, wellness behaviors, and risks of chronic disease are not measured directly or solely by BMI. Relying on BMI alone would misclassify millions of individuals as either metabolically healthy or unhealthy. Assessment of well-being and health status should include a review of every patient's diet, physical activity, family history, and cardiometabolic health irrespective of BMI.

**2. A) The test correctly identifies 80% of individuals who do not have the disease (true negatives)**

The specificity of a test refers to the likelihood that the test will correctly identify those without the condition for which the screening was designed. A highly specific test is one in which there are few false-positive results. A screening test that is 80% specific will correctly identify 80% of those who do not have the disease, i.e., true negatives. This also signifies that 20% of individuals without the disease are incorrectly identified as positive by the screening tests (false positives). Sensitivity refers to true positives and is a measure of how likely the test will correctly identify individuals who have the condition for which the tool or test was designed.

**3. A) Asking about suicidal thoughts or plan is not associated with higher likelihood of suicide**

Asking about suicidal ideation does not increase the likelihood or risk of suicide; determining the presence of suicidal ideation is significantly associated with referral for mental health support. Studies have shown that individuals are more likely to present in primary care when they are having increasing thoughts of suicide and are likely to be responsive to clinician concerns. Societal, family, and cultural factors have an impact on how individuals view mental health concerns; assessment of suicidal ideation should include assessment of the individual's perspective and support system.

**4. C) Introduce themselves**

As the care provider, the advanced practice nurse needs to establish a working rapport with the patient. He does not appear to be in acute distress, so the next step would be an introduction and then clarification of his reason for seeking care. Prior to completing the physical exam, assessing history of present illness, past medical history, family and social history, and reviewing systems would occur after clarification of chief concern, as long as the patient remains stable. If needed for the individual in this scenario, a request for collaboration could occur after the history and physical exam are completed.

**5. A) Health history including past medical history**

All wellness exams should include medication reconciliation, especially for individuals who have comorbid conditions. While completing the medication history may lead to identification of anticipatory guidance needs, assessing the use of prescribed and over-the-counter medications is considered part of the health history. Assessing medication use is not a component of the review of systems, and is not a primary prevention measure, as primary prevention measures aim to prevent disease from occurring.

**6. C) Evidence-based strategies can help individuals to self-identify protective factors and improve their safety**

The evidence-based *Stanley and Brown Patient Safety Plan* asks individuals to self-identify warning signs of suicidal ideation (SI), strategize internal coping methods, plan distractions from SI, identify support systems including family, professionals, and agencies to contact, and consider environmental changes to be made, such as removal of guns, knives, and medications; these steps increase safety and decrease risks of suicide.

All individuals, including those with mild depression or anxiety, should be screened for suicidal ideation. Those at increased risk for suicide include individuals with previous suicide attempts, family history of suicide, and/or childhood abuse, trauma, or neglect. Suicide attempt rates are more likely for individuals recently discharged from psychiatric hospitalization, especially during the immediate post-discharge time frame. Experiences of isolation, prolonged stress, access to lethal means, and the presence of mental and/or physical health conditions are risk factors.

**7. C) Secondary**

There are three levels of prevention. Secondary prevention aims to reduce the impact of disease by detecting it as early as possible; screenings are intended to improve early detection. Primary prevention aims to prevent disease from occurring; vaccines are a key example of primary prevention. Tertiary preventive measures are those aimed at decreasing the impact of illness or injury; examples include vocational and cardiac rehabilitation programs.

**8. A and B) Feeling nervous, anxious, or on edge; not being able to stop or control worrying**

The evidence-based GAD-2 screening is used to assess for anxiety symptoms. The GAD-2 is comprised of the first two questions of the GAD-7 screening, and are: Over the last 2 weeks, how often have you been bothered by the following problems? (1) Feeling nervous, anxious, or on edge and (2) not being able to stop or control worrying. In answering these two questions, the patient chooses: not at all, several days, more than half the days, or nearly every day. Asking about using alcohol is part if the CRAFT-II for adolescents in order to assess for substance use disorder. The symptoms of helplessness and hopelessness are priority questions when screening for depression.

**9. C) Limps and grimaces with ambulation**

Objective information is that which can be seen, observed, or measured by the advanced practice nurse. For example, limping and grimacing can be objectively assessed. Subjective information is data gathered from the patient. Pain, history of injury, vertigo, and the context of the patient's health history are all examples of subjective data.

**10. A) Is unable to maintain an upright stance with eyes closed**

The Romberg test assesses postural control that relies on vestibular input and proprioception when visual input is canceled. Minimal swaying is a normal finding; failure to maintain an upright stance is a positive test that indicates possible vestibular, proprioceptive, or cerebellar deficits. Nystagmus and/or nausea with position changes are assessed using the Dix-Hallpike maneuver, and are associated with benign paroxysmal positional vertigo (BPPV).

**11. D) 4+**

Clonus, repetitive involuntary muscle contractions noted with assessment of deep tendon reflexes (DTRs), are graded and documented as 4+. DTRs are scored on a 0 to 4+ scale:

- 0 No response (always abnormal)
- 1+ Sluggish or diminished response
- 2+ Active or expected response (normal)
- 3+ Brisk, slightly hyperactive
- 4+ Hyperactive, clonus (always abnormal)

**12. D) Older adults with neuropathy**

Vibratory perception declines with age and is diminished in peripheral neuropathy, diabetic neuropathy, central nervous system lesions, and spinal cord disease. Individuals with other sensory deficits (e.g., blindness, deafness) may have heightened vibratory sensation. While there are significant neurologic changes associated with adolescence, depression, pregnancy, and postpartum, these changes do not include diminished vibratory sense.

**13. B) Bell's palsy**

Bell's palsy affects the facial nerve, presents gradually, and causes peripheral facial weakness; clinical features include weakness in raising the eyebrow or furrowing the brow, difficulty or inability to close the eye, asymmetric weakness in grimacing or smiling, and flattening of the nasolabial fold. While neurologic deficits can occur with "silent" migraines, or migraines without headache pain, the presentation of significant facial weakness is not common or typical. Symptoms of ischemic stroke present abruptly over minutes or hours; resultant neurologic deficits typically affect multiple cranial nerves in addition to either motor or sensory tracts of the spinal cord. Key symptoms of stroke include weakness in an arm or leg, slurred speech, double vision, facial numbness, difficulty swallowing, incoordination, and vertigo. An allergic reaction is characterized by rash/hives, wheezing, and inflammation.

**14. B) Inattention**

The diagnosis of ADHD involves assessment for a constellation of symptoms and is understood as a spectrum of neurologic, developmental, cognitive, and genetic disorders. Individuals with ADHD show a persistent pattern of inattention and/or hyperactivity-impulsivity that interferes with function or development. While individuals may experience school failures, have difficulty with social skills, and/or exhibit compulsive behavior, these are not universal and are not required for diagnosis.

**15. A) At 20 feet what a person with normal vision can see clearly from 50 feet**

Testing visual acuity with a Snellen chart involves requiring the person to stand at a distance of 20 feet and noting the line on the chart with the smallest characters/letters that the individual can clearly see. The acuity associated with each line of the chart indicates their acuity compared to those who have normal vision. For example, an acuity of 20/50 indicates that the patient can clearly see at 20 feet what an individual with normal vision can see clearly at 50 feet. If the patient is unable to read any of the lines on the chart, an estimate of what they are capable of seeing should be assessed (e.g., ability to count fingers, detect motion, or perceive light).

**16. C) Distal muscle weakness and loss of coordination are common signs**

Peripheral neuropathy is a common complication of diabetes that usually presents first in the toes and feet. Muscle weakness, numbness, and loss of coordination are common signs. Muscle cramping and spasticity are not commonly associated with diabetes; individuals with multiple sclerosis are more likely to present with cramping, spasticity, and fatigue in addition to numbness and weakness of their extremities.

**17. D) Hearing screening**

Some of the most common complications of meningococcal disease are hearing deficits which can be partial or total. Other serious complications include cortical blindness, seizure disorders, and cranial nerve dysfunction. Older children should be assessed for hearing loss, gait problems, and memory or learning difficulties. With acute bacterial meningitis, the most serious complications are neurologic and are less likely to have respiratory, gastrointestinal, or cardiac system sequelae.

**18. A) Lumbosacral strain**

Lumbosacral strain is a stretching injury to the ligaments, tendons, or muscles of the lower back; this type of injury is common, especially within specific occupations that place high demand on the musculoskeletal system. Nerve root compression causes symptoms of radiculopathy or sciatica characterized by sharp, shooting, and/or searing pain and numbness or weakness in the leg and/or foot. A compression fracture is more likely to occur after trauma when an individual has underlying osteoporosis, which is more common in older adults. Disc herniation can lead to lumbar nerve root compression and radiculopathies and is also not as likely in the young adult age group.

**19. B) Medial collateral ligament (MCL)**

A valgus stress test helps to identify injury to the medial collateral ligament; pain or excessive laxity is considered a positive test. The varus stress test is used to assess for integrity of the LCL and is completed by applying outward or lateral pressure at the thigh and inward or medial pressure from the lateral ankle. Anterior drawer and Lachman's tests can be used to assess the integrity of the ACL and a posterior drawer test is used to assess the PCL.

**20. A) Lateral epicondylitis, B) Supraspinatus tendonitis, C) de Quervain's tenosynovitis, D) Medial epicondylitis, E) Carpal tunnel syndrome**

Special tests of the upper extremities include:

- Cozen's test to identify lateral epicondylitis, also known as "tennis elbow"
- Empty can test to identify supraspinatus weakness from a rotator cuff tear, impingement, or nerve injury
- Finkelstein test to identify tenosynovitis of the abductor pollicus longus and extensor pollicus brevis tendons, also known as de Quervain's syndrome
- Reverse Mill's test to identify medial epicondylitis, or golfer's elbow
- Tinel's test to identify compression of the ulnar nerve which causes carpal tunnel syndrome

**21. C) A 50-year-old male who drinks two to six beers daily**

Gout is typically related to an excessive amount of uric acid production; the uric acid crystalizes and deposits in synovial fluid, causing exquisitely painful joints. Gout is commonly seen in middle-aged men who have a genetic predisposition; alcohol use and diets high in purines can trigger flare-ups. Purine-rich foods include beer, red meat, pork, organ meats, and seafood, especially shrimp, lobster, anchovies, and sardines. The joint pain associated with ulcerative colitis and rheumatoid arthritis are associated with inflammation, not uric acid crystal deposits; plant-based diets are lower in purines and help to lower the recurrence of gout.

**22. C) The adolescent may be experiencing mania associated with mood disorder**

Individuals with bipolar disorder will have unusual shifts in mood, energy, and activity levels. They may have a pattern of depressive episodes mixed with hypomanic or manic episodes. Mania and hypomania symptoms include racing thoughts, irritability, aggressive or angry outbursts, insomnia, and/or excessive involvement in reckless activities. In individuals with bipolar disorder, SSRIs and other antidepressants carry a risk of inducing mania. Before increasing the medication dose or switching medications, consideration of undiagnosed bipolar disorder is warranted. False assumptions that teens cannot develop bipolar disorder or that substance use underlies the diagnosis could cause delayed treatment and poorer outcomes.

**23. C) Depression**

Symptoms of depression include persistent sadness, depressed mood, sleep disturbances (insomnia or hypersomnia), fatigue, loss of interest in most or all normal activities, feelings of worthlessness or guilt, slowed thinking or trouble concentrating, change in appetite, and thoughts of suicide. Anorexia is the abnormal loss of appetite or loss of interest in food that can occur with depression. Individuals with anorexia nervosa present first with food aversion and disordered eating; the chronic condition leads to loss of appetite. Concussion symptoms can include fatigue, loss of appetite, and sleep disturbances, but are not likely to include feelings of hopelessness and helplessness. Psychosis is defined by impaired thoughts and perceptions; symptoms include delusions and hallucinations.

**24. B) Physical violence perpetrated by intimate partners is often associated with controlling behaviors**

Physical violence of intimate partners is often accompanied by emotionally abusive and controlling behavior. Pregnancy is associated with increased risk of intimate partner violence (IPV). Due to underreporting and lack of recognition, IPV may occur more commonly among pregnant individuals than conditions for which they are currently being screened, including gestational diabetes and preeclampsia. Rates of IPV, abuse, and neglect are higher in families with young children. Screening is effective in increasing the safety of those experiencing trauma and violence.

**25. A) Characterized by reoccurring, intense, distressing dreams**

Posttraumatic stress disorder (PTSD) is a mental health disorder that may occur in individuals who have experienced or witnessed a traumatic event, including natural disasters, serious accidents, terrorist attacks, war, violent acts, or life-threatening illnesses. Studies indicate that more than half of adults have been or will be exposed to at least one incident of trauma in their lifetime. Those who develop PTSD in response experience symptoms including:

- Intrusive thoughts; reoccurring, intense, distressing dreams, or flashbacks
- Detachment; avoidance of people, places, and situations that may trigger distress
- Alterations in cognition, including distorted thoughts, shame, fear, anger, and guilt
- Alterations in arousal and reactivity, including problems concentrating and sleeping

**26. B) Lack of physical activity**

There are many biological and physiological factors that are associated with an increased risk for substance use disorder (SUD) including adverse childhood events and untreated mental illness. Although lack of physical activity can impact mood and overall health, it is not considered a risk factor for SUD.

**27. A) Adults who have had one or more motor vehicle crashes, regardless of cause**

The USPSTF recommends screening for unhealthy alcohol use in primary care settings in all adults 18 years or older, including pregnant women. While the task force recommends providing persons engaged in risky or hazardous drinking with brief behavioral counseling interventions to reduce unhealthy alcohol use, screening is not limited to those who have had motor vehicle crashes. Screening is not limited by gender, socioeconomic status, family history, or comorbid conditions.

**28. A) Tobacco**

Cigarette smoking is responsible for nearly half a million deaths per year in the United States and is the single greatest cause of preventable deaths globally. Excessive alcohol use is responsible for nearly 100,000 deaths in the United States per year, and in 2018, opioids accounted for >46,000 deaths. There is insufficient evidence to support or refute a statistical association between self-reported cannabis use and all-cause mortality.

### 29. C) Screen for substance use at this visit and assess her management of pain

An empathetic, evidence-based approach to the individual who has chronic pain, and a history of substance use disorder requires recognition that substance use disorder is a complex disease that is not a moral failing. Individuals with a history of substance use disorder can be treated for chronic pain without threats, shaming, or avoidant behavior. Awareness of comorbid conditions, and adequate assessments are key for clinicians involved in providing management for co-existing disorders.

### 30. C) Norepinephrine

A key effect that psychoactive substances cause is a dramatic increase in dopamine, which directly causes euphoria and indirectly creates desire to repeat the experience. The brain responds to repeated, massive dopamine surges by reducing the number of dopamine receptors and the amount of dopamine produced. This alleviates the overstimulation of the dopamine system, but also contributes to dependence, as the reduction in dopamine receptors can cause an individual to have difficulty in experiencing feelings of normal enjoyment during withdrawal from the substance and during long-term recovery. With depression disorders, an individual can have depletion of serotonin, norepinephrine, and dopamine. Serotonin is associated with mood, appetite, sleep, and anxiety. Norepinephrine is associated with an individual's energy, focus, and initiative; along with epinephrine, it is active in response to fear, anger, or threat. Dopamine is associated with pleasure, reward, motivation, and movement.

### 31. A) Freckles, B) Insect bites, C) Impetigo, D) Shingles, E) Lipomas, F) Psoriasis

Macules are flat (non-palpable) discrete lesions that are 1 cm in diameter or less.

- Papules are solid, raised (palpable) lesions less than 1 cm diameter.
- Pustules are circumscribed, elevated skin lesions containing purulent fluid, and are less than 1 cm in dimeter.
- Vesicles are circumscribed, elevated, fluid-containing lesions, less than 1 cm in diameter.
- Nodules are defined as raised, elevated, and firm lesions less than 2 cm in diameter. They are deeper in the dermis than papules.
- Plaques are elevated, solid, superficial lesions, typically more than 1 cm in diameter.

### 32. C) Furuncle

Furuncles are deep-seated skin infections of the pilosebaceous unit. Furuncles are boils or skin abscesses that affect the entire pilosebaceous unit; a group of furuncles can join to form a larger carbuncle. The infection and inflammation associated with folliculitis are in the hair follicle only. Cellulitis, an acute, scattered, and diffuse infection of the subcutaneous tissue is also not as deep as furuncles or carbuncles. Acrochordon (skin tags) are small, soft, benign, skin-colored papules with a narrow stalk that usually appear on the neck, chest, and underarms.

**33. A) II optic**

Testing the function of the optic nerve or cranial nerve II (CN II) includes assessing distant and near vison, performing an ophthalmoscopic exam of optic fundi, and testing visual fields by confrontation and extinction. The oculomotor (CN III), trochlear (CN IV), and abducens (CN VI) nerves are tested by assessing the movement of both eyes through the six cardinal points of gaze and by visualization of pupil size, shape, response to light, and accommodation.

**34. D) Stereognosis**

Discriminatory sensory function tests assess a person's ability to interpret sensation. These include:

- Stereognosis, which tests a person's ability to identify a familiar object by touch
- Graphesthesia, which tests a person's ability to identify symbols when traced on the skin
- Extinction phenomenon, which occurs when the sensation from two simultaneous stimulations are felt as only one sensation from an area of the body that is otherwise not numb on exam
- Point localization, which refers to the ability to locate a point on the skin that is stimulated

**35. D) Proteinuria can be benign and transient, or may indicate renal disease**

Increased levels of protein in the urine may indicate kidney damage associated with chronic illnesses, medications, or renal failure; however, proteinuria can also be benign and transient. Mild to moderate proteinuria during pregnancy may indicate preeclampsia. For individuals who present with proteinuria, further evaluation of symptoms, physical exam, and lab results would be indicated.

**36. D) Urinary frequency and pelvic pain**

Signs and symptoms of interstitial cystitis (IC) include pelvic pain, urgency to urinate, and frequent urination. IC is frequently misdiagnosed as urinary tract infection, however, it is not associated with acute, asymptomatic, or recurrent bladder or kidney infections. Urinary hesitancy and urge incontinence are more likely associated with benign prostatic hypertrophy in men, or pelvic organ prolapse in women. Numerous and overlapping factors are thought to cause the epithelial lining damage of the bladder wall associated with IC, including autoimmune disorders, trauma to the bladder, pelvic floor dysfunction, and mast cell abnormalities.

**37. B) Increased blood glucose and dry mucous membranes**

Blood glucose levels rise during acute illnesses, causing increased likelihood of diabetic ketoacidosis (DKA); this is complicated when an individual is unable to have adequate oral intake. Symptoms of dehydration include dry mucosa (especially mouth/tongue/lips), concentrated urine with high specific gravity. The individual with T1DM is likely to need an increased dosage of insulin to compensate; assessing for red flags of dehydration and early DKA are key to preventing complications.

**38. B) Renovascular hypertension**

Secondary hypertension can result from renal artery stenosis. While the presence of an abdominal bruit can be benign, when the finding is continuous, and the individual presents with stage 2 hypertension, renovascular hypertension is a key consideration. Note that critical stenosis of renal arteries is likely to cause resistant, severe hypertension, unlike transient elevations associated with white coat syndrome or anxiety. Essential hypertension usually presents asymptomatically with normal findings on physical exam; the younger age of the patient in this case suggests a secondary cause. Substance use is not likely to cause a bruit and should not be assumed.

**39. C) *Helicobacter pylori (H. pylori)***

Infection with *H. pylori* is a common cause of peptic ulcer disease, reflux, and gastritis; use of non-steroidal anti-inflammatories (NSAIDs) increases the risk. Symptoms of infection include gnawing pain, nausea, bloating, and abdominal discomfort. While cholelithiasis also causes nausea and abdominal pain, the pain is more likely to be in the right upper quadrant with radiation to the upper back; pain is often exacerbated with eating. With ischemic colitis, the individual is more likely to have lower quadrant or generalized abdominal pain with bloody stools as the characteristic presentation.

**40. D) Viral, bacterial, or parasitic infections**

Infections are the most common cause of acute and persistent diarrhea; these include viral causes (norovirus, rotavirus), bacterial infections (*E. coli*, salmonella, shigella), and parasitic causes (giardia). Other causes of diarrhea, especially chronic diarrhea, include long-term use of medications (antibiotics), food allergies or intolerances (lactose intolerance), and digestive tract problems (irritable bowel syndrome, inflammatory bowel disease, celiac disease).

**41. D) The spleen that is normal in size, shape, and contour is easy to palpate and percuss**

The spleen is typically difficult to palpate and percuss. Easily palpating or percussing the spleen increases the likelihood of splenomegaly; splenic enlargement is associated with infectious, inflammatory, or neoplastic processes, including hepatitis, lupus, leukemia, or mononucleosis. Dullness of the spleen to percussion is typically noted just posterior to the left mid-axillary line, from the sixth to tenth rib.

**42. C) Low fiber and limited calcium**

Low levels of dietary calcium and fiber are linked to an increased risk of colorectal cancer. To decrease the risks of colorectal cancer, individuals can increase the intake of fiber, whole grains, fruits, vegetables, and healthy fats, while limiting intake of processed foods, red meats, and saturated fats.

**43. A) Microcytic anemia**

Microcytic anemia is defined as the presence of small, often hypochromic, red blood cells in a peripheral blood smear and is usually characterized by a low mean cell volume (MCV). Iron deficiency, anemia of chronic disease, thalassemia, hemoglobinopathies, and lead poisoning all lead to microcytic anemia. Macrocytic anemias are caused by increase reticulocyte count (hemorrhage), vitamin B12, and folate deficiencies. Hemolytic anemias are inherited (e.g., sickle cell anemia, and metabolic disorders). Thrombocytopenia refers to low platelet count, which can occur with leukemia, autoimmune disorders, and sepsis.

**44. D) Urge incontinence**

Urge incontinence, or overactive bladder, is a condition characterized by detrusor muscle contractions; causes include advancing age, medications, and neurologic insults from stroke, surgery, or disease processes. Stress incontinence is characterized by pelvic floor laxity that allows for the leakage of urine with physical exertion that increases abdominal pressure (e.g., jumping, coughing, or laughing). Overflow incontinence is urine leakage without the feeling of urgency; this condition occurs more frequently in men related to prostate enlargement. Painful bladder syndrome, interstitial cystitis, is caused by damage to the epithelial lining of the bladder wall that results in pelvic pain, urinary urgency, and frequency of urination.

**45. C) Is not immune to hepatitis B**

The negative HBsAg (hepatitis B surface antigen) indicates that the individual is not infectious. The lack of anti-HBs (hepatitis B surface antibody) indicates that the individual has not developed antibodies or immunity by having been infected or through vaccination. The negative anti-HBc (hepatitis B core antibody) indicates that the individual has not had an acute response to hepatitis. The negative results to all three of these lab tests indicate that the individual is susceptible to infection by the hepatitis B virus; if this person is at risk for hepatitis B infection during pregnancy, vaccine would be recommended.

**46. A) Pain on passive internal rotation of flexed hip, B) Pain on passive extension of the right thigh, C) Bruising around umbilicus, D) Bruising at flank, E) Palpation of left lower quadrant causes right-sided pain, F) Referred pain to the left shoulder**

Obturator, poas, and Rovsing's signs indicate possible appendicitis. Cullen, Turner, and Kehr's signs indicate internal abdominal bleeding or irritation from the bleeding.

**47. A) Education to support breast cancer awareness**

Routine SBE and CBE in asymptomatic women at average risk for breast cancer are not currently considered evidence-based recommendations. CBE is recommended for physical evaluation of the breast in high-risk and symptomatic women. Routine genetic testing for mutations associated with breast cancer is not recommended unless a detailed history reveals the potential for an inherited cancer syndrome.

**48. A) A 4-week-old with rectal temperature of 100.8°F**

Elevated body temperature above 100.4° F (38° C) is not an expected finding in newborns, whose immune systems and temperature-regulating mechanisms are immature. Infants under 2 months of age should be evaluated urgently for sepsis if their rectal temperature is above 100.4° F. Fevers are otherwise common and usually self-limiting in children. One example of a common childhood illness associated with fever is roseola; classic presentation is in children 6 to 24 months of age who develop a blanchable rash after resolution of a high fever.

**49. D) 5 years old**

Gross and fine motor developmental milestones for 5-year-olds include prints letters and numbers; draws triangles; draws a person with at least six body parts; stands on one foot for 10 seconds or longer; swings, climbs, hops, jumps, skips, and runs. Gross and fine motor developmental expectations for 4-year-olds include climbing stairs while alternating feet, hopping, catching a bounced ball most of the time, and drawing a person with two to four body parts. 3-year-olds climb and run, can copy a circle, use buttons, and turn book pages. 2-year-olds can typically stand on tiptoe and kick a ball; they are just beginning to run and climb onto and down from furniture without help.

**50. C) 5-year-old with vesicular rash from varicella whose fever has resolved**

Individuals (including children) with varicella are contagious 24 to 48 hours prior to onset of the rash, and until all of the lesions have crusted; resolution of the fever does not indicate lack of contagion. Varicella is highly contagious and is spread by direct contact and inhalation of aerosolized secretions. Children with otitis media and children who have been vaccinated are not considered contagious. Individuals exposed to viruses are considered contagious for 10 to 14 days after exposure; whether viral shedding can begin within the first 24 hours is not known.

**51. A) Acute myocardial infarction**

Diseases that commonly present differently in older adults include acute myocardial infarction (MI), pneumonia, acute appendicitis, urinary tract infection, and depression. Atypical presentation of acute MI includes mild or no chest pain, confusion, weakness, and dizziness. Any new onset of confusion, malaise, anorexia, or diffuse pain should be further investigated in an older adult. While hypertension, osteoporosis, and incontinence are also common, the presentation of these illnesses is more typical.

**52. B) Fever**

While fevers in adults are common, presentation of fever in an older adult is a worrisome sign. Temperature elevation of even 2°F can signal serious infection. History of anorexia can also be a concern, although less emergent than fever. History of constipation and/or use of laxatives may warrant further assessment but are not solely indicative of concerning physiologic processes.

**53. B and E) Gastrointestinal and renal**

Physiological changes of aging worsen the side-effect profile of NSAIDs in older adults. Gastrointestinal side effects such as ulcers and bleeding are the most prevalent and life-threatening problems associated with NSAIDs. In addition, older adults are more at risk for developing nephrotoxicity. These risks, when added to the increased potential for drug interactions in older adults, lead to a much greater risk for adverse outcomes when NSAIDs are used by an older adult.

**54. C) XI spinal accessory**

The spinal accessory nerve, CN XI, innervates the trapezius and sternocleidomastoid muscles; injury or impairment of this cranial nerve may be assessed as muscular atrophy, or limitations in strength against resistance as the individual turns their head and as they shrug their shoulders. Damage to CN V, the trigeminal nerve, results in trigeminal neuralgia characterized by severe repeated bursts of stabbing pain. Trauma to the abducens cranial nerve results in nerve palsy that limits eye movement. Damage to the hypoglossal cranial nerve can cause weakness and paralysis of the tongue muscles.

**55. B) Axillary lymphadenopathy without skin changes**

Physical exam alone is insufficient to adequately assess the cause of axillary lymphadenopathy, which can be a sign of malignancy. Breast size asymmetry, bilateral nipple retraction, and symmetric breast tissue density without palpable masses are all expected findings and of less concern than lymph node enlargement.

**56. B) An 8-year-old with glandular tissue in sub-areolar region; breast and nipple project as single mound**

Precocious puberty is defined as the development of secondary sex characteristics, or physical signs of sexual maturity, in girls before the age of 8 and in boys before the age of 9. Tanner stage 1, elevation of the nipple with no palpable glandular tissue or areolar pigmentation, is expected prior to puberty. Tanner stage 2, the presence of glandular tissue in sub-areolar region, with breast and nipple projection as single mound, is not expected before age 10 to 12 years of age in females, and can be classified as precocious puberty. Tanner stage 4, enlargement of the areola and increased areolar pigmentation, is typically noted in girls at ages 12 to 14 years. Tanner stage 5, completion of breast development, is typically not assessed until ages 13 to 17 years of age; reaching this final developmental phase early, however, does not meet the definition of precocious puberty.

**57. A) Ask all individuals of reproductive age about their intentions for pregnancy or parenthood**

Asking all individuals of reproductive age to reflect on their intentions for parenthood is an evidence-based strategy that improves preconception health and wellness and decreases unintended pregnancies and adverse pregnancy outcomes. The CDC and national organizations have developed reproductive life planning tools for patients and clinicians. "Reminding" only select population groups or providing information about unplanned pregnancy risks are not evidence-based strategies that improve wellness.

**58. B) Bacterial vaginosis**

Recurrent yeast vaginitis is highly correlated with diabetes mellitus type I or type II, as elevated blood glucose levels predispose individuals to be bacterial and fungal infections. While pruritus associated with vaginitis can increase anxiety, vulvovaginal candidiasis (VVC) is not linked to anxiety disorders. Bacterial vaginosis (BV) and VVC are distinctly different, although both disrupt vaginal pH and flora. Atrophic vaginitis is more likely postmenopause than recurrent VVC.

**59. B) Excessive androgen, insulin resistance, and unopposed estrogen**

Polycystic ovarian syndrome (PCOS) is a complex endocrine disorder characterized by excessive androgen, insulin resistance, and unopposed estrogen; menstrual irregularity, hirsutism, acne, and infertility can result. Premature ovarian failure with elevated FSH and LH levels, or ovarian insufficiency resulting in menopausal symptoms are more likely linked to genetic disorders, radiation therapy, chemotherapy, or autoimmune disorders. Dysmenorrhea, constipation, and chronic pelvic pain are highly associated with endometriosis.

**60. C) Infertility**

Pelvic inflammatory disease (PID) involves infection and inflammation of the upper genital tract organs, including the uterus and/or fallopian tubes. Gonorrheal and chlamydial infections account for almost one-half of all cases. PID can lead to infertility as a result of the damage to the genital tract organs. Adenomyosis and endometriosis are both endometrial tissue disorders; with adenomyosis, endometrial tissue implants in the myometrium of the uterus, and in endometriosis, the tissue implants outside of the uterus. Pyelonephritis is inflammation and infection of the kidney that is often a complication of asymptomatic or untreated bladder infection.

**61. D) The squamocolumnar junction**

The squamocolumnar junction, or transformation zone, is an important anatomic landmark, as the area where the squamous epithelial cells and the columnar epithelial cells meet is where most cervical cancers originate. The dark-red tissue is a normal finding of eversion onto the surface of the cervix. While HPV and/or chlamydial infections are often asymptomatic, if the tissue is friable, bleeds easily, or if lesions or discharge are present, these concerns are more likely. An endocervical polyp would appear as an overgrowth that protrudes from the endometrium.

**62. A) Pelvic inflammatory disease**

The individual's history and physical exam are suggestive of a sexually transmitted infection (STI), (i.e., new partner, abdominal pain, discharge, and friable cervix); the tenderness of the cervix with motion suggests that the infection and inflammation are in the upper genital tract, which is consistent of pelvic inflammatory disease (PID). Because PID can lead to infertility and increase the chance of ectopic pregnancy subsequent to the infection, this diagnosis has the highest priority. Pregnancy is not likely, as the individual has an IUD in place, and had a negative pregnancy test. The need for contraception has been met as IUDs are one of the most effective forms of birth control. The friability of the cervix indicates STI, and not a bleeding disorder.

**63. C) Heart disease**

Nearly a third of women develop cardiovascular disease after menopause. Heart disease is the leading cause of death for women. Risks for breast cancer, osteoporosis, and Alzheimer's dementia do increase with advancing age post-menopause. On average, one in eight women will develop breast cancer over an 80-year life span. The prevalence of osteoporosis is approximately 10% for women after menopause, and nearly 8% of the population over 60 have dementia at a given time.

**64. A) Endometrial cancer**

Postmenopausal vaginal bleeding can be a sign of endometrial cancer. Uterine fibroids and endometrial polyps are less likely to cause vaginal bleeding after menopause. While endometrial atrophy or thinning of the uterine lining is a common cause of vaginal bleeding, malignancy is the priority concern and must be considered for early intervention.

**65. B) Fever, fatigue, rash, pharyngitis**

Individuals with acute retroviral syndrome, or primary human immunodeficiency virus (HIV) infection, present with fever, fatigue, rash, and pharyngitis. Acute retroviral syndrome should be considered for any individual with possible HIV exposure who presents with fever. While fever, fatigue, rash, and pharyngitis are the most common findings, individuals may also present with headache, lymphadenopathy, myalgia, nausea, oral ulcers, and night sweats. Abdominal pain, cough, chest pain, and pruritus are not common or expected symptoms.

**66. A) Reddish pink, well-demarcated macules, papules, and plaques with a silvery scale**

Plaque psoriasis is a chronic, systemic illness that presents as reddish-pink, well-demarcated macules, papules, and plaques with a silvery scale. Atopic dermatitis, or eczema, is more likely to begin in early childhood, and presents as pruritic, inflamed lesions. Contact dermatitis, notably poison ivy, appears as vesicular lesions on an erythematous base; allergic or contact dermatitis results from exposure to allergens. Flares of plaque psoriasis can be related to stress, diet, illness, and environmental triggers.

**67. C) Herberden nodes**

Bony nodules at the distal interphalangeal (DIP) joints are known as "Heberden's nodes." Overgrowths at the proximal interphalangeal (PIP) joints are known as "Bouchard's nodes." Both Heberden's and Bouchard's nodes are signs of osteoarthritis. Swan-neck deformities, characterized by hyperextension of the PIP and flexion of the DIP joints, are seen in cases of rheumatoid arthritis. Ganglion cysts are small fluid-filled sacs that form around a joint or tendon, most often the wrist.

**68. D) Inability to actively resist adduction**

Physical findings consistent with a rotator cuff tear include decreased range of motion in the affected shoulder, including forward flexion and internal and/or external rotation, decreased shoulder strength, and inability to actively resist adduction, which is a positive Empty Can test. Pain over the lateral epicondyle of humerus indicates epicondylitis or "tennis elbow." Pain and edema over the radial styloid can indicate wrist fracture or tenosynovitis. Decreased grip strength is more likely to indicate carpal tunnel syndrome.

**69. A) Osteoarthritis**

Osteoarthritis is often found in older adults; pain is typically isolated to a single joint, improves with mild to moderate activity throughout the day, and worsens with prolonged activity. In contrast, rheumatoid arthritis persists throughout the day and is systemic; presentation typically includes fever, flu-like symptoms, and fatigue. Osteoporosis has few symptoms yet predisposes individuals to fracture. A torn meniscus would limit weight bearing and prevent any kneeling, deep squatting, or heavy lifting.

**70. C) Flat pinpoint lesions**

Petechiae are non-blanchable, small, pinpoint vascular lesions located in the dermal or subdermal layers of the skin. Macular lesions that blanch are not vascular. Ecchymotic lesions are associated with bruising; patches would be more likely purpura than petechiae. Rashes that are both papular and pustular are more likely associated with acne or folliculitis.

**71. C) Centripetal**

Centripetal rashes start and are more concentrated on the trunk; varicella is an example of a rash with a centripetal distribution. Centrifugal rashes (e.g., smallpox) start and are more concentrated on the extremities and then spread to the trunk. Confluent rashes are those in which the lesions merge or overlap. Dermatomal rashes follow dermatomes, which are segments of skin innervated by a spinal nerve.

**72. B) Asthma**

Atopic dermatitis is associated with numerous atopic and allergic comorbidities, including asthma, contact dermatitis, allergic rhinitis, and eosinophilic esophagitis. The patient burden related to atopic dermatitis or eczema can be significant and lead to depression. Secondary infections, such as impetigo or cellulitis can occur, but are not as common as the asthma association. Clubbing, a physical sign of chronic hypoxia characterized by bulbous enlargement of fingers or toes, is not as commonly associated with atopy.

**73. B) Did you use any type of new product, shampoo, or soap in the shower?**

Wheals are raised, pruritic, irregular lesions that are an overt sign of allergy. The sudden appearance after showering suggests an exposure to an allergen. Additional questions important to note would be past history of allergic or contact dermatitis, history of allergies, and any exposures. Outdoor or family exposures and recent illness symptoms are excellent history questions; however, these are not as likely to be the cause of urticaria based on the patient's history.

**74. C) Several are irregular in shape and color**

A nevi that is suspicious for melanoma carries the traits of an irregular or asymmetric border, multiple colors, asymmetry, and has changes that evolve over time. A nevi with a smooth, uniform border would not be suspicious for melanoma. Uniformity of color, unchanged lesions are also not suspicious. When examining skin lesions, consider ABCDE = Asymmetry, Border, Color, Diameter and Evolving as a tool to assess whether or not skin lesion might need further evaluation to determine the possibility of skin cancer.

**75. B) Onychomycosis**

Onychomycosis is a fungal infection of the nails that causes discoloration, thickening, and separation from the nail bed; this condition is more prevalent in individuals over the age of 60 and who have comorbid conditions of diabetes, obesity, and tobacco use disorder. Psoriasis can also affect nailbeds, although this will appear more as pitting than thickened discoloration. Like onychomycosis, tinea corporis is a fungal infection; tinea corporis, or ringworm, infection is more superficial and can affect any part of the body. Actinic keratoses are rough, scaly patches on the skin that develop from prolonged sun exposure and are more likely to appear on sun-exposed skin.

**76. A) Basal cell carcinoma**

Basal cell carcinoma (BCC) is the most common type of skin cancer; linked to sun exposure or indoor tanning, BCCs are common on the head, neck, and arms but can form anywhere. Squamous cell carcinoma is the second most common type of skin cancer; also linked to sun exposure, early diagnosis and treatment prevents deep growth and spread. Cutaneous T-cell lymphoma is a rare type of cancer that causes rash-like skin redness, and slightly raised or scaly round patches on the skin. Malignant melanoma is the most serious skin cancer because of its tendency to metastasize.

**77. C) Post-herpetic neuralgia**

The case presentation is classic for herpes zoster, or shingles. Post-herpetic neuralgia is the most common complication of shingles and can be debilitating; prevention requires beginning anti-viral medication within the first 72 hours of the outbreak. Herpes zoster is reactivation of the varicella virus; concerns about limiting pain management to avoid opioid dependence are not a priority for the individual presenting with acute pain from shingles. The shingles rash can become infected, resulting in a cellulitis, but this is not as common or urgent of an occurrence.

**78. D) Thinning of the skin or cutaneous atrophy**

Steroid-induced thinning of the skin results from prolonged use; in most cases the epidermis also begins to atrophy. Vitiligo is depigmentation caused primarily by autoimmune or genetic factors. Scarring is caused by trauma. Lichenification is likely to result from scratching or rubbing.

**79. D) IgM**

IgM is the first immunoglobulin expressed during B cell development and is associated with a primary immune response. IgG and IgA are markers of immune response associated with chronic disease. IgE is elevated with hypersensitivity and allergic responses.

**80. A) Supraclavicular, B) Occipital, C) Preauricular, D) Submandibular, E) Anterior Cervical**

Location of lymphadenopathy is a key consideration for disease processes that involve infection and/or inflammation. 75% of all peripheral lymphadenopathies are localized to one area; over half of these cases involve the superficial lymph nodes of the head and neck.

**81. D) This is concerning; the adolescent should be evaluated for meningeal irritation**

Complications of rhinosinusitis include meningitis and brain abscess; the symptoms reported are signs of meningeal irritation, which should be evaluated for suspicion of CNS involvement immediately. New onset of fever with an exacerbation of symptoms is not the expected course of the illness and does not indicate that the original diagnosis and/or treatment were incorrect.

**82. C) Cough**

The Centor criteria for pharyngitis caused by group A beta-hemolytic streptococcus (GABHS) consists of tonsillar exudate, anterior cervical lymphadenopathy, fever, and absence of cough. Having all four of the Centor Criteria is highly indicative of having strep pharyngitis.

**83. B) Subacute sinusitis**

Subacute sinusitis is inflammation of the sinuses that persists for approximately 4 to 8 weeks, with an overall duration of less than 3 months. Acute sinusitis is an infection lasting 3 to 4 weeks. Recurrent sinusitis is defined as three or more episodes per year. Chronic sinusitis is an infection/inflammation that persists for more than 3 months. Sinusitis is inflammation of the sinuses; the etiology can be infectious (bacterial, viral, or fungal) or noninfectious (allergy). This inflammation leads to blockade of normal sinus drainage pathways, which leads to congestion, decreased mucociliary clearance, and predisposition to bacterial growth.

**84. C) Pulmonary function study results show FEV1/FVC ratio of <70%**

The most important diagnostic test for COPD is spirometry, or pulmonary function studies. The definition of airflow limitation (which is the hallmark finding of COPD) is an FEV1/FVC less than 0.70. While hyperinflation and a flattened diaphragm are chest x-ray findings consistent with COPD, these findings are not essential to the diagnosis. The FVC of <30% may be an indicator of severe COPD, although could also indicate restrictive airway disease, such as pulmonary fibrosis.

**85. D) Strep pharyngitis**

Scarlet fever is characterized by strep pharyngitis and a "sandpaper rash" consisting of small, bright, erythematous lesions that begin on the trunk and spread all over the body. Cough and coryza, inflammation of nasal passages, are more likely associated with upper respiratory infections; cough, coryza, and conjunctivitis are the classic symptoms of rubeola, or measles.

**86. C) Congenital melanocytosis**

Congenital melanocytosis, previously known as "Mongolian spots," is a very common condition in dark-skinned infants. These pigmented lesions are not ecchymosis (bruising), acrocyanosis (dusky, mottled discoloration cause by vasospasm), or purpura (vascular lesions), and usually resolve by school age.

**87. C) Rosacea**

Rosacea commonly affects middle-aged women with fair skin and is confused for acne. While the cause is unknown, trademark symptoms include macular-papular-pustular lesions triggered by stress, exercise, spicy foods, and alcohol. Cystic acne is more likely to present in teens and young adults, and less likely to have environmental triggers. Cellulitis is a superficial skin infection and not likely to be chronic. Senile keratosis is a common, waxy, scaly, elevated skin growth, more common in older adults.

**88. D) Thunderclap**

Thunderclap headaches are those that present suddenly and severely; although the pain typically resolves in less than 5 minutes, the consequences of the headache can be significant. Causes of thunderclap headaches include stroke, head injury, subarachnoid hemorrhage, hypertensive crisis, artery dissections, vasospasm, and vasculitis. Additional, urgent evaluation of severe, sudden, thunderclap headaches is indicated. Migraines with/without aura, rebound headaches, and tension-type headaches generally have a gradual onset and a history of recurrence.

**89. B) Unilateral pain**

The main symptom of a migraine most often experienced by adolescents and adults is intense unilateral headache. While auras, dizziness, and photophobia (extreme sensitivity to light) are common symptoms, not all individuals will experience these symptoms.

**90. B) Small, mobile, soft anterior cervical nodes**

Lymph nodes should be soft, mobile, and <1 cm in size; the anterior, posterior, and deep cervical chain areas are the most likely regions to palpate lymph nodes. Red flags during an examination of lymph nodes include assessment of nodes that are hard, fixed, matted, >1 cm in size, unilateral, non-resolving, generalized (throughout the body), and/or located in the supraclavicular, popliteal, iliac, or epitrochlear regions.

**91. A) Temporal**

The temporal lobe houses the Wernicke's area that is responsible for allowing a person to understand spoken and written language. Damage to the Wernicke's area can result in aphasia and cause a loss of articulation of words and may be unaware of the mistakes in their speech. The frontal lobe houses the motor cortex area and the Broca area, which is responsible for motor control of speech formation. The occipital lobe is the visual processing center, and the parietal lobe is responsible for receiving and processing sensory data.

**92. D) Multiple myeloma**

Multiple myeloma are cancers of the immune system that begin in plasma cells; the proliferation of the plasma cells damages the bone marrow, leading to bone pain, fractures, fatigue, and anemia. Leukemia is cancer of white blood cells; symptoms include fatigue, fever, dyspnea, weight loss, and lymphadenopathy. Carcinoma is a cancer that begins in epithelial tissues. Sarcoma is a malignancy that begins in connective tissues.

**93. B) Handwashing, food safety, and travel precautions**

Individuals who are immunocompromised should be advised to take precautions to prevent infections, which include hand washing, safe food handling and storage, limiting exposure to environmental toxins, handling animals safely, practicing safe sex, and taking extra care when traveling. Isolating from children and older adults, refraining from intimacy, or using strong cleansers are not safe or sustainable practices.

**94. C) Spleen**

The spleen is located just below the diaphragm in the left upper quadrant of the abdomen. The reference to the student experiencing fatigue is suggestive of mononucleosis; 50% of individuals experiencing mononucleosis are likely to have splenomegaly, which would cause the spleen to be enlarged and tender. Hepatomegaly can also occur with infectious mono; liver enlargement would be palpated in the right upper quadrant. Pyelonephritis (infection in the kidneys) is best assessed using fist percussion at the area of the costovertebral angle; deep palpation of the left flank can also be used. The thymus is not palpable, as it is located below the sternum in the upper chest.

**95. A) Dullness to percussion and decreased breath sounds to auscultation.**

Assessment findings attributed to both pleural effusion and lobar pneumonia include dullness to percussion and decreased breath sounds to auscultation. Increased tactile fremitus is found with pneumonia; decreased tactile fremitus with pleural effusion. Adventitious breath sounds are less likely with these disease processes because the sounds are muffled.

**96. D) Chlamydia trachomatis**

NAAT can be performed using urine samples for chlamydia trachomatis and *neisseria gonorrhoeae*, which is less expensive and less invasive than collection of genital swabs and is highly sensitive and specific. Serum lab testing and saliva point of care tests are available for HIV detection; blood specimens are required to screen for hepatitis. Viral cultures and/or serum specimens are needed to test for herpes simplex type 2.

**97. A) Vesicular**

Vesicular breath sounds are soft, low-pitched breath sounds normally heard over most lung fields. Bronchovesicular breath sounds are heard over major bronchi in the mid-chest (suprasternal area and between scapulae) of moderate pitch. Bronchial breath sounds are louder, higher pitch heard over the lower aspect of the trachea. Tracheal are high pitch and the loudest breath sounds, which are heard over the trachea.

**98. A) Discontinuous crackles on inspiration that do not clear with coughing**

Crackles (rales) are adventitious breath sounds that are discontinuous, heard upon inspiration, not cleared with coughing, and associated with heart failure exacerbations as pulmonary congestion increases. Inspiratory, expiratory, audible, and scattered wheezing is caused by airway obstruction in disease states that include asthma, COPD, or acute bronchitis. Stridor is indicative of laryngeal or tracheal spasm and is more common in children. Rhonchi, sonorous or rumbling breath sounds, are more commonly associated with COPD, chronic bronchitis, or pneumonia; a unilateral finding suggests lobar obstruction.

**99. B) Spirometry measures the ability of a person to inhale and exhale air respective to time**

Spirometry measures the ability of a person to inhale and exhale air respective to time to better assess pulmonary function. Determined by spirometry, the measure of forced expiratory volume over 1 second (FEV1) is especially useful in diagnosing obstructive lung diseases like asthma or chronic obstructive pulmonary disease (COPD). The ratio between FEV1 and forced vital capacity (FVC) differentiates between obstructive and restrictive lung diseases. Spirometry does not indicate whether a disease is viral or bacterial and differs from use of peak flow meters and incentive spirometers. Use of an incentive spirometer is a strategy to encourage deep inhalation. Peak flow meters are portable devices used to help with asthma management.

**100. C) Pneumonia**

Tactile fremitus, vibrations created by the voice, can be palpated on the chest wall (typically while the individual repeats a phrase such as ninety-nine). Tactile fremitus should be felt equal bilaterally. Increased fremitus is caused by a consolidation replacing healthy lung tissue, as with pneumonia. Decreased fremitus is caused by excess air in the lungs, increased distance between the lungs and chest wall, or obstruction in the bronchus; asthma, chronic bronchitis, COPD, emphysema, pleural effusions, and pneumothorax are more likely to cause decreased fremitus.

**101. B) Young adult with 3 days of cough, chest discomfort, sore throat, and malaise**

Acute bronchitis commonly causes cough, fatigue or malaise, rhinorrhea, congestion, sore throat, slight fever, and chest pain or discomfort. Asthma should be considered more likely for the pediatric patient who has recurrent wheezing. Morning cough is a common symptom of smoking cessation. Pneumonia should be the priority consideration for an older adult with fever, fatigue, cough, and tachypnea.

**102. C) Midaxillary area**

Auscultation of the lungs should occur in a systematic manner from apex to base, and comparing side to side, being certain to auscultate above the clavicle to assess upper lobes, laterally in the midaxillary area to assess the right middle lobe, and posteriorly to assess lower lobes.

**103. C) Dyspnea**

Dyspnea, or shortness of breath, is the key presenting symptom of a significant pleural effusion. Causes of pleural effusion are numerous, and include cancer (malignant effusion), heart failure, pneumonia, kidney failure, or sepsis; pleural effusions typically cause anxiety, tachypnea, and pleuritic chest pain because the fluid limits lung compliance. Older adults are less likely to have fever in response to illnesses and are more likely to present with confusion.

**104. A) A 6-month-old who is healthy and unvaccinated**

Unvaccinated infants are at highest risk of significant morbidity and/or mortality from pertussis. When anyone presents with a whoop-type cough, important assessments include immunization history and contacts with known cases of pertussis. Being up to date on vaccinations helps to mitigate the risk of exposure. Adolescents and adults can contract pertussis, but usually in a milder form. Those who are pregnant are not at risk for severe or significant disease; however, experts recommend vaccination during the third trimester of pregnancy to prevent exposing newborns to pertussis.

**105. B) Unable to arouse easily from sleep**

The most common symptom of obstructive sleep apnea (OSA) is unexplained daytime sleepiness. Other symptoms include loud snoring, frequent arousals, disruption of sleep, and presence of associated adverse clinical outcomes, which can include hypertension, heart disease, and diabetes. The most common physical finding associated with OSA is obesity.

**106. C) Maintaining the health of athletes, including their safe participation in sports**

The overall goal of a preparticipation physical evaluation is to maintain the health of an athlete, including their safe participation in sports. Although studies have not found that the evaluation prevents morbidity and mortality associated with sports participation, it may detect conditions that predispose the athlete to injury or illness and can provide strategies to prevent injuries. Clearance depends on the outcome of the evaluation and the sport in which the athlete participates. The overall goal is not exclusion from participation or screening for mental health disorders. The exam should focus on the cardiovascular and musculoskeletal systems. Further evaluation should be considered for individuals with heart or lung disease, bleeding disorders, musculoskeletal problems, history of concussion, or other neurologic disorders.

**107. C) Scoliosis**

Scoliosis, lateral curvature of the spine, causes asymmetry in shoulder heights, and in the level of the iliac spines; with forward bending, asymmetry can be observed in scapulae and rib cage, depending on the severity of the curvature. Spondylolysis is a vertebral stress fracture that can be assessed in young athletes as a result of overuse syndrome or other strenuous activities; typical presentation includes persistent back pain. Lordosis is excessive inward curvature of the lower back. Kyphosis is an excessive outward curvature of the upper back.

**108. B) This injury is very common in young children**

Radial head subluxation, or "nursemaid's elbow," is a common injury in young children. The radial head can slip under the annular ligament when a child is pulled or swung by their arm(s), resulting in pain and inability to supinate the forearm. Resolving the problem takes a few seconds; once the elbow is properly reduced and the annular ligament is in proper position, the pain resolves and the child is able to use their arm without limitation. No casting or additional testing is needed.

**109. A) New onset of urinary incontinence**

Cauda equina syndrome results from spinal nerve compression and is a medical emergency; delays in treatment can lead to permanent loss of bladder or bowel control, paresthesia, and paralysis. An individual who presents with back pain should be assessed for saddle anesthesia, motor weakness in legs, and recent onset of bladder or bowel dysfunction. Pain at greater than 7 degrees with straight leg raising is indicative of musculoskeletal tightness and is not likely neurologic. Previous history of muscle spasm is common. Although not considered an emergency, weakness with dorsiflexion may indicate L5 nerve root compression or neuropathy and should be further evaluated.

**110. B) 128/88 mm/Hg**

According to the AHA/ACC guidelines, a normal blood pressure reading is defined as systolic blood pressure (SBP) less than 120 and diastolic blood pressure (DBP) less than 80. Elevated BP is SBP between 120-129 and DBP less than 80. Stage 1 hypertension (HTN) is defined as SBP 130-139 and/or DBP 80-89. Stage 2 HTN is defined as SBP 140 or above and/or DBP 90 or above. Hypertensive crisis is when SBP is over 180 and/or DBP is over 120.

**111. C) Moderate pain and swelling, decreased range of motion**

Ankle sprains are classified according to the level of ligament injury. **Grade 1:** Partial tear causes include mild swelling and tenderness. **Grade II:** Incomplete tear causes moderate pain and selling with some loss of function. **Grade III:** Complete tear causes severe swelling, ecchymosis, instability, loss of function.

**112. C) Lack of weight-bearing exercise**

Osteoporosis is a condition that causes a decline in bone density which predisposes an individual to fracture. Risk factors include smoking, a diet low in calcium and/or vitamin D, female gender, age, certain medications, and lack of weight-bearing exercise.

**113. B) Increased limb length**

Individuals with Marfan syndrome are typically very tall with disproportionately long, thin limbs, arachnodactyly, and a long, narrow face. Key physical findings include myopia, mitral valve prolapse, pectus deformities, joint hyper-flexibility or laxity, and scoliosis. Kyphosis is not associated specifically with Marfan syndrome, is commonly postural, and may be associated with spinal arthritis. Webbed-neck deformities are usually congenital and associated with Noonan and Turner syndromes.

**114. C) Osgood-Schlatter disease**

Symptoms of Osgood Schlatter disease include anterior knee pain with swelling and tenderness to palpation of the tibial tuberosity just below the patella, where the patellar tendon attaches to the tibia. Genu varum is an outward bowing of the knees. Metatarsus adductus is a common foot deformity of infancy. Tibial torsion is an inward twisting of the tibia that causes in-toeing.

**115. A) Cholesteatoma**

Cholesteatoma is an epidermal inclusion cyst formation in the middle ear and mastoid cavity; the tumor is aggressive, causing bone erosion and infection that lead to mastoiditis, facial nerve paralysis, and/or labyrinthitis. The other ear disorders listed can cause ear pain, hearing loss, and/or vertigo, although are less likely to cause mastoiditis and severe sequelae. External otitis causes conductive hearing loss when the ear canal is swollen. Impaction of cerumen impedes the movement of air needed to vibrate the tympanic membrane. Otitis media with effusion involves fluid in the middle ear, which causes conductive hearing loss.

**116. D) Ultraviolet light, dust, and wind**

A pterygium is a benign growth of the conjunctiva. Pterygia are thought to be caused by chronic dry eyes, and chronic exposure to wind, dust, and ultraviolet light. While exposure to cigarette smoke has significant impact on health, development of pterygia is not one of them. Elevated blood glucose is associated with diabetic retinopathy. Elevated lipid levels can lead to the development of xanthelasma. Contact lens wearers are more susceptible to bacterial conjunctivitis, corneal abrasions, and other acute ocular disorders.

**117. A) Red dot = aortic; B. Blue dot = pulmonic; C. Green dot = tricuspid; D. Purple dot = mitral**

The primary auscultatory locations:

- Aortic valve area: 2nd intercostal space (ICS) at the right sternal border
- Pulmonic valve area: 2nd left ICS at the left sternal border
- Tricuspid valve area: 4th left ICS at the left sternal border
- Mitral valve area: 5th left ICS at the midclavicular line.

**118. D) Narrow angle glaucoma**

Narrow angle glaucoma is a medical emergency; symptoms include severe headache, eye pain, nausea/vomiting, blurred vision, halos around lights, and eye erythema. This is different that open angle glaucoma, which is chronic with a gradual onset. Symptoms include blind spots in both peripheral and central vision. A subconjunctival hemorrhage is not an emergency and usually clears on its own. Macular degeneration is a non-emergent condition that is age related and involves loss of central vision.

**119. B) Strabismus**

Strabismus is defined as improper alignment of the eyes when looking at an object. The Hirschberg corneal light reflex test involves observing for alignment and screening for strabismus by noting the symmetry of the light reflection in both eyes. Exophthalmos is anterior protrusion of one or both eyes, assessed by observing for bulging eyes. Assessing extraocular eye movements (EOMs) would support the diagnosis of exophthalmia or nystagmus. Nystagmus is found when eyes make repetitive or uncontrolled movements when tracking an object. Cataracts are clouding of the lens of the eye, resulting in decreased visual acuity.

**120. D) Left midclavicular line, 5th intercostal space**
The PMI is best palpated at the apex of the heart, which is located at or just medial to the left midclavicular line, 5th intercostal space (ICS). If the PMI is significantly displaced, this can indicate cardiomegaly. This location (5th ICS at the midclavicular line) is also the location where S1 can be auscultated most clearly.

**121. A) Can indicate a serious diagnosis like retinoblastoma or cataracts**
Eliciting the red reflex is a quick and noninvasive way to assess for sight and life-threatening abnormalities, including retinoblastoma, and congenital cataracts. The purpose of the assessment is to identify those who need immediate referral, so assuming inexperience or waiting to reassess would be inappropriate.

**122. A) Acute otitis media**
Diagnostic criteria for acute otitis media include rapid onset of symptoms, bulging tympanic membrane, limited or absent mobility of the membrane, and erythema of the tympanic membrane or ear pain affecting sleep or normal activity. Otitis media with effusion is diagnosed based on findings of visible amber fluid bubbles. Eustachian tube dysfunction findings include a dull or retracted tympanic membrane. Otitis externa is associated with inflammation of the ear canal, which causes pain with palpation of the pinna and tragus.

**123. C) 2+**
2+ would be considered a normal pulse. 0 would describe an absent pulse, which would indicate lack of blood flow (e.g., from cardiac arrest, shock, or thrombus). The grade of 1+ describes a weak pulse, which may indicate decreased cardiac output. The scoring of 3+ describes a bounding pulse (e.g., from exercise, anxiety, fever, anemia, or aortic valve regurgitation).

**124. A) Convergence of the eyes when shifting focus to objects that are near**
Convergence is the ability of the eyes to simultaneously demonstrate inward movement toward each other, which allows for better focus on near objects clearer. To also help with near vision, pupils should constrict to increase the depth of focus of the eye by blocking the light scattered by the periphery of the cornea. Accommodation reflexes include convergence and pupil constriction when an object is moved closer to the face; ciliary muscles are responsible for the lens accommodation response. When an object is moved further from the face, pupils dilate, and the eyes diverge.

**125. C) Hordeolum**
Commonly referred to as a stye, a hordeolum is an acute infection of the eyelid margin that presents as an erythematous, tender, papule or pustule. An internal hordeolum

can evolve into a chalazion, a chronic lesion that presents as a firm, rubbery, non-tender nodule within the eyelid. These differ from xanthelasma lesions, which are elevated plaques of cholesterol that appear as oval, irregularly shaped, yellow-tinted lesions on periorbital tissue. When an individual presents with redness and crusting of the entire eyelid, the condition is more likely blepharitis, inflammation of eyelids, which can be caused by infection or systemic illnesses, such as seborrheic dermatitis, rosacea, or dry eye syndrome.

**126. A, B, and D) Obtain the blood pressure reading while the person is seated; rest the individual's arm at the level of their heart; have the individual uncross their legs and place feet flat on the floor**

When obtaining a person's blood pressure reading, ensure the individual is quietly seated in a chair with legs uncrossed and feet flat on the floor, allowing them to relax for 3 to 5 minutes before obtaining the reading. Do not talk to the person before or during the reading, as studies have shown that this increases blood pressure readings in a manner similar to white coat syndrome. Always have the patient remove their arm from a shirt sleeve and place the blood pressure cuff directly on the skin to ensure an accurate reading.

**127. B) Upper respiratory infection**

While an individual with a history of diabetes is more at risk for bacterial infection, the case presentation suggests viral upper respiratory tract infection (URI) related to duration (less than 10 days), and severity of illness (no cough, malaise, or fever noted). URIs symptoms commonly include congestion, rhinorrhea, and pharyngitis. An older adult with bronchitis is more likely to present with cough and fatigue. History of hypertension and older age increase this individual's risk of heart failure; however, the acute nature of the symptoms would not be a typical presentation. Symptoms of heart failure include fatigue and dyspnea.

**128. A) Trismus**

Trismus is the reduced ability to open the mouth, caused by spasms of the muscles of mastication. Trismus can occur as a result of trauma (surgery), infection (peritonsillar abscess), cancer, or radiation treatment. Peritonsillar abscesses can also cause muscle spasms of the neck that cause the head to tile or twist to one side, or torticollis. Tetanus, an infection caused by *Clostridium tetani*, will cause severe trismus and dysphagia, or difficulty swallowing.

**129. C) Most inguinal hernias cause a dull ache and fullness that worsens with straining**

Most inguinal hernias cause swelling or fullness, and an aching sensation; hernias enlarge or bulge with increasing intra-abdominal pressure (straining, standing, exercising, and/or coughing). Incarcerated hernias cannot be reduced manually or spontaneously through the defect; the incarceration of a hernia requires urgent surgical referral. Inguinal hernias are common in older adults and are often perceived intermittently.

**130. D) Malignancy or carcinoma.**

Painless, unilateral nodularity is suggestive of prostate cancer. Palpation typically reveals a smooth prostate with firm lobes and a distinct sulcus. Adenocarcinoma of the prostate typically begins in the posterior lobe. With malignancy, the prostate gland becomes asymmetrical and hard or nodular; often the sulcus is no longer palpable. With prostatitis, prostate gland palpation is tender or painful. Hypertrophy of the prostate is commonly palpated as bogginess with increased width, length, or thickness.

**131. D) Hypopigmentation of the nipples and areolae**

During pregnancy, a number of skin changes occur. These include skin darkening (hyper-, not hypo-pigmentation) of the nipples, areolae, and axillae; hyperpigmentation of the face, known as "chloasma," "melasma," or "mask of pregnancy"; palms of hands and soles of feet may have diffuse redness due to increased vascularity and increased estrogen production; and a dark pigmented line (linea nigra) may be present on the abdomen, extending midline from the symphysis pubis to the top of the fundus

**132. B) If your child is a boy, there is a 50% risk that he will have hemophilia**

The genes associated with hemophilia are located on the X chromosome; daughters of fathers with hemophilia are obligate carriers of the hemophilia gene since they inherited his X chromosome. When mothers are carriers of the gene (as in this case), there is a 50% chance that her male children will have hemophilia, and a 50% chance that her female children will be carriers.

**133. C) Pyelonephritis can result if UTIs are not diagnosed and adequately treated**

Pyelonephritis, infection of the kidney and upper urinary tract, is a common, serious condition in pregnancy, resulting from undiagnosed or inadequately treated UTIs. Simple cystitis (i.e., infection of the bladder and lower urinary tract) in women who are not pregnant can be treated without physical exam or lab testing. Cystitis in pregnancy, however, is considered complicated or complex, as physiologic changes predispose women to pyelonephritis. Symptoms of UTIs during pregnancy are obscured by the symptoms of pregnancy (i.e., urinary frequency and urgency) are likely to be perceived as related to the pregnancy, and not signs of infection. Asymptomatic bacteriuria is also more common in pregnant women, which increases the likelihood of pyelonephritis.

**134. B) Heart disease and cancer**

The top ten leading causes of mortality for all ages:

1. Heart disease
2. Cancer
3. Unintentional injuries or accidents
4. Chronic lower respiratory disorders
5. Stroke or cerebrovascular diseases
6. Alzheimer's disease
7. Diabetes

8. Nephritis, nephrosis, nephrotic syndrome
9. Influenza and pneumonia
10. Intentional self-harm

**135. C) Individuals who have experienced trauma have greater health risks**
Exposure to abuse, neglect, violence, discrimination, and other adverse experiences increase potential for serious health problems, even when those experiences were during childhood. Implementing a trauma-informed approach care requires creating a safe environment; recognizing the signs and symptoms of trauma in individuals, families, and staff; and integrating knowledge in practice while actively resisting retraumatization. Access to care, patient empowerment, safety, and collaboration are key to improving health outcomes.

**136. A) Black men have the highest incidence and mortality rates of prostate cancer**
Black men and women have the highest mortality rates for most cancers in the United States. Black men also have the highest cancer incidence rate, which includes prostate cancer. The causes of these inequalities are complex and reflect socioeconomic disparities and differences in access to high-quality health care more than biological differences. For all populations in the United States, including Hispanic women, lung cancer has the highest mortality rate of all cancers.

**137. B) Sitting more than 8 hours daily is associated with obesity, hypertension, and diabetes**
Studies have linked sitting for more than 8 hours daily with a number of health risks, including hypertension, diabetes, hyperlipidemia, and obesity. For individuals who are overweight or obese, modest weight loss of 5% of total body weight is likely to produce health benefits. Diet has a significant impact on health; while exercise is important for cardiovascular health, the positive effects do not erase the impact of dietary choices. Smoking cessation can be effectively supported with pharmacologic agents.

**138. D) Why do you continue to smoke knowing that your health will deteriorate?**
Judgment places a negative value on the individual and their health challenges; asking why behaviors continue despite efforts or desire to change minimizes the individual's ability to cope and is a blame-shifting strategy inconsistent with trust and rapport. Asking permission to discuss difficult topics, paraphrasing, and exploring challenges to smoking cessation are therapeutic communication technique that can be used to provide individual support.

**139. A) Being attentive to verbal and non-verbal communication**
Best practice includes attention to verbal and non-verbal communication; observation and inspection are key assessment techniques used when care is completed by telehealth. Assessments can include general survey, mental health status, and specific body systems; individuals can be engaged to provide important history and physical

exam details. Reimbursement for care managed using telehealth technologies continues to expand. While there are limitations, individuals can have access to evidence-based, confidential, high-quality care through telehealth.

**140. A) Aortic stenosis**

Aortic stenosis results from narrowing of the aortic valve, which keeps the valve from opening fully, reducing blood flow to the body; hypertension and older age are risk factors. The stenosis causes a harsh, crescendo-decrescendo murmur during systole that is best auscultated at the 2nd or 3rd intercostal space, right sternal border, especially when the patient is seated and leaning forward. Aortic regurgitation and mitral stenosis are both diastolic murmurs. Mitral regurgitation is a systolic murmur heard at the apex, augmented when the person is supine and side-lying.

**141. D) Mitral regurgitation**

Mitral regurgitation causes the backflow of blood from a noncompliant mitral valve; the resultant murmur is best heard at the apex, is holosystolic (continuous between S1 and S2), and has a medium/high pitch and harsh sound quality. While the murmur associated with mitral stenosis is also best auscultated at the apex of the heart, the murmur is diastolic. Aortic regurgitation is best heard in the left 2nd/3rd intercostal space during diastole and is high-pitched and blowing. Aortic stenosis murmurs are mid-systolic, best heard at the right 2nd/3rd ICS, and have a crescendo-decrescendo quality.

**142. A) Rumbling diastolic murmur heard best at the apex using the bell of the stethoscope**

The diastolic murmur associated with mitral stenosis is best auscultated using the bell of the stethoscope at the apex of the heart. Aortic stenosis causes a harsh mid-systolic murmur heard best at the 2nd and 3rd intercostal spaces, right sternal border. Aortic regurgitation is best assessed by auscultation in the left 2nd/3rd intercostal space during diastole; the murmur is high-pitched and blowing. Mitral regurgitation causes a harsh, holosystolic murmur with a medium/high pitch that is best heard at the apex.

**143. C) 3+**

Pitting edema is graded as:

- 1+ mild pitting with only slight indentation and no appreciable distortion or edema
- 2+ moderate pitting, thumb indentation resolves rapidly
- 3+ deep pitting, indentation remains for brief period, noticeable edema is present
- 4+ severe pitting that remains indented for minutes, edema causes significant distortion

**144. C) Palpate the left and right carotid arteries simultaneously at the carotid sinus**

When assessing carotid pulses, palpate the right and left carotid arteries in turn; do not apply firm pressure or palpate both carotids at the same time as this can compromise blood flow to the brain, causing syncope. Also avoid palpating near the top of the thyroid cartilage, the location of the carotid sinus, as pressure on this may cause slowing of the heart rate. A thorough and comprehensive cardiovascular exam does include palpation of the radial pulse in conjunction with auscultation of the apical pulse, auscultating the apical pulse while gently palpating the carotid artery, and palpating over the heart region to determine any thrills, lifts, or heaves.

**145. C) S3**

S3 occurs as a result of early ventricular filling associated with decreased compliance of the left ventricle and volume overload and is described as a "ventricular gallop." S4, referred to as an "atrial gallop," is a late diastolic sound that occurs during atrial contraction due to a stiff ventricle and increased afterload. S1 is a normal heart sound indicating the beginning of systole; S1 is heard as "lub" and coincides with the carotid artery pulse. S2 is a normal heart sound indicating the beginning of diastole; S2 is heard as "dub" and occurs with the closure of aortic and pulmonic valves (semilunar valves).

**146. B) A 65-year-old who recently quit smoking**

The presence of an S3 heart sound is normal in children, athletes, and pregnant women in their third trimester. An S3 heart sound in an individual over 40 years old is a concerning finding and could indicate volume overload due to heart failure. Smoking is a risk factor for heart disease.

**147. A) Deformity that changes angle of nailbed; B) Nontender maculae on the palms and soles; C) Painful, erythematous, raised lesions; D) Dark-red, linear lesions in the nailbeds; E) Reddening at the thenar and hypothenar eminences**

Thorough inspection of the hands for signs includes assessments associated with underlying causes of cardiovascular and peripheral vascular disorders, including infective endocarditis (Janeway lesions, Osler's nodes, splinter hemorrhages), heart failure (clubbing), or other systemic pathology (palmar erythema).

**148. C) Prolonged QT interval**

Low calcium levels or hypocalcemia causes prolongation of the QT interval, which can lead to ventricular dysrhythmias; hypocalcemia also causes decreased myocardial contractility, which can lead to heart failure and hypotension. Causes of ST segment elevation include acute myocardial infarction, coronary vasospasm, pericarditis, left ventricular hypertrophy, and left bundle branch blocks. Causes of ST segment depression include myocardial ischemia, hypokalemia, and medications. Prominent Q waves are commonly associated with myocardial infarction, although can also be non-pathologic.

**149. A) Sternal depression causing abdominal contour of the chest wall**

Pectus excavatum and carinatum are a group of chest wall deformities, where there is an abnormal contour to the shape of the chest and the sternum in particular. Pectus excavatum, which is more common, is an indentation or depression of the chest, where the center part of the sternum is pushed backward by several centimeters; pectus excavatum is sometimes called a "sunken chest." With pectus carinatum, the sternum actually projects too far forward or protrudes anteriorly. Barrel chest is characterized by an increased anteroposterior diameter of the chest. Chest wall trauma causes flail chest, or paradoxical movement of a chest segment during respiration.

**150. B) Homeless, currently staying in local shelter**

Cues to the diagnosis of pulmonary tuberculosis include productive cough, mucopurulent sputum, hemoptysis, dyspnea, weight loss, anorexia, fever, night sweats, and malaise; symptoms typically have a gradual onset. A high index of suspicion is needed for those who are immigrants, elderly, immunocompromised, or are in poor living conditions, including those who are homeless or living in shelters. Cinnamon odor to breath has been noted in some patients with pulmonary tuberculosis. Fruity breath or breath that smells like acetone is more likely associated with ketosis, which can be associated with diabetic ketoacidosis and/or nutritional deficiencies.

# Practice Test II: Assessment and Diagnosis of Pediatric Patients

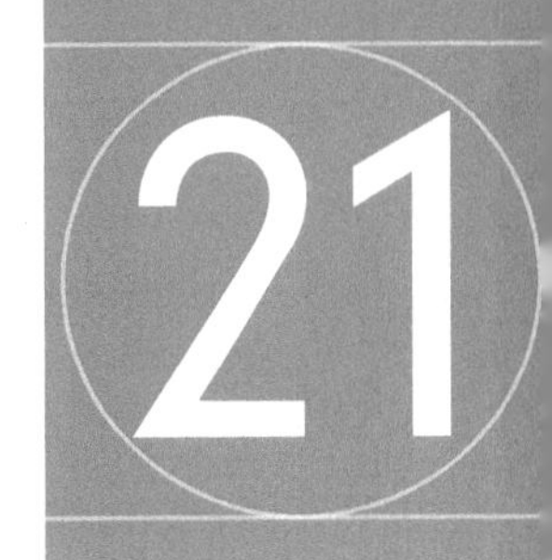


1. A father is concerned about his 9-month-old's diaper rash and explains that the rash is deep red and has not improved after using zinc oxide for a week. The infant had thrush as a newborn and has otherwise been healthy. The advanced practice nurse notes that the infant's erythematous lesions are primarily in the skin folds, is localized to the diaper area, and satellite lesions are present. Which diagnosis is MOST LIKELY?

   **A.** Atopic dermatitis or eczema
   **B.** Candidal diaper dermatitis
   **C.** Child abuse or neglect
   **D.** Impetigo bacterial infection

2. Characteristic facial features in a child with fetal alcohol syndrome include:

   **A.** Battle's sign, raccoon eyes, dilated pupils
   **B.** Allergic shiners, nasal crease, chapped lips
   **C.** Almond-shaped eyes with upward slanting palpebral fissures
   **D.** Short, upturned nose; thin upper lip; indistinct philtrum

3. An infant has 8 to 10 café au lait spots greater than 5mm in diameter. This should raise suspicion for which differential diagnosis?

   **A.** Cystic fibrosis
   **B.** Multiple sclerosis
   **C.** Neurofibromatosis
   **D.** Sickle cell anemia

4. When examining the skull of a 4-month-old, the advanced practice nurse would normally find:

   **A.** Closure of the posterior fontanel
   **B.** Ossification of the sutures
   **C.** Molding of cranial bones
   **D.** Closure of the anterior fontanel

5. Which statement is true regarding the Apgar scoring system as a component of newborn assessment? The Apgar score is derived from:

   **A.** Estimates of the gestational age of a newborn based on neuromuscular maturity
   **B.** Maternal risk factors, pregnancy-related complications, and maternal outcomes
   **C.** Assessments of the infant's heart rate, reflexes, muscle tone, respirations, and color
   **D.** Rapid assessments completed at 5 and 10 minutes of age and repeated every hour

6. Advanced practice nursing students are observed performing physical assessments. Which maneuver warrants additional instruction from their preceptor or faculty?

   **A.** Auscultating the lung sounds of an older child using a side-to-side comparison pattern
   **B.** Pulling the pinna up and back to inspect the tympanic membrane of a 5-year-old
   **C.** Using a tongue depressor to inspect when a child presents with sore throat and drooling
   **D.** Wearing personal protective equipment when collecting a throat swab for culture

7. The triad presentation typical of Henoch-Schonlein purpura (HSP) includes:

   **A.** Abdominal pain, arthritis, and palpable purpura
   **B.** High fever, conjunctivitis, polymorphous rash
   **C.** Nonspecific symptoms of fever, easy bleeding, and petechiae
   **D.** Headache, fever, and centripetal rash that is often petechial

8. Which statement describes the BEST approach to examining infants and young children?

   **A.** The "head-to-toe" sequence is the most effective and efficient for children
   **B.** Physical exams should always take place on the exam table
   **C.** The exam of a sleeping infant can be started while they are swaddled
   **D.** When children are apprehensive, complete the exam as quickly as possible

9. Factors associated with exacerbations of atopic dermatitis in children include:

   **A.** Elevated serum IgG levels
   **B.** Food or environmental allergens
   **C.** Frequent baths or showers
   **D.** Topical steroid use

**10.** A 4-year-old male is presenting to the clinic today with a purpuric rash on his upper and lower extremities. The advanced practice nurse notes that the child generally appears well. His mother reports that he has been bruising more than normal and believes this to be from rough playing. He has not had fevers, abdominal pain, or fatigue. Last visit to the office was 3 weeks ago for a well-child exam and immunizations. What is the MOST LIKELY diagnosis?

**A.** Bacterial endocarditis
**B.** Immune thrombocytopenic purpura
**C.** Hemolytic uremic syndrome
**D.** Systemic lupus erythematosus

**11.** The advanced practice nurse believes that a child has pseudoesotropia. If this assessment is accurate, performing the cover-uncover test will result in:

**A.** The covered eye re-fixating when the cover is removed
**B.** The uncovered eye re-fixating when the cover is removed
**C.** No shift in fixation when either eye is covered
**D.** Nystagmus when both eyes are covered and uncovered

**12.** Which of the following is true regarding sickle cell disease?

**A.** In children, sickle cell trait and anemia are the same condition
**B.** Individuals with sickle cell disease need more frequent ophthalmology referrals
**C.** Only infants with African ancestry carry the sickle cell trait or disease
**D.** Sickle cell disease affects children differently, and does NOT always includes pain

**13.** A parent wonders if their child has seasonal allergies because they develop eye redness every spring. Which additional assessment would MOST confirm the mother's suspicion of seasonal allergic conjunctivitis?

**A.** Copious amount of yellow eye drainage
**B.** Bilateral eyelid edema with watery discharge
**C.** Bilateral eye pain with photophobia and itching
**D.** Small bump and inflammation on lower eyelash line

**14.** Physical exam findings indicative of a coarctation of the aorta in older children include:

**A.** Circumoral, central, and peripheral cyanosis at rest
**B.** Diaphoresis, tachypnea, and retractions with activity
**C.** Diastolic cardiac murmur with bounding pulses in the lower extremities
**D.** Systolic hypertension in the upper extremities and low arterial pressure in the lower extremities

**15.** A school-aged child presents to the pediatric urgent care with a muffled "hot potato" voice and significant pharyngitis. On exam, the advanced practice nurse notes that the child has trismus, lymphadenopathy, and uvular deviation. Which diagnosis is MOST LIKELY?

**A.** Epiglottitis
**B.** Peritonsillar abscess
**C.** Strep pharyngitis
**D.** Viral pharyngitis

**16.** A young child who has strep pharyngitis is likely to have a sore throat and which associated symptoms?

**A.** Cough and runny nose
**B.** Fever and abdominal discomfort
**C.** Itchy vesicular rash and joint pain
**D.** Vasomotor rhinitis and conjunctivitis

**17.** A 12-year-old presents after an episode of syncope. Which assessment is MOST concerning and indicates the need for a cardiology follow-up?

**A.** Experienced dizziness and lightheadedness prior to syncope
**B.** Experienced nausea and diaphoresis prior to syncope
**C.** States had no prodromal symptoms at all prior to episode
**D.** States was emotionally stressed prior to syncopal episode

**18.** Which presentation of ear pain is indicative of an emergent condition?

**A.** A 1-year-old with fever, unilateral otitis, postauricular erythema and tenderness
**B.** A 2-year-old with rapid onset of ear pain, decreased mobility of the tympanic membranes
**C.** A 3-year-old with conjunctivitis and bilateral bulging, erythematous tympanic membranes
**D.** A 7-year-old with unilateral ear drainage, and pain with palpation of the tragus

**19.** The most frequent systemic disorder associated with uveitis in children is:

**A.** Bacterial conjunctivitis
**B.** Juvenile idiopathic arthritis
**C.** Ocular trauma
**D.** Type II diabetes mellitus

**20.** For children under 2 years old, the MOST sensitive indicator of acute otitis media is:

**A.** Amber fluid bubbles behind the tympanic membrane
**B.** Immobility of the tympanic membrane
**C.** Erythema of the tympanic membrane
**D.** Dull or retracted tympanic membrane

**21.** Which statement about how a child's airways responds to allergens is most accurate?

**A.** An early allergic response occurs within minutes following inhalation of an allergen
**B.** The early allergic response peaks within four minutes following allergen inhalation
**C.** A late allergic response to an allergen may occur 24 to 48 hours following inhalation
**D.** A late allergic response to an allergen is only seen in children who also have rhinitis

**22.** During the physical exam of a 2-month-old, which finding would be indicative of developmental dysplasia of the hip (DDH)?

**A.** Limited hip adduction
**B.** Negative Galeazzi sign
**C.** Positive Barlow maneuver
**D.** Symmetric gluteal folds

**23.** Which infant's presentation is MOST concerning?

**A.** 3-month-old who has 1 hour of crying every evening
**B.** 3-month-old who has a weak cry and floppy muscle tone
**C.** 6-month-old with respiratory rate of 30 breaths/minute at rest
**D.** 6-month-old with respiratory rate of 40 breaths/minute with crying

**24.** A 3-year-old male presents with hip pain after resolution of a recent upper respiratory infection. Upon exam, the child is afebrile, limping, and has pain with hip abduction and external rotation; the hip and leg are non-tender to palpation. CBC and ESR are normal; hip x-ray is normal. Based on the history and exam findings the MOST LIKELY diagnosis is:

**A.** Juvenile idiopathic arthritis
**B.** Osteomyelitis
**C.** Septic arthritis
**D.** Transient synovitis

**25.** For which pediatric patient are pulmonary function tests MOST recommended?

**A.** Infant with respiratory syncytial virus
**B.** Child with upper respiratory infection
**C.** Child with suspected asthma
**D.** Adolescent athlete

**26.** A 1-year-old presents with bronchiolitis. Which signs and symptoms are most ominous for impending respiratory failure?

**A.** Fever, expiratory wheezing, and waking at night
**B.** Fussiness, flushed face, and decreased oral intake
**C.** Irritability, intercostal retractions, and coughing spasms
**D.** Lethargy, retractions, and diminished air movement

**27.** Which child with a fever is most at risk for a febrile seizure?

**A.** 9-month-old who has a history of prematurity
**B.** 15-month-old whose mother had febrile seizures as a child
**C.** 24-month-old who had a fever for 4 days associated with otitis
**D.** 9-year-old who recently completed antibiotics

**28.** A toddler who has had a recent onset of fever and upper respiratory symptoms develops laryngitis, stridor, and a "barking" cough that is worse at night. Which diagnosis is MOST LIKELY for this toddler?

**A.** Croup
**B.** Foreign object aspiration
**C.** Laryngomalacia
**D.** Pertussis

**29.** The mother of a 3-year-old male tells the advanced practice nurse that she suspects her child has attention deficit hyperactivity disorder (ADHD) because he often ignores her and has difficulty following directions "just like his father." Which assessment is the FIRST priority?

**A.** Audiometry
**B.** Genetic testing
**C.** Conners Behavior Rating Scale (CBRS)
**D.** Vanderbilt assessment scale

**30.** An adolescent presents with significant headache pain and fever. The advanced practice nurse is concerned about meningitis, asks the teen to lie flat, and assesses for a positive Kernig's sign, which is:

**A.** Inability to bring the chin to the chest
**B.** Inability to flex the neck muscles or turn head to either side
**C.** Involuntary flexion of the knees and hips caused when head is lifted
**D.** Resistance or pain with passive extension of flexed knees

**31.** Which statement is true regarding urinary tract infections (UTIs) in children?

**A.** Children under 2 years old with a fever that has no obvious cause should be evaluated for UTI

**B.** Children 2 to 24 months old who are diagnosed with UTI should be hospitalized

**C.** Imaging studies are indicated for any child 3 to 7 years old who is diagnosed with cystitis

**D.** Children of any age should be treated for suspected abuse if UTI is diagnosed

**32.** Which complication is correlated with undiagnosed or untreated chlamydial infection?

**A.** Arthritis

**B.** Disseminated infection

**C.** Interstitial cystitis

**D.** Infertility

**33.** Which symptoms are MOST LIKELY when older children present with new onset of type I diabetes?

**A.** Constipation, acne, and weight gain

**B.** Frequent urination, thirst, and weight loss

**C.** Inattention and poor academic performance

**D.** Irritability, insomnia, and anxiety symptoms

**34.** Which is true regarding sexually transmitted infections (STIs) including human immunodeficiency virus (HIV) in the adolescent population?

**A.** Adolescents are not likely to be exposed to STIs including HIV if monogamous

**B.** Confidential testing for STIs is not approved for the adolescent population.

**C.** STI testing for teens should include testing for gonorrhea, chlamydia, and HIV

**D.** Teens who use condoms and are asymptomatic do not require STI screening

**35.** A 15-month-old male presents with acute onset of 103° F fever, irritability, and refusal to walk. The child was seen last week for a well-child exam and was healthy. Physical exam today reveals significant warmth, swelling, and pain with palpation of right hip and thigh. Range of motion is limited. The child appears toxic. Which would be the best next step for the advanced practice nurse?

**A.** Advise the parent that this is likely an adverse reaction to vaccinations

**B.** Advise the parent that this presentation can be treated with antibiotics

**C.** Recognize the signs and symptoms as red flags for septic arthritis

**D.** Recognize that the child has a viral illness and this will resolve quickly

**36.** An advanced practice nurse suspects a diagnosis of acute pyelonephritis for a 17-year-old female who presented with urinary urgency, frequency, and burning. Which additional assessments support this diagnosis?

**A.** Abundant white blood cells on vaginal wet prep
**B.** Fever, flank pain, and costovertebral angle tenderness
**C.** Patient admits to taking frequent prolonged bubble baths
**D.** Urine dipstick shows small amount of leukocytes and nitrites

**37.** During a 2-year-old male's well-child exam, his mother shares that he continues to have four or more watery or loose stools a day; he has no other symptoms. The 2-year-old is developmentally on track, growing well, and gaining weight; his height and weight have consistently been at the 50th percentile on the growth chart. Which diagnosis is MOST LIKELY for this child?

**A.** Constipation
**B.** Irritable bowel syndrome
**C.** Inflammatory bowel disease
**D.** Toddler's diarrhea

**38.** What findings on a radiograph would be indicative of osteosarcoma in a child?

**A.** Decrease in bone density
**B.** Fractures in various stages of healing
**C.** Sunburst sign or pattern
**D.** Decrease in joint cartilage

**39.** A 5-year-old with no history of trauma presents with fever, right shoulder and back pain, vomiting, and abdominal pain. On exam, the child has right upper quadrant pain with palpation, rebound tenderness, and guarding. Which imaging study would be the next step in assessing the cause of the child's symptoms?

**A.** Abdominal x-ray
**B.** Abdominal ultrasound
**C.** Computed tomography (CT) scan
**D.** Voiding cystourethrogram

**40.** Which viral pathogen is the primary cause of acute gastroenteritis in infants?

**A.** Norovirus
**B.** Adenovirus
**C.** Rotavirus
**D.** Sapovirus

**41.** Which history question related to child safety, or risks to safety, is the MOST appropriate for age?

**A.** Asking parents of a 2-month-old: "Have you installed latches, locks, and gates in your home?"
**B.** Asking parents of a 2-year-old: "Is you water heater temperature set at <100°F?"
**C.** Asking a 7-year-old: "Do you have someone at school who you are attracted to as a boyfriend or girlfriend?"
**D.** Asking a 15-year-old: "Have you ever ridden in a car driven by someone who had been using alcohol or drugs?"

**42.** Physical characteristics and comorbidities associated with Marfan syndrome include:

**A.** Allergic shiners, wheezing, and eczema
**B.** Myopia, mitral valve prolapse, and joint hyper-flexibility
**C.** Wheezing, dyspnea, and irritant cough
**D.** Shortened limb length despite height, and diminished hearing

**43.** A healthy 4-month-old should be expected to:

**A.** Sit without support
**B.** Smile spontaneously
**C.** Roll from back to front
**D.** Have object permanence

**44.** Which characteristics would the advanced practice nurse expect to find when examining a newborn recently diagnosed with Down syndrome?

**A.** Epicanthal folds, hypotonia, and Brushfield spots on the iris
**B.** Rocker bottom feet, low-set ears, and prominent occiput
**C.** Short neck with webbed appearance, low hairline, low-set ears
**D.** Thin, translucent skin that bruises very easily, prominent eyes

**45.** During adolescence, which glands are responsible for increased axillary perspiration and a change in body odor?

**A.** Sebaceous glands
**B.** Apocrine glands
**C.** Eccrine glands
**D.** Ceruminous glands

**46.** Which statement is true regarding nutrition for children who are "picky eaters?"

**A.** These children need as much whole milk as possible to provide additional calories

**B.** These children are more likely to be overweight or obese as adolescents and as adults

**C.** Tips for parents include avoid introducing new foods and prepare favorite foods

**D.** Tips for parents include set realistic expectations and enjoy family meals together

**47.** Which statement is true regarding assessments related to the introduction of solid foods for healthy infants?

**A.** Babies demonstrate readiness for solid food when they have a strong tongue thrust

**B.** Babies born vaginally should have table food very early to help their gut microbiome

**C.** Foods such as cow's milk and honey should not be introduced until after 1 year of age

**D.** Foods such as rice cereal can be mixed with formula or breast milk and given by bottle

**48.** Which question is MOST appropriate when screening a preteen for disordered eating?

**A.** Are you happy with how incredibly thin you are?

**B.** Are you unhappy because you are starting to become overweight?

**C.** Do you believe yourself to be fat when others say you are too thin?

**D.** Would you like to lose more than 15 pounds?

**49.** Parents of a 2-year-old express concern about their child's language development. Which assessment MOST indicates that the child may have a language delay? The child:

**A.** Can name six of ten pictures in their favorite book

**B.** Can put two words together, but not three

**C.** Has a vocabulary of about five words

**D.** Has speech that is 75% understandable

**50.** The mother of a 4-month-old is concerned because the infant "spits up too much." Before developing a plan, which assessments are MOST important?

**A.** Family history of allergies and mother's intake of milk

**B.** Pattern of length and weight noted on the infant's growth chart

**C.** Sleep-wake patterns noticed by parents and other caregivers

**D.** Time spent breast and/or bottle feeding in a 24-hour period

# Practice Test II: Answers and Rationales

**1. B) Candidal diaper dermatisis**

Candidal diaper dermatitis begins as deep red papules and pustules that later coalesce into a beefy red confluent rash with sharp borders; satellite lesions frequently are found beyond these borders, and skin folds commonly are involved. Because the rash is caused by yeast (candida), the diaper rash is likely to persist despite over-the-counter treatment and is associated with a history of thrush. Infants with eczema also have lesions on the face and extremities. Impetigo presents as vesicles and pustules with erosions. Diaper dermatitis can persist despite frequent diaper changes; the case presentation is not consistent with neglect or abuse of the child.

**2. D) Short, upturned nose; thin upper lip; indistinct philtrum**

Distinctive facial features characteristic of fetal alcohol syndrome include small eyes; short, upturned nose; very thin upper lip; and indistinct or smooth philtrum. Children with allergic disease may have allergic shiners (dark circles around the eyes that appear as bruises with puffiness), chapped lips from mouth breathing, and a nasal crease caused by repeated rubbing of the nose. Basilar skull fractures can cause bruising behind the ear (Battle's sign) or bruising around the eyes (raccoon eyes); dilated pupils are a red flag sign indicating serious head injury or trauma. Almond-shaped eyes with upward slanting palpebral fissures and Brushfield spots are characteristic features in a child with Down syndrome.

**3. C) Neurofibromatosis**

The presence of numerous café au lait macules should raise the suspicion of a genetic disorder. The most common associated systemic disorder is neurofibromatosis type 1 (NF1). The diagnostic criteria for NF1 includes the presence of six or more café au lait spots larger than 5mm in greatest diameter in prepubertal individuals, freckling in the axillary or inguinal regions, and two or more Lisch nodules (iris hamartomas). Cystic fibrosis, multiple sclerosis, and sickle cell anemia do not have café au lait as a manifestation; other genetic disorders that do include McCune-Albright syndrome, Fanconi anemia, tuberous sclerosis, and basal cell nevus syndrome.

**4. A) Closure of the posterior fontanel**

At birth, the pliable skull of a newborn has six fontanels and unfused skull bones that allowed for molding or overlap of cranial bones during passage through the birth canal. Molding usually resolves within 3 to 5 days after birth. The posterior fontanel usually closes during the first 2 months of life. The larger anterior fontanel usually closes by 15 months of age. Early ossification or premature closure of one of more cranial sutures causes asymmetry of the head, or craniosynostosis.

**5. C) Assessments of the infant's heart rate, reflexes, muscle one, respirations, and color**

Apgar scoring has five components: 1) color, 2) heart rate, 3) reflexes, 4) muscle tone, and 5) respiration, each of which is given a score of 0, 1, or 2. Apgar scores quantify clinical signs of neonatal depression such as cyanosis or pallor, bradycardia, depressed reflexes, hypotonia, and apnea or gasping respirations. The score is reported at 1 minute and 5 minutes after birth for all infants, and at 5-minute intervals until 20 minutes for infants with a score less than 7. The Apgar score is affected by many factors, including prematurity, maternal medications, resuscitation, and neurologic conditions; however, the score is not a measure of gestational age or maternal outcomes, and predictive of infant outcomes.

**6. C) Using a tongue depressor to inspect when a child presents with sore throat and drooling**

A child presenting with a sore throat and drooling could indicate epiglottitis which is a medical emergency; inspection of the throat should be avoided in this case as it could cause airway obstruction. The lungs should be auscultated in a Greek key pattern (side-to-side) to compare sounds bilaterally. In children over 3 years old, the pinna should be pulled up and back to best visualize the ear canal and tympanic membranes. Wearing appropriate personal protective equipment is a priority consideration.

**7. A) Abdominal pain, arthritis, and palpable purpura**

The classic triad of HSP includes palpable purpura without thrombocytopenia, abdominal pain that is colicky in nature, and migratory arthritis. This triad of symptoms is caused by IgA-mediated, acute, systemic vasculitis. Most cases occur in children under 10 years old after resolution of an upper respiratory infection; fatigue and low-grade fever are common. Other causes of purpura include Kawasaki disease (presents with high fever, conjunctivitis, polymorphous rash); leukemia (causes nonspecific symptoms of fever, easy bleeding, and petechiae); and Rocky Mountain spotted fever (presents with headache, fever, and centripetal rash that is often petechial).

**8. C) The exam of a sleeping infant can be started while they are swaddled**

To examine infants and young children use the "quiet to active" approach; any aspects of the physical exam that necessitate the most cooperation, or may be potentially uncomfortable, should be performed last. Modify the order of the exam according to the child's comfort or cooperation level. For example, the clinician can start an exam by auscultating heart and lung sounds of a sleeping infant while swaddled, or for the child who is apprehensive about the ear exam, can save it for last and have the parent hold the child during the exam. Any assessment technique that may make the child cry should be postponed until the end of the exam; once an infant or child is distressed and crying, it is very difficult to auscultate heart and lung sounds or perform an eye exam.

**9. B) Food or environmental allergens**

Atopic dermatitis is a chronic, pruritic inflammatory skin condition; primary physical findings include dry skin, lichenification, and inflammatory lesions. Children experience a constellation of symptoms that are relieved with frequent baths or showers with tepid water, and application of moisturizers and topical steroids. Triggers include food or environmental allergens, stress, heat, and immune compromise; family history of asthma and allergies and elevated IgE levels are often associated.

**10. B) Immune thrombocytopenic purpura**

Immune thrombocytopenic purpura (ITP) typically presents with a purpuric rash on both upper and lower extremities in a child who is overall healthy. A history of increase in bruising is common, as ITP involves accelerated platelet destruction. In children, ITP is usually preceded by a viral illness or immunization,, (e.g., measles, mumps, and rubella [MMR] vaccine). Bacterial endocarditis, hemolytic uremic syndrome, and systemic lupus erythematosus are less likely in this case because the child appears healthy, and does not present with fever, flu-like symptoms, lethargy, or musculoskeletal complaints.

**11. C) No shift in fixation when either eye is covered**

The cover-uncover test is used to assess for strabismus as occluding binocular vision reveals eye muscle weaknesses and misalignment. Diplopia (not nystagmus) is likely to occur during the assessment when the child has strabismus. With true esotropia, the child has an inward turning of the eye; re-fixating will occur in the affected eye during the assessment. Occasionally children may appear to have esotropia without evidence of true strabismus; this pseudoesotropia or pseudostrabismus is usually due to the shape of the eyelids and/or nasal bridge. With pseudoesotropia, the cover-uncover test is normal, and no shift in fixation occurs.

**12. B) Individuals with sickle cell disease need more frequent ophthalmology referrals**

The term "sickle-cell disease" includes all manifestations of the hemoglobin variant, HbS. Hemoglobinopathies are among the most common inherited diseases around the world, and sickle cell disease is the most serious. In the United States, one in three individuals with sickle cell disease have African ancestry. Sickle cell disease causes pain crises as a result of the sickling of the hemoglobin; complications include stroke, chronic pain, retinal detachment, gallstones, pulmonary hypertension, splenomegaly, avascular necrosis, and liver failure. Individuals with sickle cell disease need more frequent ophthalmology, cardiology, and genetic counseling referrals. Individuals with sickle cell trait have inherited one copy of the sickle cell gene, so the disease is not expressed; carriers have a 50% chance of passing the gene to offspring.

**13. B) Bilateral eyelid edema with watery discharge**

Allergic conjunctivitis is likely bilateral and with clear discharge; symptoms typically include eyelid edema. While seasonal allergic conjunctivitis is associated with itching and discomfort, bilateral eye pain is unlikely, and is more indicative of keratoconjunctivitis or corneal trauma. A small, raised lesion with associated inflammation on lower eyelash line is more likely a hordeolum or stye.

**14. D) Systolic hypertension in the upper extremities and low arterial pressure in the lower extremities**

The classic findings of coarctation of the aorta include systolic hypertension in the upper extremities, diminished or delayed femoral pulses, and low arterial pressure in the lower extremities. With coarctation of the aorta, the narrowing of the aortic arch creates symptoms of decreased blood pressure and blood flow distal to the area of narrowing, generally the lower extremities, and increased blood pressure and sometimes bounding pulses prior to the narrowing, generally the upper extremities. Cardiac auscultation may be normal, or a systolic murmur may be heard. Diagnosis of coarctation of the aorta is often delayed in older infants and children because physical findings are subtle and because most patients are asymptomatic.

**15. B) Peritonsillar abscess**

Children with peritonsillar abscess may present with severe sore throat, trismus (difficulty opening their mouth), and dysphonia (muffled "hot potato" voice); on exam, individuals with a peritonsillar abscess typically have unilateral tonsillar enlargement and uvular deviation. Children with epiglottitis are more likely to present with fever, restlessness, stridor, and drooling. Those with viral or bacterial pharyngitis without an abscess are more likely to have bilateral tonsillar enlargement and will not have significant uvular deviation or trismus. Viral and strep pharyngitis cause symptoms of fever, pain with swallowing, and lymphadenopathy.

**16. B) Fever and abdominal discomfort**

Group A Beta Hemolytic Strep (GABHS), or strep pharyngitis, commonly causes sudden onset of sore throat, fever, lymphadenopathy, tonsillar hypertrophy, and pain with swallowing. Other symptoms include headache, abdominal pain, nausea, and vomiting, especially in children. Strep pharyngitis is not associated with cough, rhinorrhea, conjunctivitis, vesicular rashes, or rhinitis; these symptoms suggest viral or allergic etiology. Individuals who present with strep pharyngitis and pinpoint macular rash are likely to have scarlet fever; painful joints after GABHS may indicate rheumatic fever.

**17. C) States had no prodromal symptoms at all prior to episode**

Absence of prodromal symptoms prior to a syncopal episode requires referral to cardiology for further evaluation, as it suggests cardiogenic syncope, which can be life-threatening and includes primary electrical disturbances and structural heart diseases. Vasovagal syncope (i.e., neuro-cardiogenic or reflex fainting), is the most common cause of syncope in children and teens. Typical features of vasovagal syncope include a precipitating event and a prodrome. Precipitating events include emotional stress. Prodrome symptoms may include lightheadedness, dizziness, visual changes, nausea, pallor, and diaphoresis.

**18. A) A 1-year-old with fever, unilateral otitis, postauricular erythema and tenderness**

Mastoiditis is a complication of acute otitis media that causes inflammation of a portion of the temporal bone. Children with mastoiditis present with fever, otitis, and postauricular erythema, tenderness and warmth; complications if untreated can be life-threatening and include meningitis and intracranial abscess. Children with acute otitis media present with rapid onset of ear pain and erythematous tympanic membranes with decreased mobility. Unilateral ear drainage and pain with palpation of the tragus correlates with otitis externa, or swimmer's ear. Acute otitis media and otitis externa can be managed outpatient with either observation or antibiotic therapy.

**19. B) Juvenile idiopathic arthritis**

Juvenile idiopathic arthritis (JIA) is the most common systemic disorder associated with uveitis; JIA leads to significant polyarticular joint inflammation. While bacterial infections and ocular trauma (e.g., hyphema, foreign body, or corneal abrasions) can cause severe conjunctivitis that mimics uveitis, distinguishing the two is important. Uveitis can lead to vision loss. While type II diabetes is also a systemic disorder with ocular manifestations, the most common complications associated are glaucoma, dry eye syndrome, cataracts, and diabetic retinopathy.

**20. B) Immobility of the tympanic membrane**

Diagnostic criteria for acute otitis media include rapid onset of symptoms, bulging tympanic membrane (TM), limited or absent mobility of the membrane, and erythema of the TM or ear pain affecting sleep or normal activity. Because crying can cause erythema of the TMs, pneumatic otoscopy to determine mobility is more reliable, sensitive, and specific for acute otitis media than plain otoscopy. Visible amber fluid bubbles are suggestive of otitis media with effusion. Dull or retracted TM more likely indicates eustachian tube dysfunction.

**21. A) An early allergic response occurs within minutes following inhalation of an allergen**

Studies have shown that an early allergic response occurs within minutes after inhalation of an allergen and peaks at 20 minutes. A late allergic response may occur 4 to 10 hours later. Late allergic responses are characterized by infiltration of inflammatory cells into the airway and are thought to be caused by activation of lymphocytes and eosinophils.

**22. C) Positive Barlow maneuver**

The Barlow maneuver is an exam technique using gentle downward force while the infant's hip is adducted to identify an unstable hip that can be passively dislocated. Other identifiers of DDH include limited hip abduction, asymmetric gluteal folds, positive Galeazzi sign (asymmetric height of knees when flexed), and positive Ortolani maneuver. The Ortolani maneuver is an exam technique using gentle upward force while the infant's hip is abducted; the sensation of a palpable clunk is a positive sign that indicates reduction of a dislocated hip.

**23. B) 3-month-old who has a weak cry and floppy muscle tone**

Lethargy and weak cry are significant, emergent symptoms during infancy and are red flags for serious conditions including sepsis, respiratory failure, hypoglycemia, dehydration, and cardiovascular collapse. Poor feeding is often associated as an early sign. Periodic crying is normal in infancy as a way of communicating hunger, discomfort, or sleepiness; persistent crying or irritably is unexpected and can be a sign of illness. Tachypnea at rest is an indicator of infectious disease in infants; the normal respiratory rate for infants from 6 to 12 months of age is 25 to 40 breaths/minute.

**24. D) Transient synovitis**

Transient synovitis (TS) is an acute, non-specific, inflammatory process affecting the joint synovium; while the exact etiology is unknown, children typically present with a history of viral symptoms, unilateral limb disuse, and mild range of motion restrictions. With septic arthritis, juvenile idiopathic arthritis, and osteomyelitis, the child would likely present with fever, and labs and/or x-rays would be indicative of the disease processes. TS is a diagnosis of exclusion based on history and physical exam.

**25. C) Child with suspected asthma**

Pulmonary function testing (PFT) is used to assess lung function and is essential to the diagnosis and treatment of asthma, cystic fibrosis, bronchopulmonary dysplasia, and other chronic respiratory conditions. PFT is not used as a screening for acute illness, or as an evaluative tool in otherwise healthy athletes.

**26. D) Lethargy, retractions, and diminished air movement**

Diminished movement of air causes poor oxygen exchange leading to hypoxemia. Retractions are one of the child's compensatory mechanisms to promote lung expansion and oxygen exchange; lethargy is a worrisome sign that the child has been unable to compensate for the hypoxia. Diminished air movement, retractions, and lethargy combined are ominous for impending respiratory failure and the need supplemental oxygen or ventilation support. Fever, flushed face, decreased intake, wheezing, coughing, irritability, fussiness, and waking at night are all signs and symptoms of bronchiolitis that require further assessment and monitoring.

**27. B) 15-month-old whose mother had febrile seizures as a child**

Febrile seizures are more common in infants and children under 5-years-old, associated more frequently with viral illnesses, and are more likely in the first 24-hours of an illness. A genetic predisposition to febrile seizures exists; in some patients and families, the tendency for febrile seizures is an early sign of epilepsy.

**28. A) Croup**

Croup is a viral respiratory infection that begins with cold symptoms and progresses to laryngeal swelling that causes hoarseness, stridor, and a characteristic barking cough. While laryngomalacia and foreign object aspiration can also cause inspiratory stridor, neither would have associated upper respiratory tract symptoms. Pertussis does not result in stridor; this lower respiratory tract infection that can persist for months causes uncontrolled spasms of coughing with a characteristic whooping sound that lead to vomiting, gasping, and hypoxia.

**29. A) Audiometry**

Inattentiveness and difficulty following directions are developmentally appropriate for preschoolers; however, these traits can be exacerbated by hearing loss. While there are inherited disorders that can cause inattention and/or hearing loss, before referring for genetic testing, audiometry to assess hearing is needed. ADHD can be understood in the context of family, although less likely to diagnosed in young children; the Vanderbilt and Conners assessment tools are intended for screening children over 6 years old.

**30. D) Resistance or pain with passive extension of flexed knees**

To assess for Kernig's sign, an individual should lie supine with the thighs flexed on the abdomen and the knees flexed; the examiner then passively extends the legs. In the presence of meningeal irritation, the individual is likely to have a positive Kernig's sign (i.e., will resist leg extension or have significant pain in their back/thighs). A positive Brudzinski sign, or involuntary flexion of the knees and hips caused when head is lifted, is also indicative of meningeal irritation. Nuchal rigidity can also result from meningitis, which causes an individual to bring their chin to their chest by adequately flexing neck muscles.

**31. A) Children under 2 years old with a fever that has no obvious cause should be evaluated for UTI**

Urinary tract infections are relatively common in children; because children under 2 years old may present with only fever, any presentation of fever with unknown cause should be evaluated for UTI. Children under 2 months of age with UTI require hospitalization for treatment to avoid/manage sepsis. Imaging studies may not be indicated for girls over 7 years old who are afebrile; guidelines based on observational studies and expert opinion recommend that all boys, girls younger than 3 years, and girls 3 to 7 years of age with a temperature of 101.3°F (38.5°C) or greater receive cystography and ultrasonography with a first-time UTI. (https://www.aafp.org/afp/2011/0215/p409.html)

**32. D) Infertility**

Untreated chlamydia can lead to pelvic inflammatory disease, infertility, epididymitis, and urethritis. Untreated gonorrhea, syphilis, and genital herpes can result in disseminated infections that cause arthritis, rashes, fatigue, and nerve and organ damage. The exact cause of interstitial cystitis is not known, although autoimmune reactions are contributing factors.

**33. B) Frequent urination, thirst, and weight loss**

Hyperglycemia causes polyuria, polydipsia, polyphagia, and weight loss in children who develop type I diabetes. These children will present appearing ill, are prone to dehydration, and may have vague nonspecific complaints, such as lethargy; typically, these children are more sluggish than irritable, inattentive, or anxious. Type I diabetes is characterized by insulin deficiency; weight loss despite oral intake is a physiologic consequence.

**34. C) STI testing for teens should include testing for gonorrhea, chlamydia, and HIV**

STIs are common in adolescents. Routine screening for chlamydia and gonorrhea is recommend annually for those under 25 years old who are sexually active. HIV screening is recommended at least once during adolescence. Additionally, HPV vaccination is recommended in this age group if not already received as teens are at high-risk. All 50 states and the District of Columbia allow minors (generally at age 12 to 14) to consent to testing and treatment for STIs.

**35. C) Recognize the signs and symptoms as red flags for septic arthritis**

The most likely diagnosis for a febrile, toxic child with swelling, warmth, and limited range of motion of the hip is septic arthritis which is an orthopedic emergency. Transient synovitis, which is benign and resolves without intervention, would be more likely if the child was afebrile and non-toxic. Assuming that this is a cellulitis or infection that resulted from trauma or vaccination could lead to a significant delay in treatment.

**36. B) Fever, flank pain, and costovertebral angle tenderness**

The diagnosis of acute pyelonephritis relies on assessment for infection in the urinary tract that has ascended into the upper tract including kidney(s). Signs and symptoms of pyelonephritis include fever, chills, flank pain, nausea, vomiting, and costovertebral angle tenderness. Symptoms of cystitis, or infection of the bladder and lower urinary tract include urinalysis positive for small amount of leukocytes, blood, and nitrites. Prolonged or frequent bubble baths are a risk factor for cystitis. Findings that support a diagnosis of pelvic inflammatory disease (PID) include abundant white blood cells on wet prep of vaginal secretions, lower abdominal or pelvic pain, and cervical motion tenderness.

**37. D) Toddler's diarrhea**

Toddler's diarrhea, also called "functional diarrhea" or "chronic nonspecific diarrhea of childhood," is a common cause of chronic diarrhea in toddlers and preschoolers. Children with toddler's diarrhea have three or more watery or loose stools a day and have no other symptoms. They typically are growing well, gaining weight, and are healthy. Children with constipation typically have infrequent bowel movements or hard, dry stools that are difficulty to pass. They can have watery stools with constipation, however abdominal pain and discomfort are associated. Irritable bowel syndrome and inflammatory bowel diseases are more common in older children and teens, and typically cause pain and other symptoms.

**38. C) Sunburst sign or pattern**

Osteosarcoma is a type of bone cancer in which tumor cells produce immature bone. Radiologic images will show the formation of new bone in a "sunburst" pattern; this sunburst sign, in addition to the appearance of a white cloud-like lesion or "cumulus cloud" sign indicate the likelihood of osteosarcoma. Decreases in bone density, joint cartilage, or healing fractures are not likely with this malignancy.

**39. B) Abdominal ultrasound**

Abdominal ultrasound scans are useful in evaluating pain in the right upper quadrant (likely caused by cholecystitis or cholelithiasis). Ultrasound is also recommended to evaluate suspected appendicitis (which is usually RLQ, but may be considered in this case as the child presents with fever and guarding). X-ray and CT scans have higher radiation exposure risks and are not recommended as initial imaging studies. A voiding cystourethrogram is indicated in children between 2 and 24 months of age after an initial urinary tract infection if ultrasound reveals hydronephrosis, scarring, or findings that suggest vesicoureteral reflux or obstruction.

**40. C) Rotavirus**

Infants who develop acute gastroenteritis are more likely to have an infection from rotavirus than other viral pathogens. Rotavirus infection is universal among humans; despite widespread use of the vaccine in developed countries, rotavirus is still the leading cause of infantile diarrheal illness. Norovirus is a frequent cause of outbreaks of acute gastroenteritis in schools and residential facilities, as the virus can withstand common disinfectant products. Because of its relative stability in the environment, norovirus is implicated in nearly 50% of all foodborne outbreaks. Other viral causes include adenovirus, sapovirus, and astrovirus; each of these viruses can cause approximately 5% of viral gastroenteritis cases.

**41. D) Asking a 15-year-old: "Have you ever ridden in a car driven by someone who had been using alcohol or drugs?"**

Assessment of safety risks should be guided by age. For newborns and infants, having a safe sleeping environment is the priority. It is important for infants and young children that water heaters in the home are set to 120°F; above this temperature can cause burns, and below this temperature risks bacterial growth. During middle childhood, assess for anxiety, school phobia, and bullying; same-sex friendships at this age are important to social development more than expressions of sexual identity. Asking history questions about alcohol and drug use, including asking about whether they have ever been in a car with a person under the influence, is appropriate when assessing adolescent safety risks; this question is part of the evidence-based CRAFFT screening tool.

**42. B) Myopia, mitral valve prolapse, and joint hyper-flexibility**
Marfan syndrome is characterized by tall, thin stature. Other signs, symptoms or risks include ocular hypertension; flexible joints; high, arched neck; disproportionately long arms and legs; intraocular lens dislocation; crowded teeth; pectus carinatum or pectus excavatum; stretch marks; long fingers; flat feet; and scoliosis. Assessing for Marfan syndrome is key to identification of associated heart and blood vessel complications including aortic dilation, aortic aneurysm, aortic dissection, and pneumothorax. Leg length discrepancies and hearing issues are more often seen in those who have genetic syndromes that cause short stature. Wheezing, dyspnea, irritant cough, allergic shiners, and a history of eczema are all associated with asthma.

**43. B) Smile spontaneously**
Developmental expectations for 4-month-olds include smiles spontaneously, begins to babble, responds to affection, and rolls from front to back. 6-month-olds can be expected to roll from back to front and begin sitting without support. 9-month-olds develop object permanence and will look for things that are out of sight.

**44. A) Epicanthal folds, hypotonia, and Brushfield spots on the iris**
The most common physical manifestations of Down syndrome include hypotonia, a flat nasal bridge, epicanthal folds, up-slanting palpebral fissures, Brushfield spots, a small mouth, head and ears, excessive skin at nape of neck, transverse palmar crease, and a short, curved fifth finger. Infants with Trisomy 18 have rocker bottom feet, low-set malformed ears, and prominent occiput. Females with Turner syndrome have distinctive physical features which include short neck with webbed appearance, low hairline, and low-set ears. Children with vascular Ehlers-Danlos syndrome have a thin nose, thin upper lip, prominent eyes, and thin, translucent skin that bruises very easily.

**45. B) Apocrine glands**
Apocrine glands are scent glands located primarily in the axillary and anogenital areas that remain inactive until puberty. Once the glands' secretions combine with bacteria on the skin's surface, body odor is produced. Sebaceous glands are small oil-producing glands that develop along the hair follicle. Eccrine glands are sweat glands controlled by the sympathetic nervous system. Ceruminous glands are modified apocrine glands that produce cerumen or ear wax.

**46. D) Tips for parents include set realistic expectations and enjoy family meals together**
Being a "picky eater" (i.e., favoring just a couple of foods or not wanting foods to touch on the plate) is developmentally normal for toddlers and preschoolers. These children are not more likely to become obese. Setting realistic expectations, introducing new foods while preparing favorites, offering choices, preparing meals together, and being focused on enjoyment during family mealtimes are important tips for parents.

**47. C) Foods such as cow's milk and honey should not be introduced until after 1 year of age**

Children under 12 months of age should not be given honey or any food containing honey, unpasteurized foods, or fortified cow's milk, as these products can cause serious harm. Assessments for the readiness of solid foods include good head control, ability to sit up with minimal support, and disappearance of the tongue thrust. Breastfeeding supports the development of a healthy microbiome in infancy, not the introduction of table food. Adding rice cereal to a bottle of formula or breast milk is not likely to improve sleep, can lead to over-feeding, and is not recommended for healthy infants.

**48. C) Do you believe yourself to be fat when others say you are too thin?**

Clinicians can assess eating and weight-related topics in an authentic and sensitive manner and must avoid implicit bias. Asking about satisfaction with body weight and shape without assumptions or negativity is key. The SCOFF questionnaire is a five-question screening measure to assess the possible presence of an eating disorder; questions include:

- Do you make yourself **S**ick (induce vomiting) because you feel uncomfortably full?
- Do you worry you have lost **C**ontrol over how much you eat?
- Have you recently lost more than **O**ne stone [approximately fifteen pounds] in a 3-month period?
- Do you believe yourself to be **F**at when others say you are too thin?
- Would you say that **F**ood dominates your life?

**49. C) Has a vocabulary of about five words**

At 2 years of age, developmental expectations for speech include using sentences of two to four words, following simple commands, and pointing to body parts, pictures in a book, and common objects. Typically, speech is about 50% understandable at this age, and children will have a vocabulary of 50 to 100 words. Additional assessments for developmental delay are needed if 2-year-olds are not meeting these milestones.

**50. B) Pattern of length and weight noted on the infant's growth chart**

Accurate and reliable growth measures are essential for determining health in children. Infants with poor weight gain or growth measurements that trend downward or fall below the 3rd percentile may have a failure to thrive and the cause should be investigated. Infants with a reassuring pattern of weight gain and growth measurements are not likely to be experiencing malnutrition or organic disease. While family history of allergies, sleep-wake patterns, and amount of infant feedings are important assessments, the key indicator that the child is not having adverse effects from spitting up is an adequate pattern of growth. Spitting up is common in infants related to immaturity of the lower esophageal sphincter; forceful vomiting causing failure to gain weight requires further investigation for pyloric stenosis, obstruction, gastroenteritis, and other illnesses.

# Index

**NOTE:** Page numbers followed by "f" and "t" refer to figures and tables, respectively.